SEVENTH EDITION

MEDICAL LAW, ETHICS, & BIOETHICS

for the HEALTH PROFESSIONS

Marcia (Marti) Lewis (deceased), EdD, RN, CMA-AC (AAMA)
Former Associate Dean for Nursing Programs,
Dean of Mathematics, Engineering, Science, and Health
Adjunct Instructor, Medical Assisting
Olympic College
Bremerton, Washington

Carol D. Tamparo, PhD, CMA-A (AAMA)
Former Dean, Business and Allied Health
Lake Washington Institute of Technology
Kirkland, Washington
Coordinator, Medical Assistant Program
Highline Community College
Des Moines, Washington

Brenda M. Tatro
Assistant Professor
Director of Medical Assisting
Medical Office and Coding & Billing Programs
Mount Wachusett Community College
Gardner, Massachusetts

F.A. Davis Company • Philadelphia

F. A. Davis Company
1915 Arch Street
Philadelphia, PA 19103
www.fadavis.com

Copyright © 2012 by F. A. Davis Company

Printed in the United States of America

Last digit indicates print number: 10 9 8

Senior Acquisitions Editor: Andy McPhee
Manager of Content Development: George Lang
Developmental Editor: Julie Munden
Manager of Art and Design: Carolyn O'Brien

As new scientific information becomes available through basic and clinical research, recommended treatments and drug therapies undergo changes. The author(s) and publisher have done everything possible to make this book accurate, up to date, and in accord with accepted standards at the time of publication. The author(s), editors, and publisher are not responsible for errors or omissions or for consequences from application of the book, and make no warranty, expressed or implied, in regard to the contents of the book. Any practice described in this book should be applied by the reader in accordance with professional standards of care used in regard to the unique circumstances that may apply in each situation. The reader is advised always to check product information (package inserts) for changes and new information regarding dose and contraindications before administering any drug. Caution is especially urged when using new or infrequently ordered drugs.

Library of Congress Cataloging-in-Publication Data

Lewis, Marcia A.
    Medical law, ethics & bioethics for the health professions / Marcia (Marti) Lewis, Carol D. Tamparo, Brenda M. Tatro. — 7th ed.
        p. cm.
    Medical law, ethics, and bioethics for the health professions
    Rev. ed. of: Medical law, ethics, and bioethics for the health professions. 6th ed. c2002.
    Includes bibliographical references and index.
    ISBN 978-0-8036-2706-2 (pbk. : alk. paper)
    1. Medical laws and legislation—United States. 2. Ambulatory medical care—Law and legislation—United States. 3. Medical ethics—United States. I. Tamparo, Carol D., 1940- II. Tatro, Brenda M. III. Lewis, Marcia A. Medical law, ethics, and bioethics for the health professions. IV. Title. V. Title: Medical law, ethics, and bioethics for the health professions.
    [DNLM: 1. Ambulatory Care—legislation & jurisprudence—United States. 2. Ethics, Clinical—United States. WB 33 AA1]
    KF3821.L485 2012
    344.7304'1—dc23
2011025925

"The way a book is read—which is to say, the qualities a reader brings to a book—can have as much to do with its worth as anything the author puts into it."

Norman Cousins

It is imperative that any health-care professional have knowledge of medical law, ethics, and bioethics so that clients are treated with understanding, sensitivity, and compassion. No matter what the professional's education, experience, or position, any client contact involves ethical and legal responsibility. It also is imperative that this knowledge be used to provide the best possible service for the provider and employer. Our goal is to provide the health-care professional with an adequate resource for the study of medical law, ethics, and bioethics.

Although the material is applicable to all health-care professionals in any setting, our emphasis continues to be on the ambulatory health-care setting rather than on the hospital or long-term-care setting. For example, we do not address such legal and bioethical issues as whether to feed an anencephalic newborn in the neonatal center of the hospital. We realize, however, that all the bioethical issues affect ambulatory health-care personnel directly or indirectly. Continued enthusiastic feedback from instructors, students, and reviewers is gratifying and has resulted in many changes that will make this Seventh Edition more useful than the first six. We are reminded of the truth, which comes from our colleagues in community and technical colleges, that no matter how many times a piece is written, it can always be improved.

The continuing evolution of health care, of legal and, especially, bioethical issues, necessitates this revision. The material has been updated throughout to reflect the latest developments and emerging ethical issues. The newest developments in stem cell research for treating disease and for creating new organs and tissue are included in the Genetic Engineering chapter as the legal and ethical debate "rages." The chapter introducing the reader to the cultural perspectives of health care continues to heighten one's awareness of the importance of culture in health care. The chapter on reproductive health issues has been greatly enhanced. Abortion is still covered as an important element in reproductive health, but many new topics have been added.

The authors and their editors have made every attempt to ensure currency and pertinence of the material. However, some bioethical issues change almost daily as lawmakers and the public become actively involved and press for legislation. Even as this edition goes into production, the coauthors struggle to be current as federal and state legislations clash. Furthermore, funding and morality issues are being addressed in the political arena, sometimes bringing research and advancement in medicine to a standstill. For ease of reference, pertinent codes of ethics appear in Appendix I. Appendix II offers samples of some of the legal documents clients may use in implementing decisions about health care, life, and death.

A thought-provoking vignette appears in each chapter. The vignettes are adapted from case law or from actual situations. Learning outcomes designed for the educational setting precede each chapter. The Seventh Edition places case studies throughout the chapters. The case studies are for reflection rather than a test of chapter contents. CAAHEP and ABHES competencies also appear at the beginning of each chapter to help students and faculty identify competencies necessary for accreditation and certification in the content area of medical law and ethics.

For students' benefit, we have included questions for review at the end of each chapter for increased learning. Classroom exercises and Internet activities will whet the appetite, stimulate discussion, and highlight the most pressing legal, ethical, and bioethical issues faced by ambulatory care employees. Lastly, Web resources are provided to help the reader in further research on the Internet.

DavisPlus offers many additional resources and exercises for both the student and the instructor. Videos are available for classroom use or small-group discussions. The videos will require students to put themselves in the place of making legal and ethical decisions.

"Have a Care!" has been updated. It continues to be one of the most popular pieces of this textbook. Because nearly every person has a "Have a Care" moment in his or her life and experiences with the medical community, it is our hope that it will always be a part of any upcoming edition. However, this particular "Have a Care" ends with the death of Marcia (Marti) Lewis, the primary person in this story. It took much courage for Marti to agree to its inclusion in the First Edition, but gradually in subsequent editions she was more comfortable revealing herself as the main character and allowing the readers to fully experience her frustration and discomfort.

A new author has been added for this edition. It is not easy to come into an already established author relationship (especially where one is grieving the loss of the other) and make one's mark. Brenda Tatro did so with grace, understanding, humor, and the willingness to interject a new dimension into the writing.

We hope that from this book you will derive a great sense of pride for your professional position in health care.

Marti A. Lewis
Carol D. Tamparo
Brenda M. Tatro

OF SPECIAL NOTE
The term "provider" rather than "physician" has been used throughout the text unless the reference is directly that of a medical doctor (MD) or a doctor of osteopathy (DO) This change is made to reflect the increasing numbers of other providers giving primary care. Also, the term "client" continues to be used in preference to "patient." The term patient is reserved for an individual receiving care in a hospital. It is also a term that denotes an "unequal" relationship between two individuals—doctor and patient or provider and patient. The best of medical care today places emphasis upon the participation of the person receiving the care; therefore, "client" becomes the appropriate term. It may be helpful to recognize that the majority of nursing texts use the term client rather than patient for the same reasons.

REVIEWERS

Jean Cuppet, RN, MSN
Professor, Department Chair
Health Professions
Pennsylvania Highlands Community College
Johnstown, Pennsylvania

Dolly Horton, CMA(AAMA), BS, Med
Chairperson of Medical Assisting, Interim Dean of
    Allied Health
Allied Health Department
Asheville Buncombe Technical Community College
Asheville, North Carolina

Christine M. King, AAS, CMA(AAMA)
Program Chair/Instructor
Medical Assisting Technology
Hinds Community College
Pearl, Mississippi

Sandra Moaney-Wright, BS, Med, RMA(AMT)
CEO, Moaney-Wright & Associates, LLC
Palmetto, Georgia

Marilyn S. Pooler, RN, RMA, MEd
Retired Professor, Medical Assisting
Springfield Technical Community College
Springfield, Massachusetts

Wendy Sammons, CMA(AAMA), LPN, AAT
Instructor
Medical Assisting Department
Lanier Technical College
Oakwood, Georgia

Janice Vermiglio-Smith, RN, MS, PhD
Division Chair, Health Careers
Health and Science Department
Central Arizona College
Apache Junction, Arizona

ACKNOWLEDGMENTS

It is never possible to acknowledge all the people who make contributions to the authors of a book. Completing a book requires assistance from so many individuals and sources. We wish to thank, however, a few who were especially helpful. Without them, the book would have been impossible to create.

F.A. Davis has a fine cadre of individuals who make a writing project pleasant. Each individual's desire for excellence and thoroughness helps to create the final product. Margaret Biblis, Publisher, and Andy McPhee, Senior Acquisitions Editor, refresh our thoughts and goals with new ideas and discerning eyes. With the assistance of Julie Munden, Developmental Editor; Yvonne N. Gillam, Developmental Editor; and George W. Lang, Manager of Content Development, our thoughts, ideas, text, and presentation have all been pulled together into the book you hold in your hands. Elizabeth Stepchin, Developmental Associate, monitors our budget and provides direction and support as necessary. All these people have been positive, encouraging, and helpful to us in all matters. Our relationship with F.A. Davis for over 33 years has always been one of high professionalism and integrity.

Students continually offer critical thought and information on legal, ethical, and bioethical issues and act as a sounding board for all ideas. Their input and comments have influenced this product. Students continue to be our inspiration and the reason for this book!

The support of families and friends has been an essential ingredient from the inception of the First Edition to the completion of this Seventh Edition. Thanks to Tom Tamparo, Jayne Bloomberg, and Duuana Warden and their families. Many thanks to Dick Tatro, Kim Perry, Mike Tatro, Matt Tatro, and their families. They relinquished their time with us so we could write. Lester and Martiann Lewis remained supportive throughout the writing of this edition as well. These family members and dear friends provided encouragement when we were discouraged and celebrated with us when we were successful. Thanks; we love you all!

CONTENTS IN BRIEF

CONTENTS

Understanding the Basics

CHAPTER 1

Medical Law, Ethics, and Bioethics

"The aim of education is the knowledge, not of facts, but of values." —William Ralph Inge (1860-1954); Church of England clergyman, scholar, and critic

KEY TERMS

hospitalist Individual who assumes the care of hospitalized individuals in place of their primary care provider.

internal milieu Internal environment.

pluralistic Referring to numerous distinct ethnic, religious, and cultural groups that coexist in society.

LEARNING OUTCOMES

Upon successful completion of this chapter, you will be able to:

1.1 Define key terms.
1.2 Compare medical law, ethics, and bioethics.
1.3 Discuss some bioethical issues in medicine.
1.4 Explain the importance of medical law, ethics, and bioethics in the practice of medicine.
1.5 List and discuss at least three ethical codes.
1.6 Describe the American Association of Medical Assistants (AAMA) Code of Ethics.
1.7 Interpret the AAMA Creed.
1.8 Compare/contrast the AAMA and the American Medical Association (AMA) codes of ethics.
1.9 Describe the Patient Bill of Rights.
1.10 Explain the Ethics Check questions.
1.11 Describe characteristics that are important for a professional health-care employee.

COMPETENCIES

COMMISSION ON ACCREDITATION OF ALLIED HEALTH EDUCATION PROGRAMS (CAAHEP)

- Summarize the Patient Bill of Rights. (CAAHEP IX.C.4)
- Differentiate between legal, ethical, and moral issues affecting health care. (CAAHEP X.C.1)
- Compare personal, professional, and organizational ethics. (CAAHEP X.C.2)
- Identify the effect personal ethics may have on professional performance. (CAAHEP X.C.5)
- Incorporate the Patient's Bill of Rights into personal practice and medical office policies and procedures. (CAAHEP IX.P.5)

- Develop a plan for separation of personal and professional ethics. (CAAHEP X.P.2)
- Apply ethical behaviors, including honesty/integrity in performance of medical assisting practice. (CAAHEP X.A.1)
- Examine the impact personal ethics and morals may have on the individual's practice. (CAAHEP X.A.2)

ACCREDITING BUREAU OF HEALTH EDUCATION SCHOOLS (ABHES)
- Being cognizant of ethical boundaries. (ABHES 11.b.4)
- Analyze the effect of hereditary, cultural and environmental influences. (ABHES 5.g)

VIGNETTE

Are You a Professional?

A certified medical assistant (CMA) employed by an obstetrician/gynecologist calls her former medical assistant instructor to inform her of an opening for a clinical assistant in the obstetrics and gynecology (OB-GYN) clinic. After describing the position and its responsibilities, the CMA says, "We really need another person in the clinical area. I'm the doctor's only nurse."

Surprised by the comment, the instructor inquires, "When did you go back to school to become a nurse?"

She replies, "Oh, I didn't, but everyone thinks I am his nurse. I do everything a nurse does."

The title of this text, *Medical Law, Ethics, and Bioethics for the Health Professions,* presents three distinct topics: medical law, ethics, and bioethics. Such distinction, however, is for the sake of clarity. Discussion of any one of these topics will include the others. Any study of health law will surface themes of ethics and bioethics. Conversely, discussing ethics and bioethics without considering the law is futile.

 ## LAW

Laws are societal rules or regulations that are prudent or obligatory to observe. Failure to observe the law is punishable by the government and/or law enforcement agencies. Laws are designed to protect the welfare and safety of society and to resolve conflicts in an orderly and nonviolent manner. They constantly evolve in accordance with an increasingly pluralistic society. Laws have governed humankind and the practice of medicine for thousands of years. Today federal and state governments have constitutional authority to create and enforce laws. A brief look at these laws, their sources, and their definitions appears in subsequent chapters.

Medical law is essential in regulating licensure of health-care professionals and institutions, providing for client safety, protecting the client-provider relationship, and identifying liability for health-care professionals and institutions. Health law also regulates insurance and managed care as well as federal public health programs. It also has established standards for reproduction and birth issues as well as life and death decisions.

 ## ETHICS

Ethics is a set of moral standards or a code for behavior to govern an individual's interactions with other individuals and within society. Joseph Fletcher (1905–1991), an American professor who pioneered in the field of bioethics, differentiates *morals* from ethics, stating, "'morality' is what people do in fact believe to be right and good, while 'ethics' is a critical reflection about morality and the rational analysis of it." According to Fletcher, for example, "Should I terminate pregnancy?" is a moral question, whereas "How should I go about deciding?" is an ethical concern.

Although laws are more apt to be rules applied to and observed by all, different cultures have different moral codes. Cultural differences exist relative to age, gender, sexual orientation, ethnic heritage, educational preparation, life experiences, spiritual influences, role models and mentors, economics, values, internal milieu, and health and illness. Every standard for ethics is culture-bound. Therefore, there are few if any universal truths in ethics because it is difficult to identify customs as being either correct or incorrect. It is also true that one person's moral code has no special status relative to another person's moral code; it is only one among many. See Chapter 12, A Cultural Perspective for Health Professionals, for further discussion on the influence of culture.

Ethical standards can be personal, organizational, institutional, or worldwide. Ethics refers to the various codes of conduct that have been established through the years by members of many professional organizations, including the medical profession. A number of medical codes appear in the appendices and on Davis*Plus*.

BIOETHICS

Bioethics refers to the ethical implications of biomedical technology and its practices. *Bio* refers to life, and issues in bioethics are often life-and-death issues. Edmund D. Pellegrino, Professor Emeritus of Medicine and Medical Ethics at Georgetown University, states that "bioethics, still in its infancy, is routinely called on by the government to provide political cover for controversial public health decisions involving the life and death of Americans." In other words, political leaders often look to bioethical discussions to guide them in making decisions regarding controversial public health issues. Specialists in the field of bioethics provide the platform for this decision making.

Since former President Clinton established a National Bioethics Advisory Commission (NBAC) in 1995, subsequent presidents have established their own commission to provide input to the president and national leaders on issues of bioethics. In April 2010, President Barack Obama appointed members to his Presidential Commission for the Study of Bioethical Issues. Obama mandated that this Commission address potential bioethical issues through advancements in biomedicine and "related areas of science and technology." The Commission plays a key role in keeping the President informed about bioethical issues.

The challenge to bioethics created by modern medicine and research in the past few decades is staggering. Rapid changes in medicine and technology offer unique and sometimes overwhelming choices to clients and their families. Consumers more actively involved in their health care and quite knowledgeable of medical technology and its implications question medical professionals as they have never before been questioned. The public carefully scrutinizes medical technology and how it relates to their daily lives. Thus, the application of bioethics in everyday life provides opportunities, challenges, enthusiasm, and sometimes difficult choices.

COMPARING MEDICAL LAW, ETHICS, AND BIOETHICS

Law, ethics, and bioethics are different yet related concepts. Laws are mandatory rules to which all citizens must adhere or risk civil or criminal liability. Ethics often relate to morals and set forth universal goals to try to meet, but there is no temporal penalty for failing to meet ethical goals as there is apt to be in law. However, law in the United States has been and continues to be a driving force in shaping ethics.

Confusion over the interpretation of law, ethics, and bioethics is understandable. They sometimes conflict. Consider the following example for further clarification:

The U.S. Supreme Court addressed the issue of abortion in *Roe v Wade,* 410 U.S. 113, 1973. The *law* states that during the first trimester, pregnant women have a constitutional right to abortions, and the state has no vested interest in regulating them at this time. During the second trimester, the state may regulate abortions and insist on reasonable standards of medical practice if an abortion is to be performed. During the third trimester, the state's interests override pregnant women's rights to abortions, and the state may deny abortion except when necessary to preserve the health or life of the mother.

The personal *ethics* of a provider or health-care professional may dictate nonparticipation in an abortion or any abortion-related activities. *Bioethics* and the allocation of scarce resources are evidenced by some state statutes that have denied the use of state funds for an abortion or strive to make abortions less available. As demonstrated by this example, sometimes law, ethics, and bioethics conflict.

IN THE NEWS

As a result of two U.S. Supreme Court rulings that prohibit parents from having absolute veto over their daughters' decision to have an abortion, many state legislatures rushed to tighten controls on abortions. As of 2011, only Washington, Oregon, New York, Vermont, Connecticut, Hawaii, Maine, and Washington DC had no parental notification or consent laws related to minors seeking abortion (see Fig. 1-1). Thirty-six states require some involvement in a minor's decision; 22 states require parental consent, 10 states require only parental notification, and 4 states require both parental consent and notification. This information changes yearly as state legislative bodies struggle to exercise control over abortions in their state. Sometimes, such legislation is later overturned by the U.S. Supreme Court. Legal attempts continue the move to rescind *Roe v Wade*.

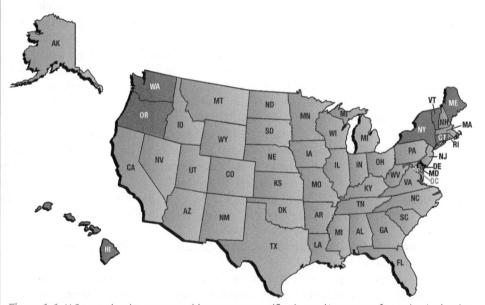

Figure 1-1. U.S. map showing states requiring no parent notification and/or consent for a minor's abortion.

THE IMPORTANCE OF MEDICAL LAW, ETHICS, AND BIOETHICS

There are many reasons that make medical law, ethics, and bioethics important for health-care professionals. It is necessary to follow health-care laws and to examine one's actions in light of both laws and ethics. It is helpful to learn more from the bioethical issues that clients face and to appreciate differences in moral reasoning among individuals and various cultures. Also, there is the need to confront personal biases and bigotry.

In addition, there are political and economic factors that are relevant to the importance of medical law, ethics, and bioethics. They include:

- Demands of society for quality health care at minimal personal cost
- The debate over whether health care is a right or a privilege
- The equality of the distribution of and access to emerging medical technology
- The controversy among the political arena, national health-care reform, and the consumer over who pays for health care and how it is paid
- The powerful role of medical insurance and managed care.

Thoughtful consideration of the reasons identified here as well as the political and economic factors fosters mature decision making and quality health care for clients.

TODAY'S HEALTH-CARE CLIMATE

There is much in today's health-care environment to challenge any health-care professional's ethics, values, and practices. Just a few are identified here for reflection.

- *Consumers are bombarded with medical information.* The media, both printed and electronic, report on many aspects of health care. This immediate access of information empowers consumers to ask more questions of medical professionals, allowing them to be better informed about choices.
- *Increasingly, hospitals and ambulatory care centers are establishing ethics committees and/or institutional review boards (IRBs)* that enable community resource persons, educators, and providers to grapple with ethical dilemmas both before and after they occur in the clinical setting. Laws and ethical standards designed to protect clients and establish guidelines for the medical community represent an effort to create a climate for an equitable exchange between client and provider. The primary goal of an ethics committee is to have a plan in place before a crisis occurs. IRBs have been empowered by the U.S. Food and Drug Administration (FDA) and the Department of Health and Human Services (DHHS) to monitor, review, and oversee any medical research involving human subjects. An IRB is required if there is either direct or indirect support from the DHHS.
- *Medical technology is advancing at a more rapid rate than legal and ethical standards can address.* Consider the time without antibiotics, when premature infants died due to lack of neonatal intensive care and when invasive surgery rather than a computed tomography scan was the only method to reveal problems with internal organs. There are a number of medical advances likely to occur in the next decade. Many may come with a flurry of ethical and bioethical implications that will create debate in the medical community. They include:
  - Restoring irreversibly damaged hearts by replacing dead heart muscle with new laboratory-grown muscle after a heart attack
  - Using harvested skin cells obtained through a small biopsy and suspended in a solution to be sprayed directly onto a major burn area. These cells rapidly divide to cover the wound up to 80 times larger than the donor site
  - Using computer-assisted therapy sessions to identify depression and excessively negative thoughts in the treatment of clients
  - Using high-technology brain scans to detect the earliest signs of both plaques and tangles found in Alzheimer disease and using a vaccine to stimulate the body's own immune response to wipe out the plaques once identified
- *Increasing numbers of specialists in medicine make it more difficult to coordinate client care.* It is quite conceivable that a client has a primary care provider, a neurologist, a nephrologist, and an oncologist, all providing care. If hospitalization is necessary, is the primary care provider or a hospitalist in charge? Who coordinates, and who approves care? Who decides the appropriate course of action in the case of conflicting medical opinions?

Although specialization may enhance quality health care, it demands greater coordination for clients to benefit, and it increases the cost of medical care. Managed care policies and providers will in part dictate how medical choices are made.

• *Costs of medical care have risen exponentially.* In 1940, a normal infant delivery cost $35 for 10 days of inpatient hospital care. The delivering physician received an additional $35. In 1990, a normal delivery cost an average of $3300 for a 2- to 3-day inpatient hospital stay. In 2005, hospitalization for normal delivery and a 1- to 2-day hospital stay was $5200. The factors affecting the cost of a birth are: whether it is a vaginal or cesarean delivery, if there are complications, and the length of the hospital stay. Infant delivery is most expensive in the Northeast and on the West coast and least expensive in the South. In 2010, the typical cost of a vaginal delivery without complications ranged from about $9000 to $17,000 or more. The typical cost for a cesarean delivery without complications or a vaginal delivery with complications ranged from $14,000 to $25,000 or more.

The importance of these issues is further evidenced by the struggle that has been made through the past couple of decades to pass some form of a national health-care reform in the nation's capital. It finally happened in 2010, but not without a great deal of political maneuvering and posturing.

ETHICAL ISSUES IN MODERN MEDICINE

Many situations arise in the practice of medicine and in medical research that present problems requiring moral decisions. A few of these can be illustrated by the following questions.

Should a parent be able to refuse a mandated immunization for his or her child? Does public safety supersede an individual's right? Is basic health care a right or a privilege? Who dictates client care—the client, the provider, or the health insurance company? Who pays for the care of children with very serious and life-threatening birth defects? Should more medical attention be paid to a "cure" or for "prevention?" How should legal abortions be funded? Is it important that everyone receive equal treatment in medical care? What are the issues related to prolonging life or assisted death for individuals with terminal illnesses? What criteria determine who receives donor organs? Should stem cell research be limited or advanced?

None of these questions has an easy answer, and most individuals do not even think about them unless suddenly and personally faced with one or more of them. These questions and other possibilities are the reason for entering into a discussion of pertinent bioethical issues. For some, answers can be found in ethical codes.

CODES OF ETHICS

For generations ethical codes have been written to further clarify medical law and ethics. Many codes have become law. Professional codes have evolved throughout history as practitioners grappled with various ethical and bioethical issues. Increasingly, groups of medical professionals have defined how members of their profession ought to behave. Below are a few examples.

The *Hippocratic Oath* (see Appendix 1), although not prominent in medical schools today, still carries significant weight among the medical community. The oath, which was first written in the fifth century B.C., was Christianized in the 10th or 11th century A.D. to eliminate reference to pagan gods. The Hippocratic Oath protected the rights of clients and appealed to the inner and finer instincts of the physician without imposing penalties.

The *Geneva Convention Code of Medical Ethics,* established by the World Medical Association in 1949, is similar to the Hippocratic Oath. This code refers to colleagues as brothers and states that religion, race, and other such factors are not a consideration for care of the total person. This code reflects the fact that medicine was becoming available to all during this era.

The *Nuremberg Code* was established between 1946 and 1949 as a result of the trials of war criminals after World War II. This code suggests guidelines for human experimentation and is directed to the world. The writers hoped that the code would ensure the safety of humans in the years to come.

The *Declaration of Helsinki,* written between 1964 and 1975, is an update on human experimentation. Much more detailed than the Nuremberg Code, it includes guidelines for both therapeutic and scientific clinical research. Unlike the Nuremberg Code, the Declaration of Helsinki is directed to the world of medicine rather than the world at large.

The American Medical Association (AMA) established the *Principles of Medical Ethics* in 1847 and updated it in 1957, 1980, and again in 2001 (see Appendix 1). The preamble and nine principles have served as guidelines for physicians for many years. The document "Current Opinions of the Judicial Council of the American Medical Association" is intended as an adjunct to the revised Principles of Medical Ethics. Both documents are pertinent to physicians and their assistants today.

The number of professional medical organizations with written ethics codes is numerous. The codes are available on the Internet by searching the particular association and then for its code of ethics. A few are identified here:

- American Academy of Professional Coders (AAPC)
- International Medical Informatics Association (IMIA)
- National Association of Emergency Medical Technicians (NAEMT)
- American Osteopathic Association (AOA)
- American Association of Naturopathic Physicians (AANP)
- American Chiropractic Association (ACA)
- National Certification Commission for Acupuncture and Oriental Medicine (NCCAOM)
- National Medical Association (NMA)
- American Nurses Association (ANA)

By far the most important code directed to the ambulatory care professional is the *AAMA Medical Assistant Code of Ethics* and AAMA Medical Assistant Creed directed to the medical assistant (MA) in the ambulatory setting (see Appendix 1). The code was adopted by the American Association of Medical Assistants and appears in its constitution and bylaws. It provides guidelines to assist MAs in serving their profession in an ethical and professional manner. This code, as well as most other ethical codes, identifies to society at large what the standards are for the profession.

A number of codes have appeared that deal more with the rights of clients than the responsibilities and guidelines for health-care providers. They include numerous Patient Bill of Rights established by the American Hospital Association (AHA) and federal and state governments as well as individual hospitals and institutions. Contact the hospital nearest you for a sample of a patient bill of rights, or refer to Davis*Plus* for the sample from the AHA; they are all quite similar in content. Increasing in popularity are patient bills of rights specific for ambulatory health care. They are usually written by specific clinics and generally include the right to be respected, right to access your medical record, right to receive a second opinion, right to participate in your health care, and the right to have your privacy protected at all times. A number of samples can be seen on the Internet by searching for entities such as the Cleveland Clinic and the Mayo Clinic.

The 2010 Healthcare Reform Bill includes a Patient Bill of Rights that has an entirely different scope. This portion of the bill is designed to ensure that there is affordable health care for everyone; it is designed to put consumers back in charge of their health coverage and prevent insurance carriers from certain practices to ban clients from coverage. The purpose of any patient bill of rights is to make certain clients know their rights. It can be helpful to recognize that in some cases clients always had these rights but were not aware of them.

The most challenging aspect of any ethical code is its personal application. Many books have been written on the subject, and decades of scholarly debate have sought effective criteria for making ethical decisions. No one method is the result. What is certain, however, is that how each individual makes an ethical decision is very personal. The Ethics Check questions identified below may be helpful as you begin to think about medical law, ethics, and bioethics as a health-care professional.

ETHICS CHECK

Blanchard and Peale, in *The Power of Ethical Management*, developed a set of questions to serve as an "ethics check" that is a useful tool for a person facing an ethical dilemma. These questions suggest that ethics is a very personal concept and a personal decision. Consider Blanchard and Peale's three questions to include in a personal code of ethics:

1. Is it legal or in accordance with institutional or company policy?
2. Does it promote a win–win situation with as many individuals (client/employee/employer) as possible?
3. How would I feel about myself if I read about my decision or action in the daily newspaper? How would my family feel? Could I look myself in the mirror? (Fig. 1-2.) ●

According to Blanchard and Peale, if the answer to any one of the three questions is no, consider the action unethical. If the answer to all three questions is yes, the action is ethical. The identification of such a simple personal code of ethics can help to clarify actions, and these Ethics Check questions may provide further guidelines on how to act when in a difficult situation.

An individual will have greater difficulties remaining ethical in an organization in which the highest leaders are not ethical in their actions. It helps if the leader of a group is ethical, setting the standard and making it easier for everyone else to be ethical. However, ethical actions may and should come from anyone, regardless of status.

Case Study

You are the clinic manager in a large multiprovider medical center. There is no upward mobility in this center, and you relish a new challenge. It is a rather slow day, and you use your office computer to access the Internet to do a job search. You find four jobs that are exciting, and you send your resume via the Internet. As you disconnect from the Internet, you recall that it is easy to trace access to sites on the Internet that you have just used for personal business.

Apply the Ethics Check to this case study.
What is your conclusion?

Figure 1-2. Ethics Check question: How would I feel if I saw my decision in the newspaper?

APPLYING MEDICAL LAW, ETHICS, AND BIOETHICS AS A PROFESSIONAL HEALTH-CARE EMPLOYEE

The significant conflict that often arises among medical law, ethics, and bioethics mandates that individuals choosing the health professions be people of high moral standards. They should be clear, open, and knowledgeable about their personal choices and beliefs and be able to recognize vast diversity in a pluralistic society. Health-care professionals must feel comfortable in a "servant" role while maintaining their own integrity and the respect of their clients.

Individuals employed in a service-oriented industry such as health care are expected to have certain characteristics. The health professional must always be tactful and should know instinctively when speaking is wise and when listening is better. The health-care employee is an important communication link between the client and the provider.

Anyone in a health-care profession is in a nonreciprocal relationship with clients. The professional serves the client and gives the client full respect even when the client is disrespectful. Health-care professionals will want to act and speak nonjudgmentally of their clients and their activities, offering information rather than opinions. Clients expect to be treated with courtesy and understanding. Only the most caring and sensitive of employees can handle day after day of sick, hurting, and complaining clients and remain objective yet compassionate and positive.

Physician- and provider-employers require that their employees be diligent and knowledgeable in every detail of the job. Such knowledge and training can come only through professional preparation that is demanding and exacting and continues throughout employment. Professionals who are flexible and take initiative will be an asset to their employers.

Honesty and integrity are traits required of the employee. Health-care professionals must always remember to practice only within the scope of their professional training and never misrepresent themselves. Confidentiality must be tenaciously protected, and both the clients' and the providers' best interests must be guarded.

Wise and prudent health-care employees will select employers for whom they have respect and to whom they can remain loyal. Matching your personal understanding of how to care for clients to that of your employer avoids conflicts at a later time. The majority of health-care professionals have a concern for quality health care, and that concern is often reflected in community efforts and contributions.

Refer to the following Case Law that illustrates a disregard of personal and professional ethics on the part of a medical provider.

Case Law ·

A physician in Lehi, Utah was accused in August 2009 of the following:

1. Fondling his female medical assistant (MA) while pretending to teach her how to diagnose heart murmurs (Civil Suit)
2. Two counts of forcible sex abuse (Criminal Case)
3. Two counts of voyeurism (Criminal Case)
4. One count of obstruction of justice (Criminal Case)

Dr. Steven Pack also faces an investigation by the Division of Occupational and Professional Licensing.

Dr. Pack allegedly called his 18-year-old MA to an examination room to teach her how to diagnose heart murmurs. He asked her to lie on an examination table, lifted her shirt and bra, and fondled her breasts as he told her he was "feeling" for heart murmurs. Pack allegedly again inappropriately touched the woman while teaching her how to use a heart monitor and electrocardiograph machine. The MA became upset and told a nurse practitioner at the office what happened. This civil lawsuit comes 1 day after Lehi police arrested Pack for allegedly recording with a concealed digital camera his female patients undressing in an examination room. In August 2010, Judge Samuel McVey sentenced Steven Pack to 1 year in jail without any early release and a second year with global positioning system (GPS) monitoring. Pack's license to practice was suspended by the Utah Division of Occupational and Professional Licensing. Civil suits brought by the victims were settled before the sentencing, but the civil remedies were not made public.

There are a number of ethical and legal issues in this case. Identify them.
Describe the action you might take in a similar situation.

YOU MUST DECIDE

There is no attempt in this book to determine right or wrong for any of the ethical issues in modern medicine. The purpose is to present the law and the facts that are pertinent in the ambulatory health-care setting and to raise some questions for consideration. Most everyone has decided what is right or wrong on the majority of moral issues, but the same distinction in ethics and bioethics is more complex and not so easily identified. This is partly because of lack of accurate knowledge or information on a particular issue, but accuracy, knowledge, and information are imperative. It is also important to know how and why those opinions have been formed and to look at what is acceptable according to the legal and ethical standards of today. As health professionals, the challenge is to live and act out of respect for oneself and others and to encourage others to do the same. It is important to know what we are to become and how we can become better than we are. Even when our opinions differ from those of the clients we serve, our clients always deserve respect and dignity from us. The hope is that the forthcoming discussions on "Allocation of Scarce Medical Resources," "Genetic Engineering," "Reproductive Issues," "End of Life Issues," and "Have a Care" will offer a better understanding of what *is* and what may become.

In reading the following chapters and considering their effect on you personally as well as your role as a health professional, you may find the following lines from a poem by F. A. Russel (1849-1914) helpful.

REMEMBER ... *Seek the right, perform the true,*
Raise the work and life anew.
Hearts around you sink with care;
You can help their load to bear.
You can bring inspiring light,
Arm their faltering will to fight.

SUMMARY

Knowledge of law, ethics, and bioethics is essential for all health-care professionals. The Ethics Check questions offer one approach to address these issues on a personal level. Professional codes of ethics are further guides to performance as a health-care professional. Those who have the professional traits identified in this chapter will be successful health-care employees and will find their profession rewarding and fulfilling. There is no opportunity for boredom in such a fast-paced and rapidly changing field as health care.

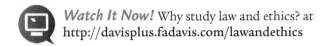 *Watch It Now!* Why study law and ethics? at
http://davisplus.fadavis.com/lawandethics

Questions for Review

SELECT THE BEST ANSWER

1. Medical law, ethics, and bioethics are necessary to understand
   a. Health law.
   b. Differences in moral reasoning among individuals and groups.
   c. The need to confront biases and bigotry.
   d. All of the above.
   e. Only a and b above.

2. Increasingly, hospitals find themselves in the ambulatory care business when
   a. Individuals are turned away from a clinic setting.
   b. Certain procedures can only be performed in the hospital.
   c. Medical technology is not available in a clinic setting.
   d. Clients prefer the added hours of service the hospital provides.
   e. Only b and c above.

3. The Hippocratic Oath
   a. Was written as a result of trials of war criminals.
   b. Protected the rights of clients and appealed to the finer instincts of the physician.
   c. Is an update on human experimentation.
   d. Is very similar to the Nuremberg Code.
   e. Only a and c above.

4. The most important code of ethics for the ambulatory care professional is the
   a. AMA Principles of Medical Ethics.
   b. AAPC Code of Ethics.
   c. AAMA Code of Ethics and AAMA Creed.
   d. Personal Ethics Check questions.
   e. Only c and d above.

5. Making an ethical and/or bioethical decision is based on
   a. An individual's religious belief for the most part.
   b. The direction of the provider-employer.
   c. State and federal law.
   d. The cost effectiveness of the particular decision to be made.
   e. Accuracy, knowledge, and information of the particular issue.

TRUE OR FALSE

T F   1. Ethics is a set of moral standards or a code of behavior.

T F   2. Bioethics relates to societal rules or regulations obligatory to observe.

T F   3. Increased numbers of specialists make it more difficult to coordinate client care.

T F   4. National Healthcare Reform of 2010 is likely the most historic domestic policy since Medicare was created in 1965.

T F   5. Blanchard and Peale identified a Patient Bill of Rights.

CLASSROOM EXERCISES

1. State in your own words what medical law, ethics, and bioethics mean to you.

2. What is the difference between law and ethics? Can a law be unethical? Can an ethic be unlawful? Justify your response.

3. What would you do if your personal code of ethics does not agree with that of your employer?

4. Do the Medical Assistant Code of Ethics and the Principles of Medical Ethics have any conflicting views? Explain.

5. In a small group discussion, tell how you as a health-care professional can show respect for a client who is rude and disrespectful to you.

6. What will you do if your opinions differ from your clients? For instance, a mother refuses inoculations for her child, and you believe they are necessary.

INTERNET ACTIVITIES

1. Using your favorite Internet search engine, key in the words "world medical ethics codes." Identify the results.

2. Research the Judicial Council of the AMA on the Internet. What is the Council's function? List two or three standards identified by this group as ethical/legal guidelines for physicians.

3. Research the 2010 Healthcare Reform Bill to determine whether the Patient Bill of Rights has been implemented, eliminated, or modified. Report your findings and identify any ethical concerns.

4. Research patient bill of rights for clinics for a number of samples. Compare with the hospital patient bill of rights. Identify the similarities and the differences.

REFERENCES

Blanchard, K., & Peale, N.V.: *The Power of Ethical Management.* New York: William Morrow, 1988.

Fletcher, J. *The Ethics of Genetic Control Ending Reproductive Roulette.* Buffalo, NY: Prometheus Books, 1988.

WEB RESOURCES

American Association of Medical Assistants (AAMA)
   www.aama-ntl.org

American Medical Association (AMA)
   www.ama-assn.org

All Business: Lawsuit Comes a Day after Physician's Arrest
   www.allbusiness.com

Medical Assistant Code of Ethics
   www.ehow.com/about_7221549_code-ethics-medical-assistants.html

State Policies in Brief, Guttmacher Institute: Parental Involvement in Minors' Abortions
   www.guttmacher.org

 DavisPlus | For additional resources please visit
http://davisplus.fadavis.com

CHAPTER 2

Medical Practice Management

"The best careers advice to give to the young is 'Find out what you like doing best and get someone to pay you for doing it.'"—Katherine Whitehorn;

English journalist and writer

KEY TERMS

bond An insurance contract by which a bonding agency guarantees payment of a specified sum to an employer in the event of a financial loss to the employer caused by the act of a specified employee; a legal obligation to pay specific sums.

capitation Health-care providers are paid a fixed monthly compensation for a range of services for each health maintenance organization (HMO) member in their care.

complementary medicine The practice of medicine that complements traditional medicine with alternative medicine.

conglomerate A corporation of a number of different companies operating in a number of different fields.

co-payment A medical expense that is a member's responsibility; usually a fixed amount of $25 or higher.

deductible A cost-sharing arrangement in which the member pays a set amount toward covered services before the insurance carrier begins to make any payments.

fee-for-service Pays providers for each service performed.

gatekeeper A term referring to managed care primary care providers responsible for referring members to specialists (usually within the same plan) with the intent of matching the client's needs and preferences with the appropriate and cost-effective use of those specialists' services.

group practice Type of business management in which three or more individuals organize to render professional service and share the same equipment and personnel.

health maintenance organization (HMO) A type of managed care plan offering health-care services from participating physicians and providers to an enrolled group of persons for a predetermined fee per member.

integrative medicine The practice of medicine that accounts for the whole person (body, mind, spirit, and lifestyle) using all appropriate therapies, both traditional and alternative.

joint venture A type of business management formed by hospitals, physicians and other providers, and clinics to offer client care.

managed care A type of health-care plan; generally one of two types, namely HMO or preferred provider organization (PPO).

opt-out option Members or clients can seek treatment from providers outside the health-care plan but pay more to do so.

partnership Type of business management involving the association of two or more individuals who are co-owners of their business.

pay for performance (P4P) A type of managed care that encourages providers to improve the quality of their clients' care; reimburses them for their progress toward a fixed goal.

preferred provider organization (PPO) A type of business agreement between a medical service provider and an insurer organization in which the fees for specific services are predetermined for an already established group of clients assigned to or selected by the provider.

professional service corporation Specific type of corporation in which licensed individuals organize to render a professional service to the public. Such licensed individuals include physicians, medical providers, lawyers, and dentists.

sole proprietorship Type of business management owned by a single individual.

LEARNING OUTCOMES

Upon successful completion of this chapter, you will be able to:

2.1 Define key terms.

2.2 Compare/contrast types of medical practice management.

2.3 List two advantages and two disadvantages of each of the types of practice management for both the provider and the employee.

2.4 Compare personnel needs in each of the types of practice management.

2.5 Discuss the role of managed care.

2.6 Describe health maintenance organizations (HMOs).

2.7 Discuss joint ventures and preferred provider organizations (PPOs).

2.8 Define the concept of general liability for providers.

2.9 Identify providers' responsibilities to employees in medical practice management.

COMPETENCIES

CAAHEP

• Define the concept of general liability for providers. (CAAHEP IX.C.6)

VIGNETTE

How Did This Happen?

It is 9:00 p.m. Thursday, and Geralyn is sitting at her desk in the Midway Medical Clinic. Everyone else has gone home. Her work is not yet done; she sits back to reflect on the past 30 years. She started as a medical assistant when the clinic was a two-physician partnership. The practice grew, and many changes were made. Soon there were five providers and multiple staff and specialists, and a corporation had been formed. Because of tenure and willingness to expand her education and responsibilities, Geralyn became the clinic manager. She really likes this job, her staff, and her employers. She is, however, continually frustrated by the fact that she has less time to do what she really enjoys as a clinic manager. Instead, she finds herself managing the practice and its finances for her employers. It is more than a full-time job just to keep track of all the insurance contracts, including federal and state reimbursement programs. As manager she wants to make sure that her employers and the clinics' clients are well served.

Graduates of today's medical schools have numerous choices to make before entering practice. Increasing numbers of graduates seek advanced education and training opportunities in a specialty area. Fewer graduates are choosing to specialize in family practices than are actually needed by society, and the last decade has seen many changes in the delivery of health care. Before that time, most graduates chose to function in private practice with a partner or a small group. Ultimately, their goal was to "fly solo" because that was where the most money could be made. Today that model has changed. Very few graduates enter into solo practice unless it is in a rural part of the country where the federal government, in cooperation with some medical schools, has set forth incentives for graduates to pay their college loans if they commit to practice in a rural area for a set amount of time. The majority of graduates will enter one of any number of different group forms of management.

Providers may function as partners with other providers, as members of health maintenance organizations (HMOs), and as shareholder/employees in professional service corporations. Increasingly, however, the majority of providers practice in a complicated combination of more than one type of medical practice management. Some serve as salaried employees in clinics sponsored by hospitals. Although fewer physicians may be practicing as sole proprietors, other providers of health care are picking up the model for their practices. Naturopaths, osteopaths, chiropractors, and acupuncturists often practice as sole proprietors. The type of business management to select is an early decision when entering practice but likely changes throughout one's career.

The type of organization for the medical practice is important to health-care employees and their work. Differences will be seen in the medical records, billing and accounting procedures, payroll, number and duties of employees, and benefits. The type of business organization will determine, in part, how health-care employees do their jobs. A brief overview of the most common medical management models is provided here, beginning with the most simple and easiest to establish.

SOLE PROPRIETORS

A sole proprietorship, or single proprietorship, is a business owned by a single individual who receives all the profits and takes all the risks (Fig. 2-1). It is the oldest form of business and is the

Figure 2-1. Sole proprietor is a practice owned by a single individual.

easiest to start, operate, and dissolve. It can be the most expensive to establish. Even sole proprietors, however, are likely to provide services under the umbrella of one or more managed care health insurance programs as preferred providers and in other types of business management. Sole proprietorships are a common management choice for the increasing number of providers in complementary and integrative medicine. There are advantages and disadvantages to this form of business management.

ADVANTAGES OF SOLE PROPRIETORSHIPS

The advantages of a sole proprietorship include having the simplicity of organization; being one's own boss; being the sole receiver of all profits that may generally be larger than any other forms of business management; and having lower organizational costs, greater flexibility in operation, and fewer government regulations than other forms of business management.

In addition, a sole proprietorship allows the provider to establish a practice in a community through the purchase or rent/lease of a facility, to make all the decisions without having to consult with any partners or other business colleagues, and to incur minimal organizational costs. This provider also will not have to divide the profits with any other person and will be able to run the practice exactly as desired. When the provider participates as a preferred provider in a managed care system, the provider must follow the guidelines of the system but is free to choose whether to participate.

DISADVANTAGES OF SOLE PROPRIETORSHIPS

The sole proprietorship does have disadvantages. For instance, providers may have difficulties raising sufficient capital to begin their business. Medical equipment is among the most expensive of any type of equipment in a new business. The sole proprietor typically performs all or most of the managerial functions in the business and works more than a standard 40-hour workweek. The profits of the business may be insufficient at a later time to allow for expansion. In addition, providers must know that if the business fails in a sole proprietorship or if a liability claim surpasses their insurance protection, their personal property may be attached, and they may lose virtually all personal savings and possessions.

Again, consider a provider who has sufficient capital when entering practice to establish business as a sole proprietorship. Initially, the system works well while the client load is light. However, the provider soon finds that time is at a premium if working 70 to 80 hours a week carrying a full client load, managing the business aspects of the practice, and having no other provider to cover weekends or vacations. Also, no one is available when the provider is ill or a family crisis must be attended to.

CONSIDERATIONS FOR THE HEALTH-CARE EMPLOYEE

The sole proprietor probably begins with just one assistant. This person needs education and training in *all* areas of administrative and clinical tasks to be performed in the health-care setting and will have variety in the work. Although some assistants enjoy the opportunity to use all their skills in the entire operation, others may find this situation less attractive and prefer that the provider have certain tasks sent outside the office for completion. These tasks may include laboratory work, transcription, correspondence, or billing and coding. The sole proprietorship often uses the services of an accountant for payroll and quarterly and yearly tax reports.

The sole proprietorship offers little if any opportunity for advancement for its employees. Therefore, providers will want to select employees carefully on the basis of their education, training, credentialing and experience; reward them sufficiently for their work; and encourage them to stay a long time with the practice. Some medical assistants will prefer the sole proprietorship because of the opportunity they have to make decisions and assume leadership responsibilities.

Case Study

The 64-year-old sole proprietor, a family practitioner, is the only physician in a rural community with a population of 3500. He has one medical assistant who has been with him for several years. The physician works 70 hours a week and many weekends. His assistant is feeling overworked also, and complains of less time with family. The physician wants very much to ease into retirement or to lessen his load.

What might the physician and his assistant do?
Identify how the plan you suggest might be implemented.

PARTNERSHIPS

A partnership is an association of two or more persons who are co-owners of a business for profit (Fig. 2-2). Partnerships may have only two or three members, but there is no maximum number of individuals who may enter into a partnership. The organization may take many forms and should be defined in a partnership agreement.

The partnership agreement should be written and reviewed by an attorney. It should include such items as the type of business to be conducted or services to be performed, the type of partnership being established, authority held by each partner, length of the partnership agreement, and capital invested by each partner. The agreement should also include a description of how profits and losses are to be shared, how each partner is to be compensated, limitations on monetary withdrawals by a partner, accounting procedures to be followed, procedures for admitting new partners, dissolution of the partnership, and, of course, the signatures of the partners involved in the agreement.

ADVANTAGES OF PARTNERSHIPS

Some advantages of partnerships are easily recognized. Generally, a partnership has more financial strength than a sole proprietorship. Partners are likely to bring additional managerial skills and

Figure 2-2. Partnership is a business agreement between two or more individuals.

share the workload. The organization of a partnership remains relatively simple, although somewhat more complicated than a sole proprietorship.

When a provider is deciding how to establish a practice, the partnership may be desirable. If the practice is already established, only a small capital investment may be required in the beginning. This investment can be increased as the provider becomes more financially secure. A sole proprietor often will turn to a partnership when the workload of the practice requires a second person to share the work.

DISADVANTAGES OF PARTNERSHIPS

A disadvantage of a partnership is that two or more people make the decisions, depending on the partnership contractual agreement. In addition, each partner is responsible for the business. If one partner lacks the personal finances to assume a full share of any loss, the other partners are required to make up for the deficit. If the partnership fails, usually one partner can be liable for all of the partnership debts, regardless of the size of the investment.

Personality differences should be considered because compatibility is important in any partnership. A trial period that allows a partner to withdraw from the association or be asked to withdraw after a given period may be advantageous. If the provider does not wish to enter a partnership agreement but needs additional help, another provider may be hired strictly on a salary basis. Although this arrangement does not constitute a partnership, a contract may be desirable for the protection of each party.

CONSIDERATIONS FOR THE HEALTH-CARE EMPLOYEE

A partnership should consider hiring more than one assistant in the health-care setting because of the increased workload. Each partner may desire an assistant, but many tasks will be common to each and are best performed by one person. Assistants must understand the partnership relationship and the line of authority. Open communication on the part of all members of the staff is essential. Otherwise, each provider may expect an assistant to function as a member of the staff but may not provide input as to how this function should be performed.

In addition, with more than one employee, both job advancement and job specialization are possible. For example, the newly formed partnership hiring a second assistant may want to name the first assistant clinic manager with a specific set of duties or to assign one assistant to administrative tasks while the other performs clinical duties.

 ## PROFESSIONAL SERVICE CORPORATIONS

A corporation is a legal entity that is granted many of the same rights enjoyed by individuals. These include the right to own, mortgage, and dispose of property, the right to manage its own affairs, and the right to sue and be sued (Fig. 2-3). Providers in a professional service corporation (PSC) remain personally liable for their acts of medical malpractice; however, they are not liable for the professional acts of their colleagues. Corporations are costly to establish, more formal than either the proprietorship or partnership, and require a legal document for formation and operation.

Professional service associations or professional corporations are designed for such professional persons as medical providers, lawyers, dentists, and accountants. These corporations can be identified by the letters SC (service corporation), PC (professional corporation), PSC, Inc. (professional service corporation, incorporated), and PA (professional association), depending on each state's law. The PSC is the most intricate of all forms of medical practice and can be formed by one or more individuals.

ADVANTAGES OF PROFESSIONAL SERVICE CORPORATIONS

Advantages of PSCs include the fact that contributions to pension or profit-sharing plans can be made for all employees as well as the provider. Such funds are deducted by the corporation from its taxable income, are invested, and accumulate in tax-free trusts until a future time of disbursement.

Figure 2-3. Medical providers often form professional service corporations.

Taxes are not paid on the funds until the time of their disbursement, usually at retirement, when the individual is in a lower tax bracket.

Another advantage of a PSC is the corporate medical reimbursement plan. Medical and dental expenses are deductible to the corporation and nontaxable to the employee. This plan can result in substantial savings to both corporation and employee. Group term life insurance on a deductible premium basis is another advantage of a professional corporation. The professional corporation also may pay the professional liability premiums for providers and their employees. Furthermore, in a corporation, providers' personal assets are protected and cannot be attached to satisfy a debt as they can be in a sole proprietorship or partnership.

DISADVANTAGES OF PROFESSIONAL SERVICE CORPORATIONS

When PSCs first became legal, many providers eagerly incorporated, only to discover the disadvantages. The complexity of the PSC and its detailed requirements call for reliable, well-informed attorneys and accountants to advise the corporation. The PSC may be more expensive to operate than other forms of organizations.

Regular meetings and agreement on organization, investments, pensions, and profit-sharing plans are important and legally required. Because more individuals generally are involved than in a sole proprietorship or most partnerships, decision making is more complicated. Providers often have problems finding the time to perform the business functions required to run a corporation.

Although a PSC usually involves two or more providers functioning in a group setting, a sole proprietor can incorporate as a PSC. The income of a single individual who incorporates needs to be sufficient to allow full participation in the benefits granted to the PSC, or such an arrangement is financially ineffective.

CONSIDERATIONS FOR THE HEALTH-CARE EMPLOYEE

The PSC generally employs more assistants than a partnership or sole proprietorship. The possibility of having medical expenses covered by the corporation is an attractive inducement to prospective employees. This form of practice usually provides ample opportunity for advancement and specialization. One person should be responsible for all personnel matters to enable a smooth-running organization.

GROUP PRACTICES

Another option of medical practice available to providers is joining a group practice. Group practice in medicine is defined as a group of medical providers who formally organize and agree to provide medical care, consultation, diagnosis, and treatment to clients. Equipment and personnel are used jointly. The income from the group is distributed according to a predetermined agreement of the members.

The provider in a group practice will either be a partner, an officer of the corporation, or an employee of the practice. Most group practices are also professional corporations or partnerships, but as the workload increases, new providers may be hired as employees.

The four main types of group practice include:

1. *Single specialty*, providing services in only one field of practice or major specialty; for example, a group of pediatricians joining together in practice
2. *Multispecialty*, providing services in two or more fields of practice or major specialties; for example, a group of obstetricians/gynecologists and pediatricians joining together in practice
3. *Primary care group*, providing services by obstetricians/gynecologists, pediatricians, family practitioners, and internists
4. *Hospital-managed medical groups*, providing all the services of a group practice, but owned by a hospital. Group practices formerly managed by providers are being sold in increasing numbers to hospitals when the members realize that the challenges of running a group are simply too costly and take too much time. Figure 2-4 illustrates this trend toward medical practices owned by hospitals.

Group medical practices operate on some form of fee-for-service basis, through insurance coverage, preferred provider arrangements, or even private pay with the same type of business arrangement as a sole proprietorship, a partnership, or a professional service corporation.

ADVANTAGES OF GROUP PRACTICE

Advantages to providers in group practice include a shared financial investment for diagnostic and therapeutic equipment, the opportunity for consultation with other providers, little administrative responsibility for the practice (a group may actually employ a medical manager for the business side of the operation), and more family and recreation time because providers in the group cover for one

Figure 2-4. A hospital-managed medical group.

another. In addition, group practice may offer informal consultations as well as the intellectual and social stimulation desired by many practitioners.

DISADVANTAGES OF GROUP PRACTICES

The disadvantages of group practices are easily identified. Not every individual has the personality to function well in a group setting. A provider cannot act totally independent of the group and may feel a loss of freedom in such a situation. Although the working hours may not be as long as in sole practice, the income, although guaranteed, also may not be as high. Working in a close relationship with colleagues on a daily basis may lead to personality clashes and differences of opinion.

CONSIDERATIONS FOR THE HEALTH-CARE EMPLOYEE

A group practice will have more employees than the other forms of medical organizations simply because of the larger staff of physicians and providers. Providers may have less responsibility for hiring and selecting personnel, which may be an advantage or a disadvantage, depending on the provider's personal preferences. An employee may choose employment in a group for many of the same reasons as those in the corporation. Depending on the number of employees, a larger group may be less personalized.

 ## HEALTH MAINTENANCE ORGANIZATIONS

The health maintenance organization (HMO) is a familiar form of medical practice management in today's society. Kaiser Foundation Health Plan is one of the largest, not-for-profit HMOs in the country. In this form of management, groups contract with clients to provide comprehensive health care and preventive medicine for premiums paid that entitle the subscriber to service during the duration of the contract.

The staff-model HMO owns and operates health-care centers, staffed by providers contractually employed directly by the plan. These health-care centers provide a broad range of services "under one roof," although perhaps in many locations.

Another form of HMO allows providers to maintain their private practices, charge their fee-for-service clients, and be reimbursed for their HMO clients by the central HMO organization. This type of HMO is really not a medical practice management model. The providers involved in this form of HMO may have clients who have prepaid for their services to any number of HMO organizations that will, in turn, pay the provider. The HMO may make use of the concept of a primary care provider (PCP) (often referred to as a gatekeeper) as a method of controlling costs. In a gatekeeper situation, all medical care sought by a client must be channeled through the PCP, and any referrals are made within the HMO provider list.

The advantage to providers who practice in a staff-model HMO is that the working hours will be regular and allow for more personal time. Also, practitioners will not have to provide the building or equipment necessary for practice.

Generally speaking, client and provider satisfaction with managed care services is based on personal experience. Some clients feel more satisfied; others feel less satisfied. Providers, forced to pay more attention to the management of their practice, are generally frustrated by this additional organizational burden.

 ## MANAGED CARE

Managed care is any arrangement for health care in which an organization, such as an insurance company, an HMO, or another type of doctor–hospital network, acts as an intermediary between the person seeking care and the provider (see Fig. 2-5). Although it is not a form of business management in the strictest sense of the word, managed care has dramatically restructured the delivery and financial aspects of health care. No provider can practice without feeling the effects of this system. In managed care, clients, too, have experienced a radical change in the delivery of their health

Figure 2-5. Managed care serves all its subscribers with an umbrella policy.

care. Some question the managed care corporation's financial interest in client care. To fully understand managed care, a brief history of insurance coverage is warranted.

In the early 1900s, consumers expected to pay for all health care from their own pockets. During the Depression, many health-care providers received little or no pay for their services. Blue Cross first provided insurance for hospital costs in the early 1930s. Blue Shield was introduced soon afterward to cover office and physician costs. Both were driven by union contracts in the automobile industry.

Soon employees expected that a part of their employment benefit package would include health insurance to cover all but a few incidental and minor expenses. Increased specialization, advancing technology, and little or no emphasis on preventive care drove health-care costs to a new all-time high. Employers began to struggle with the increased costs of offering health insurance to an all-demanding workforce. HMOs were introduced to emphasize preventive health care, assure providers they would receive payment for their services, and ultimately begin to contain costs. It was not long before nearly every health insurance carrier was offering some form of an HMO to employers as one of the available health-care plans.

Not all providers and health-care consumers were excited about HMOs, however. In some cases, consumers lost the right to choose their PCP. The choice had to be made from a list of participating providers. A common complaint from providers was their loss of control in the provider–client relationship because they felt the HMO dictated the kind and type of care to give clients. While providing basic health care to all persons was being hotly debated in Congress and across the country, HMOs continued to grow in popularity by paying close attention to preventive care, standardizing many medical practices, and eliminating unnecessary tests and procedures. Today, the largest HMOs in the country have become billion-dollar businesses; they still dictate how many medical decisions related to client care are made, and consumers are paying more for their medical coverage.

The method of payment for professional services has changed from only the fee-for-service method of payment, in which a provider is paid for each service rendered, to payment that may include a **co-payment**, a **deductible**, and/or **capitation.**

Co-payments, a specific dollar amount paid by the client or member (usually $25 or a percentage of the total bill), were established. The co-payment helps clients to realize their responsibility toward payment, but the amount is not considered exorbitant. It adds a cash flow to the provider receiving deductible amounts and the percentage paid by insurers for remaining services.

The deductible requires policyholders to pay a set amount toward covered services on a fee-for-service or preferred provider basis before the insurer begins to pay claims. Providers, however, often receive only a percentage of the cost of their services once the insurer's responsibility begins.

Another method of payment, much less popular with providers, and little known and understood by clients, is capitation. Capitation gives health-care providers a fixed monthly compensation for a range of services for each managed care or HMO member under their care rather than a fee for each service performed. The capitation models that are most successful are placing an emphasis on the quality of care and client-satisfaction targets. In some areas, capitation plans are increasing, in other areas, they are decreasing in popularity.

A more recent form of managed care is pay for performance (P4P). P4P is a plan to encourage providers to improve the quality of their clients' care, and reimburses providers for their progress toward a fixed goal. Payment is dependent on how well providers adhere to practice standards, especially in the arenas of preventive care and management of chronic illness. P4P programs vary in their approach. Some programs pay their providers from income received directly from participating employers or purchasers. Other programs, sponsored by managed care companies, reimburse providers who make their target. The reimbursement rate can be as much as 5% of revenues from sponsors or purchasers. Medicare, Blue Cross, and Blue Shield are major players in P4P. The latest research indicates, however, that client care showed no more significant improvement in quality than any other payment plan.

One can readily see the complexity of the problem faced by both providers and consumers in understanding the payment process and the cost of health care. What were seemingly subtle changes in the managed care contracts have had a great impact on providers and clients. Many found themselves in a form of managed care in which profit rather than health was the motive. Increasingly, providers must contact a third party for permission to perform certain procedures or make a referral to a specialist. Likewise, a client's health-care services are covered when obtained from a preferred provider chosen by the insurance carrier but only partially covered or not covered at all if obtained from an unaffiliated provider. Further, some managed care plans allow members to seek treatment outside the network but charge the members more to do so. This is called an opt-out option.

The problems of a business-first, client care–second system are found not only in managed care insurance. Covered fee-for-service plans have similar problems. The increased power of insurance carriers, which no longer simply collect premiums from subscribers and process claims, continues to take decision making away from providers and clients. Political influences at the state and national levels cannot be ignored either. The U.S. Congress still struggles after years of political infighting over Patient Bill of Rights legislation that would return some control, choice, and power to clients and their providers. The national Healthcare Reform Bill of 2010 may get it accomplished.

Case Study

Medicare clients find themselves in a bind. Because of a 21% reduction in Medicare reimbursements that occurred in 2010, increasing numbers of providers are opting not to provide medical care to the senior population. They simply cannot cover the loss incurred. This means that individuals with Medicare insurance will find it very difficult to select a new PCP if they move to another area (perhaps to be closer to family members) or they just wish to choose another provider. Many providers will continue to carry their current clients on Medicare, but will take no new clients.

As an employee in a practice that chooses to limit its Medicare clients to the current number, how will you respond to requests from individuals seeking a PCP?
Does the 2010 Healthcare Reform Bill address this issue? Explain your findings.

Some form of managed care or managed competition seems destined to play a role in the health-care delivery system for some time to come. Good and bad managed care plans are no different from good and bad health-care providers. Change will most likely come from informed clients, who will benefit most from their health-care providers. Information available through the Internet, television, public service programs, and print media will empower clients by giving them the information and vocabulary necessary to make themselves true partners in the client–provider relationship. Ideally, the federally mandated Healthcare Reform Bill will provide options.

 ## OTHER BUSINESS ARRANGEMENTS

Today's ambulatory health-care setting as a form of business management for medical practice continues to evolve. Larger clinics, PSCs, and conglomerates are increasingly popular.

JOINT VENTURES

Competition, marketing, and escalating costs have encouraged hospitals and providers to enter into joint ventures that may be profitable and advantageous to both entities. For example, hospitals are building ambulatory health-care settings within their service area to entice providers to rent office space and in turn refer their clients to the hospital. Hospitals may purchase a practice and staff it with one or more of their providers. Such ventures offer providers improved marketing capabilities and fewer start-up costs.

Case Law

The Sarah Bush Lincoln Health Center employed Richard Berlin, Jr., MD, in 1992 to practice medicine at the Health Center for 5 years. They entered into a written agreement whereby Dr. Berlin could terminate his employment arrangement for any reason during the 5-year period by giving 180-day advance written notice. The agreement also stipulated that he could not compete with the hospital by providing health services within a 50-mile radius of the Health Center for 2 years after the end of his employment.

On February 4, 1994, Dr. Berlin terminated his employment with the hospital (effective February 7, 1994) and immediately began employment with the Carle Clinic Association located approximately 1 mile from the Health Center.

The Health Center brought an injunction against the doctor to prohibit him from practicing so close to the hospital.

What problems surface here?
Did Dr. Berlin satisfy all elements of his agreement? Explain.

Summary Judgment: Richard Berlin, Jr., MD, filed a complaint seeking to have the restrictive covenant of his employment agreement with Sarah Bush Lincoln Health Center declared unenforceable.

The Circuit Court found in favor of Dr. Berlin on the basis that the entire employment agreement was unenforceable. A divided appellate court affirmed the district court's decision. Upon appeal, however, the Supreme Court of Illinois reversed the decision stating that the central issue was that the "corporate practice doctrine" is inapplicable to licensed hospitals.

Supreme Court of Illinois, 1997. 179 Ill.2d 1, 227 Ill. Dec. 769, 688 N.E.2d 106.

Note: Since the time of this case, many states have enacted legislation that permits licensed hospital corporations to utilize physicians as independent contractors and/or employees.

An unusual twist to the joint venture is the establishment of in-store medical clinics in chain-store markets, large and small, across the country. These chains seek such ventures to increase their customer base. The in-store clinics are providing limited medical care at decreased costs and added convenience to customers. A unique example of this is seen in the "Minute Clinics" common in CVS pharmacies that provide basic and very quick medical attention to clients. They are staffed by physician assistants (PAs) and nurse practitioners (NPs) and accept most insurance plans. Today, it is quite common to go to the pharmacy within a grocery conglomerate to receive flu vaccinations.

Physician–hospital organizations (PHOs) combine hospital and group medical practices in order to offer clients a "one-stop shopping approach." A primary reason for forming a PHO is the concept that combined services are more attractive than individual services would be. In addition, both providers and hospitals benefit one another. Clients receive more services, sometimes at a lower cost. This concept is becoming increasingly popular.

Case Study

In a joint venture arrangement, the hospital manages three satellite clinics. In one of the clinics, there is concern that a PA is spending too much time with clients. The PA is asked to log time in and time out for clients seen during a 3-week period. The PA's profitability is in question.

What do you think?
Identify circumstances that may contribute to longer periods of time with clients.

The *multiple service organization (MSO)* can be owned by providers, hospitals, a totally separate party, or any combination of the three. This organization is developed to perform office management services. For example, the MSO often provides secretarial and office services, billing and collections, group purchasing, and computer servicing. An MSO allows providers to focus on client care and permits the management service to run the business side of the organization.

PREFERRED PROVIDER ORGANIZATIONS

A provider may be a sole proprietor, a partner, or a member of a professional service corporation as well as a preferred provider for an organization. A preferred provider organization (PPO) creates a contractual agreement between an insurance carrier organization and the provider to supply medical care to an already established number of clients. For example, a provider may contract with Blue Cross's preferred provider plan to give medical care to a certain number of individuals who have subscribed to the Blue Cross preferred provider plan.

Providers considering a move into any of the integrated organizations should be certain that the business arrangement does not violate antitrust laws. Antitrust laws exist to preserve free-market competition. Consequently, under antitrust laws any activities that restrict competition are seen as unfavorable. Providers must ensure that the business arrangement does not oppose Medicare's fee-for-service reimbursement rules or violate any Medicare or Medicaid fraud and abuse laws. Because Medicare seeks a direct relationship with its providers, it may not recognize some business organizations as being eligible for Medicare reimbursement. Medicare and Medicaid laws further prohibit kickbacks and some referrals. For example, providers cannot refer Medicare or Medicaid clients to any entity in which they have any financial interest.

More and more physicians and providers are entering into a variety of business management arrangements, and they most likely will want to seek the appropriate legal advice to ensure that they are within the legal bounds of medical practice. ●

Case Study

The large medical conglomerate provides services to health-care providers in rural areas that would otherwise not have access to medical specialists. A practitioner in a rural area can send her electrocardiograph via telephone and have it read by a cardiac specialist, resulting in state-of-the-art, immediate diagnosis and treatment.

Can you think of another example in which medical care in rural areas can benefit from new technologies?

GENERAL LIABILITY

Physicians and providers engaged in business must be aware of their general liability. Unlike professional liability that relates to clients' medical treatment (see Chapter 5, Professional Liability), general liability regards business matters. These matters include liability for the building, any automobiles, theft, burglary, fire, and employees' safety. Office employees will be involved in payments of these liability insurance premiums and submission of claims. Also, they likely assist their employers in practice when making applications for business licenses.

BUSINESS LICENSE

Some communities require a business or occupational license before allowing a clinic to be opened for the practice of medicine. Providers should check with county and city clerks to determine whether a license is required and what procedures are to be followed. An annual renewal fee may be necessary; payment of the annual fees generally becomes the responsibility of an employee responsible for monitoring the activities of the business side of the practice.

BUILDING

The provider or the organization that owns the building is responsible for the building and grounds where business is conducted. If a person is injured on those premises, providers may be held legally responsible. Therefore, providers and managing organizations will carry liability insurance for the premises.

AUTOMOBILE

Aside from personal car insurance, providers may want to consider nonowner liability insurance. Such a plan protects the provider-employer if an employee has an automobile accident while performing some duty related to the business. For providers who commonly ask their employees to make a bank deposit on their drive home or to deliver the monthly statements to the post office, such protection is wise. Whose car an employee drives makes no difference.

FIRE, THEFT, AND BURGLARY

Providers should have protection against fire, theft, and burglary on the building as well as on equipment and furniture. Two types of fire insurance are most common. A coinsurance plan dictates that the owner is responsible for payment of a certain percentage of the loss, such as 20% or 30%. A second plan covers not only the loss but also the replacement costs. The replacement costs are, of course, more expensive, but more beneficial in the case of loss.

Cost of protection from burglary and theft depends on location and the amount of money or valuables kept on the premises. Large amounts of money should not be kept on the premises, even though most burglary attempts are made for the purpose of stealing narcotics. A discussion with insurance agents will identify proper protection.

Some providers may also insure their accounts receivable, which would be nearly impossible to recover in case of fire or loss. These items belong in a fireproof cabinet or safe after working hours to prevent their loss, even if insured.

EMPLOYEE SAFETY

Providers are expected to provide a safe place of employment for their employees. Safety requirements include federally mandated regulations as well as rules that vary from state to state. Some of the variables include the number of employees, the type of employment, and the safety record of the business. Check with the state agency administering such safety regulations, with workers' compensation statutes, and with the state medical association to determine responsibility in this area. Refer to Chapter 11, Employment Practices, for a discussion of Occupational Safety and Health Administration (OSHA) and other regulations to further protect employee safety.

BONDING

Providers may wish to bond employees who are handling financial records and money in the ambulatory health-care setting. Bonding is an insurance contract with a bonding agency. The purchase of a bond for a certain amount in an employee's name ensures that providers will recover the amount of the loss, up to the amount of the bond, in case the employee embezzles funds. This precaution is especially important when providers do not have the time to spot-check financial transactions made by employees. Careful employers ask prospective employees if they are bondable. It is also an advantage to a medical office employee to be bonded. Many providers will also check the credit ratings of potential employees who will be managing financial transactions if this is not included as part of the bonding process. This step is legal as long as the potential employee is informed in advance.

 ## RESPONSIBILITIES TO EMPLOYEES

Whatever the style of operation in which providers choose to practice, employers have certain business responsibilities to employees. These include federal, state, and local requirements for Social Security compensation protection and workers' compensation for all employees. Benefits can include a uniform allowance, paid parking, medical benefits, retirement benefits, profit-sharing plans, vacations, sick leave, paid holidays and personal leave time, professional improvement allowances, and professional liability insurance.

As stated previously in this chapter, providers must realize the value of appropriately qualified and educated employees and encourage employees to remain with the organization as long as possible. Specific information about providers' responsibilities to employees can be obtained from an accountant or attorney. County, state, or national medical associations have information about requirements for establishing a practice and also have guidelines for employees.

SUMMARY

Physicians and providers can open new practices, function as sole proprietors, be employed by others on a straight salary basis, establish partnerships, become part of PSCs, and practice alone or in groups. Most also will be related to some form of managed care and may participate in at least one HMO. All forms of medical practice have advantages and disadvantages. The choice depends on the individual personality and preference of the provider. None should be entered into without advice and consideration from people knowledgeable in the field.

The overriding factor for providers to consider is what type of business organization will best permit them to serve their clients. Providers must remember that the type of practice chosen will dictate their responsibilities in all areas of general liability. To be less than meticulous in this area of business can potentially mar a provider's professional reputation.

 Watch It Now! Where will you choose to work? at http://davisplus.fadavis.com/lawandethics

Questions for Review

SELECT THE BEST ANSWER

1. The sole proprietor
    a. Is owned by two or more individuals.
    b. Is the oldest form of business.
    c. Will have at least two medical assistants.
    d. Works a standard 40-hour workweek.
    e. None of the above.

2. A partnership
    a. Is an agreement that should be in writing.
    b. Has more financial strength than a sole proprietorship.
    c. Usually only has one medical assistant.
    d. Does not protect personal financial loss.
    e. Only a, b, and d are correct.

3. Professional service corporations
    a. Allow deductions from taxable income to make contributions to pension plans.
    b. Are relatively inexpensive to establish.
    c. Can only be formed with at least three providers.
    d. Are only established for multispecialty practices.
    e. Only a and c are correct.

4. A health maintenance organization
    a. Is one type of managed care.
    b. Often identifies a gatekeeper for each member.
    c. Always provides services under one roof.
    d. Only a and b are correct.
    e. None are correct.

5. Joint ventures are created
    a. To provide better insurance coverage for clients.
    b. To avoid paying taxes on shared income.
    c. Are designed to be profitable and advantageous to both entities.
    d. In order to perform office management services for providers.
    e. As a preferred provider organization.

TRUE OR FALSE

T   F   1. A co-payment is a member's medical expense paid to the provider.

T   F   2. SC, PSC, PA, and PSC, Inc. are all identification letters for professional service corporations.

T   F   3. Providers often have problems finding time to perform business functions.

T   F   4. Capitation gives providers a variable monthly fee for services provided to HMO members under their care.

T   F   5. PHOs are physician–hospital organizations designed to provide clients "one-stop shopping" for services.

CLASSROOM EXERCISES

1. What kind of business management exists in the ambulatory health-care setting where you are employed or where you would be most interested in seeking employment? Justify your response.

2. The clinic's neighborhood is changing and includes more low-income residents. The practice already has a high percentage of Medicare and Medicaid clients. The providers are considering "closing the doors" to any new clients in this category. As a receptionist, you know you will be the one to turn people away. Describe your feelings. What can you do?

3. If the number of primary care providers in family practice continues to decrease, what might ambulatory care begin to look like?

4. Why would an employer in an ambulatory health-care setting or clinic have the bookkeeper bonded?

5. In the vignette "How Did This Happen?" what options does Geralyn have? What advantages does either the partnership or corporation offer her? Personally, what gains has she made as the practice has grown, and what has she lost?

INTERNET ACTIVITIES

1. Research the Internet for "concierge medical practice." Describe your findings. Would you like to be employed in such a practice? Explain your response.

2. Visit the Web site for the Medical Group Management Association (MGMA). Browse the site to determine resources available. What do you find to add to your knowledge base related to this chapter's topics? Would it be beneficial for a member of a clinic's practice to be a member of the MGMA? Justify your response.

REFERENCES

Harris, G. More Doctors Giving Up Private Practices. www.nytimes.com

WEB RESOURCES

Agency for Healthcare Research and Quality
   www.ahrq.gov/news

American Medical Association
   www.ama-assn.org

American Medical New
   www.ama-assn.org/amednews

Healthcare Information and Management Systems Society
   www.himss.org

Kaiser Health News
   www.kaiserhealthnews.org/

DavisPlus | For additional resources please visit
http://davisplus.fadavis.com

CHAPTER 3

The Health-Care Team in the Ambulatory Setting

"The idea behind the tiny flower is that it really doesn't matter how small you are, whether in size or numbers. It doesn't matter how much you know, or how skilled you are. It doesn't matter how much education or how many credentials you have. What really matters is how you affect the world around you."—Serge Kahili King; Author, Humanitarian, Shaman of the Hawaiian Tradition

KEY TERMS

certification Documentation usually from a professional organization that an individual has met certain requirements and standards set forth by that organization.

clinic manager Person who has additional education and experience in the health-care field to manage a facility.

continuing education units (CEUs) These are awarded to professionals within a particular field after gaining additional knowledge at a workshop or seminar.

credential Evidence of having achieved a certain level of knowledge through education and experience.

endorsement An agreement in which one state recognizes the licensing procedure of another state, considers it valid, and grants a license to practice; sometimes referred to as *reciprocity*.

licensed practical nurse (LPN) or licensed vocational nurse (LVN) A graduate from a 9-month to 1-year practical nurse vocational or college program who has passed the state licensing examination for practical or vocational nurses.

licensure Legal permission, granted by state statutes, to perform specific acts; for instance, a physician is licensed to practice medicine.

medical assistant (MA) Person who assists the provider in both administrative and clinical duties; education varies from on-the-job instruction to 2 years in an accredited program for medical assisting.

medical/professional coder Person who has had education and experience in *Current Procedural Terminology, 4th Edition* (CPT-4) and *International Classification of Diseases* (ICD-9; soon to be ICD-10) coding; responsible for the correct application of codes for procedures, supplies, and diagnoses used for billing professional medical services.

medical laboratory technician (MLT) A graduate from a certificate or associate degree program who works under the supervision of a provider or medical technologist in a laboratory preparing specimens and operating automated analyzers.

medical technologist (MT) A graduate from a 4-year college or university program in medical technology that includes 1 year of clinical experience in the laboratory. MTs perform complex tests and analyses, ensure accuracy of testing, and may supervise medical laboratory technicians.

medical transcriptionist Person who may or may not have formal education; will have superior medical terminology knowledge as well as keyboarding and grammar skills; transcribes medical dictation.

nurse practitioner (NP) Nurse practitioner is an RN (usually with a bachelor of science in nursing) who has successfully completed additional education in an NP program at the master's or doctoral level.

physician A provider who is identified by law as a doctor of medicine (MD) or a doctor of osteopathic medicine (DO).

physician assistant (PA) Person with 1 to 4 years of education in an approved PA program; a PA works under the supervision of a physician.

provider Any health-care professional who examines, diagnoses, and treats individuals (includes MDs and DOs).

reciprocity An agreement by which two states recognize the licensing procedures of each other, consider them valid, and grant licenses to practice based on the other state's licensure. In some states, it is referred to as *endorsement.*

registered nurse (RN) A graduate from a 2-year associate degree, 3-year diploma, or 4- to 5-year bachelor's degree program who passed the state licensing examination for RNs. An RN works under the direction of a physician.

registration An entry in an official record listing names of persons satisfying certain requirements and level of education.

scope of practice Terminology used by state licensing boards that defines the procedures, actions, and processes that are permitted for a professional depending on their education, experience, and demonstrated competency.

tickler file A chronological file used as a reminder to do specific tasks on schedule; usually daily, weekly, or monthly.

LEARNING OUTCOMES

Upon successful completion of this chapter, you will be able to:

3.1   Define the key terms.

3.2   Discuss licensure, certification, and registration of health-care professionals.

3.3   Identify the role of the medical assistant (administrative and/or clinical) in ambulatory care.

3.4   Provide at least three examples of nonlicensed personnel in the health-care setting.

3.5   List and define the three categories of nurses found in health-care settings and compare their education and their scope of practice.

3.6   List two similarities and dissimilarities between a physician assistant and a nurse practitioner.

3.7   Describe scope of practice for ambulatory health-care personnel.

COMPETENCIES

CAAHEP

- Discuss legal scope of practice for medical assistants. (CAAHEP IX.C.1)
- Discuss licensure and certification as it applies to health-care providers. (CAAHEP IX.C.5)
- Perform within scope of practice. (CAAHEP IX.P.2)
- Demonstrate awareness of the consequences of not working within the legal scope of practice. (CAAHEP IX.A.2)

ABHES

- Compare and contrast the allied health professions and understand their relation to medical assisting. (ABHES 1.b)
- Understand medical assistant credentialing requirements and the process to obtain the credential; comprehend the importance of credentialing. (ABHES 1.c)
- Define scope of practice for the medical assistant, and comprehend the conditions for practice within the state that the medical assistant is employed. (ABHES 1.e)
- Conducting work within scope of education, training, and ability. (ABHES 11.b.9)

What Would You Do?

The receptionist in a pediatrician's clinic answers the phone and immediately hears a baby crying in the background. The caller states that her baby seems to be in pain and is pulling at her ears. The receptionist states, "Oh, she probably has an ear infection. Why don't you come right in and the doctor will see her." Discuss the issues raised by this conversation.

In any type of health-care setting there is a "team" of people who provide care to a client. The leader of the team is the provider, but the team includes every individual employed in the facility. Each member has a very important responsibility and many assigned tasks, some of which can be performed only by that individual. Even the custodian contributes to the client's care by helping to provide a safe and clean environment. All employees need to work in cooperation and collaboration as a team to provide the client with quality health care. The number and types of employees in the health-care setting will vary with the size and type of the practice. Each employee has specific skills and education level.

THE HEALTH-CARE TEAM

Employees in the health-care setting may fall into the following categories: (1) those that are certified, (2) those that are registered, and (3) those that are licensed. Some employees may be none of the three, and some more than one. The classifications of certification, registration, or licensure establish that the employee has met a minimum standard required by law or a national organization.

Certification is the most common form of regulation. It occurs when a professional organization administers a national examination to assess the knowledge and skill of its applicants. With passage of this examination, the applicant has demonstrated that he or she has met the minimum standards set forth by the organization. This certification of health-care professionals usually exceeds the standards required by any governmental agency. There is a fee associated with the exam and a membership fee for the organization. There is a process set forth for recertification that takes place every 2 to 5 years depending on the organization. Certification is a self-regulating, credentialing process that is fully voluntary. However, this does not prevent anyone without certification from practicing.

Registration is a process by which individuals in a particular health field are listed in a registry. This list is then available to health-care providers. The state has little or no power over the registration process. There are two methods of registration. One occurs when individuals list their names in an official registry of a health area in which they work. The second form of registration requires a predetermined level of education. Professional associations interested in recognizing qualified health-care professionals administer examinations that must be passed before the appropriate credential can be conferred. This formal registry is most likely seen in ambulatory care. There is a fee associated with the exam and a membership fee for the organization.

Licensure is the strongest form of regulation. It requires passing a licensing examination and paying a licensing fee as well as a fee associated with the examination. A license establishes that the employee has met minimum standards required by law. Licensure laws protect the public from unqualified practitioners, and limit and control admission to different health-care occupations. When licensure is a requirement to practice, it is illegal to practice without one. Licensed employees must obtain their licenses from the state authority in which they wish to be employed. Most licensed personnel also hold memberships in professional organizations for which there is a fee.

Renewal of certification, registration, and/or licensure usually involves a fee and proof of continuing education units (CEUs) over a certain period of time, usually 2 or 5 years.

Certified, registered, and licensed individuals may use appropriate abbreviations after their names to verify their credentials. Examples include certified medical assistant, CMA (AAMA); registered medical assistant, RMA; and licensed practical nurse, LPN. Both certification and registration are voluntary. Licensure is mandatory (Fig. 3-1).

There are a number of members of the health-care team serving in either administrative and/or clinical areas in ambulatory care that fit within the models of certification, registration, and licensure.

ADMINISTRATIVE TEAM MEMBERS

The administrative staff is most likely to schedule appointments, tend to the client flow through the clinic, and complete all of the clinic's clerical work. These team members may include receptionists or administrative assistants, insurance specialists, coders, billers, and file clerks. Most of these health professionals have additional education and experience beyond high school. Such educational experiences include community and technical colleges, private schools, and/or online course preparation. These courses include medical terminology, medical office procedures, transcription, coding and billing, and other pertinent classes. Such courses may lead to a Medical Office Certificate, Medical Receptionist/Secretary Certificate, or a Medical Support Certificate conferred by the educational institution and not to be confused with professional certification. It is this additional education that gives a prospective employee an advantage in the job market or helps an employee gain additional compensation in pay.

Among the administrative team members there are those who are apt to be certified. There are different certifications offered by professional organizations to which the employees may belong.

Within this area are medical assistants (MAs). An MA can be a graduate medical assistant, MA; certified medical assistant, CMA (AAMA); registered medical assistant, RMA; or certified medical administrative specialist, CMAS (Fig. 3-2). Upon graduation from a medical assistant program, an individual is known as an MA. The MA's versatility provides for efficient management of the entire ambulatory health-care setting. Although the MA is a generalist, the role may be highly specific, depending on the duties assigned.

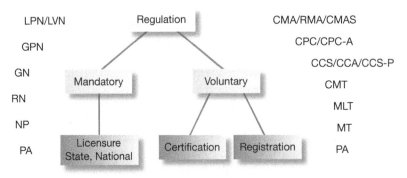

Figure 3-1. Not all professions follow the same regulations.

MEDICAL ASSISTANT PROGRAMS
in
PRIVATE AND POSTSECONDARY SCHOOLS

Recognized by the U.S. Department of Education

CAAHEP	ABHES
600 Programs	129 Programs

AAMA   AMT

National Certification Examination

CMA	RMA and CMAS
Certified Medical Assistant	Registered Medical Assistant
	Certified Medical Administrative Specialist
Requires 60 CEUs every 5 years for recertification	Requires 30 CEUs every 3 years

Figure 3-2. Education and credentialing of medical assistants.

The AAMA defines MAs in the following manner on their Web site: "Medical assistants are the only allied health professionals specifically trained to work in ambulatory settings, such as physicians' offices, clinics, and group practices. These multiskilled personnel can perform *administrative* and *clinical* procedures. Physicians value this unique versatility more and more, as managed care compels them to contain costs and manage human resources efficiently. Not surprisingly, the demand for MAs is expanding rapidly." **(www.aama-ntl.org/about/what_is_a_cma.aspx)**

Educational programs for the MA are usually 1 or 2 years in a private or postsecondary vocational/technical, community, junior, or senior college awarding a certificate, diploma, or associate's degree. Programs include academic courses and clinical experience. The MA receives education in both administrative and clinical practices.

A person who has graduated from an accredited program of either the Commission on Accreditation of Allied Health Education Program (CAAHEP) or the Accrediting Bureau of Health Education Schools (ABHES) is allowed to take a national certification examination that covers all aspects of medical assisting. There is a fee for each examination. With successful passage of the examination, the individual becomes either a certified medical assistant (CMA) through the AAMA or a registered medical assistant (RMA) through the American Medical Technologists (AMT). The RMA recertification requires 30 CEUs every 3 years. The CMA (AAMA) must renew the credential every 60 months, requiring a total of 60 CEUs. Current certified status is required to use the CMA (AAMA) credential in connection with employment.

Another certification is that of a certified medical administrative specialist (CMAS). This certification is offered by the AMT organization. A CMAS is familiar with clinical and technical concepts required to coordinate administrative functions throughout the entire clinic. This credential is often held by a clinic manager or practice manager. This person oversees the daily operation of the clinic, including all the staff, whereas medical-related issues are managed by the providers. Clinic managers will have procedures in place to monitor the certifications, registrations, and licenses of all employees. Practice-specific certifications and compliances, such as Clinical Laboratory Improvement Amendments (CLIA) and Occupational Safety and Health Administration (OSHA), and other legal requirements may also be overseen by the clinic manager. (See Chapter 10, Reimbursement and Collection Practices.)

ACCREDITATION OF MEDICAL ASSISTANT PROGRAMS

The CAAHEP awards or denies accreditation to MA programs (in addition to many other allied health programs). The AAMA, working in conjunction with the American Medical Association (AMA), defines the essential components and standards of quality that educational institutions must follow in educating MAs. Only graduates of CAAHEP-accredited MA programs are eligible to sit for the national certification examination. The AAMA believes that this safeguards the quality of care to the consumer, ensures the CMA's role in a rapidly evolving health-care delivery system, and continues to promote the identity and stature of the profession. Further, CAAHEP is recognized by the U.S. Department of Education.

The ABHES also awards and denies accreditation to MA programs in private and postsecondary institutions. The AMT, in cooperation with ABHES, defines the curriculum for the programs that prepare students for the medical assisting profession. ABHES is also recognized by the U.S. Department of Education.

Medical/professional coders are responsible for the correct application of procedures, supplies, and diagnostic codes used for billing professional medical services. Without accurate medical documentation and the correct coding, reimbursement will be lessened or even denied. There are approximately 57,000 professional coders in the country. Two associations credential professional coders:

1. American Academy of Professional Coders (AAPC), which includes certified professional coder apprentice (CPC-A) and certified professional coder (CPC) for those who work in an ambulatory setting, and certified professional coder—hospital apprentice (CPC-HA) and certified professional coder—hospital (CPC-H) for those working in a hospital.
2. American Health Information Management Association (AHIMA), which includes certified coding associate (CCA), certified coding specialist (CCS), certified coding specialist—physician based (CCS-P)

These various levels of certification can be attained with additional education and experience.

Case Study

Margie is the billing clerk at Lake Family Practice. She is working on Dr. Dillon's forms and notices that Linda Young is being billed for a complete physical examination. Margie remembers seeing Linda, a friend from the gym, and thought she had spent only a little time in the clinic with Dr. Dillon. Margie decides that she must have been mistaken.

As Margie progresses through the forms, she sees a form for Robert Brown. Mr. Brown is being charged for an expanded focus examination. Margie remembers Mr. Brown commented on his way out that he has never been in and out of the office so fast. He was happy to have had a quick appointment.

Margie becomes suspicious of Dr. Dillon's billing and checks closely the encounter forms for today, comparing them to his chart documentation. She finds more contradictions.

What would you do?
What legal ramifications does this situation present?

Medical transcriptionists may be part of the administrative team. These team members have knowledge and experience in the transcription of the provider's clinic notes, medical reports, and correspondence. Much of this work is currently outsourced to private companies. Whether located in-house or offsite, these individuals remain an important part of the health-care team. The certified medical transcriptionist or CMT is a transcriptionist who has passed the national certifying examination offered by the Association for Healthcare Documentation Integrity (AHDI) (formerly the American Association of Medical Transcription—AAMT).

There are additional certifications available to the administrative staff. These can be found at the Web sites of various organizations.

Case Law

A patient is referred to a consultant for diagnosis. The consultant's receptionist/secretary obtains the patient (client) information, including the referring physician's (provider's) name. The receptionist/secretary is not familiar with this doctor's name, looks it up in the telephone directory, and cannot locate any information on the doctor. She comments to the patient, "I cannot find your doctor's name in the directory. He must not be licensed to practice." When the patient is examined by the consultant, the consultant makes some derogatory comments about the referring physician.

The patient later tells his primary physician what the receptionist/secretary and the consultant said.

Kaplan v Goodfried, 497 SW2D 101 (1973)

CLINICAL SUPPORT TEAM MEMBERS

The clinical support staff will include members with a variety of educational experiences.

In this area you will find a CMA (AAMA) or RMA performing clinical duties as assigned by the physician or provider. Among their duties are assisting with examinations and minor surgeries, checking vital signs, and taking electrocardiograms. Providers see the value of these professionals because CMAs (AAMA) or RMAs have been educated and specifically prepared for ambulatory care settings. An MA or any other health professional must never attempt to go beyond their education and experience. Some states limit an MA's scope of practice. For example, in some states a CMA (AAMA) is not allowed to administer vaccinations even though they have been trained to do so. MAs must be aware of the laws in the state in which they wish to practice.

If there is a laboratory onsite at a health-care facility, medical laboratory technicians (MLTs) may be employed. MLTs have graduated from a certificate or associate's degree program. They work under the supervision of a physician or medical technologist in a laboratory preparing specimens and operating automated analyzers, among other tasks. Most MLTs become certified by the AMT.

Also employed in a laboratory is a medical technologist (MT) who has graduated from a 4-year college program. This education includes 1 year of clinical experience. MTs are certified through the American Society of Clinical Pathologists (ASCP). The job of an MT encompasses a wide variety of responsibilities. Most MTs work in clinical pathology laboratories where they run blood and tissue tests and analyze biological samples. Whether employed in a large independent laboratory, a hospital laboratory, or ambulatory care, this individual offers a critical piece to a client's care.

A licensed practical nurse (LPN) or a licensed vocational nurse (LVN) may be found in the clinical area of an ambulatory care setting. The terms LPN and LVN are interchangeable, depending on the geographic region of the country. These team members are licensed through the state in which they work, where they must pay a fee and pass an examination. They have completed a 1-year education course at a community agency; a public vocational/technical school; or a junior, community, or senior college. The substance of their program includes nursing practices and introductory educational courses. LPNs or LVNs care for the disabled, the sick, and the convalescent under the supervision of physicians or registered nurses (RNs). They usually provide basic bedside care in hospitals, nursing homes, and long-term care facilities. Renewal of their license requires an application, a fee, and a list of CEUs to produce if audited by the Board of Nursing.

A small number of RNs may be found in an ambulatory setting assisting with clinical duties. Graduate nurses (GNs) must take the National Council Licensure Examination (NCLEX) to be licensed as an RN. They can be graduates of a hospital-based program (very few left in the country) receiving a diploma, or they could receive an associate's or bachelor's degree.

A nurse must pass the appropriate national examination in order to use the LPN, LVN, or RN title. This license is renewed as mandated by state law. Most states require a renewal fee; some states require CEUs for license renewal. All nurses need to know their state's requirements and recommendations for license renewal. Nurses wishing to practice in another state may seek reciprocity or endorsement in that state. Reciprocity or endorsement occurs when one state recognizes the licensing procedure of another, considers it valid, and grants a license to practice based on the other's licensure. If there is no reciprocity process, the nurse must satisfy the state's licensure requirement.

Nurses may be employed in clinics (especially those clinics where surgery is performed) because of their technical expertise in clinical areas. Few nurses, however, have skills relating to the business aspect of the ambulatory health-care setting or have the desire to function in that capacity.

Case Study

An MA and an RN work side by side in a large medical setting. A recent downsizing has required assignments to be shifted. The RN is angered by the MA's appointment to an expansion of duties. There is a significant pay difference between the two salaries, with the nurse's salary being higher.

Discuss the ramifications of this situation as they apply to both the RN and the MA.

HEALTH-CARE PROVIDERS

This portion of the health-care team includes those who provide the examination, diagnosis, and treatment plan for each client. There are a variety of caregivers in this area, all with varying degrees of education.

Within the category of health-care providers is a physician assistant (PA). A PA can fit into all three models of certification, registration, and licensure. The typical PA program is 24 to 32 months and requires at least 4 years of college and some health-care experience before admission. There are more than 140 PA programs that are accredited by the Accreditation Review Commission on Education for the Physician Assistant (ARC-PA). More than 43% of PAs work in group practices or solo physician clinics, and more than one third are found in hospitals. The remaining PAs are located in rural clinics, community health centers, freestanding surgical facilities, nursing homes, school- or college-based facilities, industrial settings, and correctional systems. These individuals perform tasks usually done by physicians and work under the direction of a supervising physician. All states require PAs to pass the certification examination of the National Commission on Certification of Physician Assistants (NCCPA). Following certification, PA-Cs must meet the requirements of the state in which they wish to practice. All states except three require state licensing. Maryland and Ohio require state certification, and New York requires registration. Recertification through the NCCPA requires 100 hours of continuing medical education (CME) every 2 years and a recertification exam every 6 years. PAs are credentialed by their state medical board and fall under the medical practice act provisions. With more than 74,500 PAs in practice, these health-care providers serve a significant role in the health-care field. PAs may supervise MAs.

The nurse practitioner (NP) is a licensed RN with a bachelor's of science in nursing (BSN) degree who has successfully completed additional education in an NP program at the master's or doctoral level. Graduates are prepared for primary care practice in family medicine, women's health, neonatology, pediatrics, geriatrics, or mental health. The NP then seeks national certification, which requires written and/or oral examination. NPs are licensed in all states. They practice under the rules and regulations of the state in which they are licensed. Most NPs are nationally certified in their specialty area and are recognized as expert health-care providers. NPs may examine, diagnose, and treat clients—acts formerly performed solely by physicians.

The employment field for NPs varies. For instance, they may be found in isolated areas of the country managing a clinic and providing total client care, or they may be found in public health in charge of family planning clinics. NPs also may be found in medical clinics. They work independently and collaboratively on the health-care team. Almost half of all NPs work in family practice. There are more than 135,000 NPs practicing in the United States. Recertification requires 1500 direct patient-contact hours and 75 CEUs every 5 to 6 years. No examination is required. NPs practice under their basic RN license and fall under the Nurse Practice Act. In most states they may supervise MAs. However, in some states, such as Mississippi, NPs cannot supervise or delegate to unlicensed personnel. This fact illustrates the point that no matter what the position is in the health-care field, the rules and regulations for the geographic area in which employment is held must be known and fully understood.

Case Study

Edna Johnson came into the office for nasal congestion, cough, and a fever of 2 days. She was given one of the only available appointments open for the day with the NP. After taking Edna's vital signs, the MA told her that the NP would be in shortly. Edna became agitated and demanded to see the doctor, stating, "I want to see someone who can diagnose my condition and prescribe an antibiotic."

What is your response to Edna?
How can you reassure Ms. Johnson regarding the experience and preparation of the NP?

Also in the clinical setting is the doctor. Among these individuals are physicians (MDs), osteopaths (DOs), and naturopaths (NDs). The doctor oversees some health-care professionals directly (NP, PA, LPN, LVN, RN, MA); for others they provide clinical guidance and/or advice (clinic manager and administrative staff). The doctor is the one who sets the standard and is responsible for maintaining the medical and ethical standards of the clinic. These providers are ultimately responsible for everyone on staff. The education of MDs and DOs includes a 4-year bachelor's degree, a 4-year medical degree, and then a 2- to 8-year residency program, depending on the type of doctor and the specialty involved. Doctors are also licensed by a state medical board. (See Chapter 4, State and Federal Regulations.) Physicians may then go on to take a certification exam in their specialty area offered by their professional organization. They gain the distinction of being "board certified." This board certification is then renewed every 2 to 7 years depending on the specialty.

An ND attends a 4-year graduate-level naturopathic medical school and is educated in all of the same basic sciences as an MD, but also studies holistic and nontoxic approaches to therapy with a strong emphasis on disease prevention and optimizing wellness. NDs take professional board exams so that they may be licensed by a state as primary care general practice physicians.

CONSIDERATIONS FOR AMBULATORY CARE EMPLOYEES

It is important for ambulatory health-care employees to remember that, because of the ever-changing field of medicine, they need to continue their education. Obviously, continuing education benefits not just the individual and the employer but also, and more importantly, the welfare of the clients they serve. Many health-care professions require continuing education to maintain their certification, registration, or licensure. Employers should have a procedure for making certain all employees are up to date in their credentialing. This task is often assigned to the clinic manager, who perhaps will maintain a tickler file of all important dates to recall. These include due dates for license renewals, insurance premiums, and narcotic registrations. Established patterns must be maintained for drug inventory and accurate records. Detailed descriptions and examples of such activities in the clinic's procedure manual are most helpful. All employees, administrative and clinical, are to be encouraged to belong to and be active in a professional organization that pertains to their area of expertise. Many employers will give incentives to employees who seek certification in their area, if available. Some employers will pay membership fees as part of a benefit package. This is a win–win situation for all parties. Employees are able to keep up to date and network within their field; the employer has a well-informed and educated employee; and thus the quality of care to the client is improved.

 ## SCOPE OF PRACTICE

State regulations vary from state to state and will continue to change as medicine becomes more specialized. These state regulations are addressed in medical practice acts. These are state laws written for the express purpose of governing the practice of medicine that delineates the scope of practice for health-care professionals. "Scope of practice" is terminology used by state licensing boards to define the procedures, actions, and processes that are permitted for a professional depending on education, experience, and demonstrated competency. The scope of practice varies from one health-care professional category to the next. Even within one specific category, the scope of practice can vary from state to state. There is one constant, however, from state to state within each category: the requirement to have a doctor oversee all other health-care professionals. As stated previously, the doctor is responsible for overseeing the medical and ethical standards of the staff of the clinic. It is the doctor's responsibility to see that the staff are assigned tasks within their scope of practice. Ultimately, each staff member is responsible for his or her actions.

Case Law

East Missouri Action Agency is a federally tax-exempt, not-for-profit corporation that maintains several clinics in Missouri. The agency, specializing in family planning, obstetrics, and gynecology, services the low-income population.

Among the many staff members that the agency employs are two nurses who are licensed and have postgraduate education in the field of obstetrics and gynecology. They take histories, provide and give information about birth control, perform breast and pelvic examinations, dispense certain designated medications, and provide counseling services and community education. All acts of the nurses are performed under written standing orders and protocols signed by the physicians of the agency.

Missouri Board of Registration threatened to order the nurses and physicians to show why the nurses should not be found guilty of the unauthorized practice of medicine and the physicians guilty of aiding and abetting such practices.

The two nurses and five physicians petitioned the court for a declaratory judgment and injunction stating that the agency nurses are authorized under the nursing law of Missouri and that such practices do not constitute the unauthorized practice of medicine.

The court found that the nurses' acts were authorized and within their scope of practice to provide these services.

Sermchief v Gonzales, Supreme Court of Missouri, 1983

In some states, MAs cannot perform venipuncture or give injections. Some states also regulate who can practice radiography and who can administer medications. All states regulate laboratory procedures and protocol. An employer must understand regulations pertinent to those individuals in his or her employ. Employees also have the professional responsibility to abide by the regulations pertaining to their jobs. Practicing within the law is essential for the protection of all concerned. Employers must recognize that hiring employees with appropriate qualifications and credentials helps ensure that clients receive the optimal level of quality care and reduce risk for liability.

Case Study

The Medical Board of California in their October 2002 Action Report responded to physicians' interests about who may perform what type of cosmetic procedures. In response to who may use lasers or intense pulse light devices to remove hair, spider veins, and tattoos, they state: "Physicians may use lasers or intense pulse light devices. In addition, physician assistants and registered nurses (not licensed vocational nurses) may perform these treatments under a physician's supervision. Unlicensed medical assistants, licensed vocational nurses, cosmetologists, electrologists, or estheticians may not legally perform these treatments under any circumstances, nor may registered nurses or physician assistants perform them independently, without supervision."

In response to who may inject Botox, they state: "Physicians may inject Botox, or they may direct licensed registered nurses, licensed vocational nurses, or physician assistants to perform the injection under their supervision. No unlicensed persons such as medical assistants may inject Botox."

Watch for action in other states regarding these issues.

SUMMARY

When considering the education of various health-care professionals, one must remember that each is a vital link in the chain to quality health care. No one functions independently of any other. Each health professional has skills and responsibilities to complement every other health professional. When competition and territoriality cause conflict between professionals, quality health care is diminished. The education, knowledge, and scope of practice for each health-care professional are specifically and purposely designed to complement rather than to conflict. Because health-care delivery is changing every day, it is vital that the health-care team's needs keep changing with it.

Watch It Now! Can you be a member of the "team" in health care? at
http://davisplus.fadavis.com/lawandethics

Questions for Review

SELECT THE BEST ANSWER

1. When two states recognize the licensing procedures of each other, consider them valid, and grant licenses to practice based on the other state's licensure, this is called
   a. Reciprocity.
   b. Endorsement.
   c. Certification.
   d. Only a and b above.
   e. None of the above.

2. Which of the following are specifically prepared to work in a medical clinic/practice?
   a. LPN/LVN
   b. RN
   c. MA
   d. Only a and c above
   e. None of the above

3. A medical transcriptionist may become certified by passing a certifying examination offered by the
   a. AAMA.
   b. AHDI.
   c. AMA.
   d. AMT.
   e. NCCPA.

4. What credentialing is required of a physician assistant in all states except MD, OH, and NY?
   a. Certification
   b. Registration
   c. Licensure
   d. Only a and b above
   e. None of the above

5. Once an MD has achieved the designation of "Board Certified," he/she
   a. is certified for life.
   b. must recertify every 2 to 7 years.
   c. must recertify every 15 years.
   d. is certified in all specialties.
   e. must register the certification yearly.

TRUE OR FALSE

T **F**   1. Medical transcriptionists perform an important part of the documentation process.

T **F**   2. A clinic manager may desire the CMAS certification through the AAMA.

T **F**   3. Inclusion is another term for reciprocity.

T **F**   4. MTs are required in all ambulatory care settings.

T **F**   5. The LPN and LVN receive the same education.

CLASSROOM EXERCISES

1. 1. *Case A:* A solo family practitioner is setting up a practice in a small, rural community. *Case B:* Six providers are entering a group practice in a city of 40,000. Specialties include obstetrics/gynecology, family practice, internal medicine, and pediatrics.
   What number and kinds of employees would you recommend in case A? In case B? Explain your choices.

2. What kind of medical practice is most likely to employ a
   a. PA.
   b. MA.
   c. Nurse practitioner.

3. Discuss the difference between a CMA (AAMA) and an RMA with regard to their certification requirements.

4. Discuss the advantages of belonging to and being active in a professional organization.

5. Consider the AAMA definition of a medical assistant. Change that definition to include any state regulations particular to your area.

6. Increasingly, large health facilities are asking health-care professionals to do more with less. Some are approached about becoming a specialist in a particular area with or without additional education. For example, a CMA may be asked to become an emergency room (ER) technician with specialized, in-house education. Or the same person may be asked to be a surgical technician with the appropriate education. What are the legal and ethical implications of such requests? Discuss.

INTERNET ACTIVITIES

1. As we have learned, the scope of practice for MAs is different in each state. Search the Internet and research the scope of practice for MAs in your state. Compare what you find with the education that you have received. Will you be able to do everything that you have learned?

2. Visit the Web site for the AAMA. List the advantages of becoming a member as a student and the advantages of continuing your membership once you have graduated.

REFERENCES

American Association of Medical Assistants: What is a Medical Assistant? **www.aama-ntl.org/**

Furrow, B., Greaney, T., Johnson, S., Jost, T., & Schwartz, R.: *Health Law: Cases, Materials and Problems, 6th Edition.* St. Paul, MN: Thomson West, 2008.

WEB RESOURCES

American Academy of Nurse Practitioners (AANP)
www.aanp.org

American Academy of Physician Assistants
www.aapa.org

American Academy of Professional Coders (AAPC)
www.aapc.com

American Association of Medical Assistants (AAMA)
www.aama-ntl.org

American Health Information Management Association (AHIMA)
http://ahima.org

American Medical Technologists (AMT)
www.amtl.com

American Society of Clinical Pathology
www.ascp.org

Davis*Plus* | For additional resources please visit **http://davisplus.fadavis.com**

UNIT II

Law, Liability, and Duties

CHAPTER 4

State and Federal Regulations

"When you get right down to the root of the meaning of the word 'succeed,' you find it simply means to follow through." —F.W. Nichol; Author

KEY TERMS

administer a drug To introduce a drug into the body of a client.

Controlled Substances Act Federal law that regulates the administration, dispensing, and prescribing of particular substances that are categorized into five schedules.

dispense a drug To deliver controlled substances in a bottle, box, or some other container to a client; under the Controlled Substances Act, definition also includes the administering of controlled substances.

Drug Enforcement Administration (DEA) Branch of the Department of Justice that enforces drug laws.

drug formulary An insurance carrier's list of preferred drugs.

Health Insurance Portability and Accountability Act (HIPAA) National standards to protect health information.

medical practice acts State statutes that define the practice of medicine, describe methods of licensure, and set guidelines for suspension or revocation of a license.

National Provider Identification (NPI) A 10-digit unique number given to a health-care provider for identification purposes under HIPAA regulations.

prescribe a drug To issue a drug order for a client.

Privacy Rule A portion of HIPAA that regulates the confidentiality of a client's health record while still allowing that information to flow properly and effectively in order to treat the client.

protected health information (PHI) All the past, present, and future physical and mental conditions of an individual's health care.

LEARNING OUTCOMES

Upon successful completion of this chapter, you will be able to:

4.1 Define key terms.

4.2 Identify four common requirements for a physician to be licensed.

4.3 Identify three conditions under which a physician's license may be revoked.

4.4 Explain the purposes of the DEA and its regulations.

4.5 Identify the five controlled substances drug schedules, giving an example of each.

4.6 Discuss the role of the health professional in preventing and treating substance abuse.

4.7 Summarize the key points of HIPAA related to health care.
4.8 Explain the key points that should be provided in a clinic's Notice of Privacy.
4.9 Explain the main points of the Healthcare Reform Act of 2010.

COMPETENCIES

CAAHEP

- Explore the issue of confidentiality as it applies to the medical assistant. (CAAHEP IX.C.2)
- Describe the implications of HIPAA for the medical assistant in various medical settings. (CAAHEP IX.C.3)
- Summarize the Patient Bill of Rights. (CAAHEP IX.C.4)
- Discuss all levels of governmental legislation and regulation as they apply to medical assisting practice, including FDA and DEA regulations. (CAAHEP IX.C.13)
- Respond to issues of confidentiality. (CAAHEP IX.P.1)
- Apply HIPAA rules in regard to privacy and release of information. (CAAHEP IX.P.3)
- Incorporate the Patient Bill of Rights into personal practice and medical office policies and procedures. (CAAHEP IX.P.5)
- Apply local, state, and federal health care legislation and regulation appropriate to the medical assisting practice setting. (CAAHEP IX.P.8)
- Demonstrate sensitivity to patient rights. (CAAHEP IX.A.1)
- Recognize the importance of local, state, and federal legislation and regulations in the practice setting. (CAAHEP IX.A.3)

ABHES

- Comply with federal, state, and local health laws and regulations. (ABHES 4.f)
- Understand legal aspects of writing prescriptions, including federal and state laws. (ABHES 6.d)
- Comply with federal, state, and local health laws and regulations. (ABHES 6.e)
- Maintain confidentiality at all times. (ABHES 22.b.3)

VIGNETTE

Who Has a Right to Know?

Kelly, a first-year medical assistant (MA) student, tells her instructor that she thinks she may be pregnant and wonders what she should do. The instructor recommends that Kelly go to the campus health center for a pregnancy test. When Kelly's test is positive, she again discusses her case with her instructor. As a single woman, Kelly decides she cannot support a child now but is not sure whether to have the baby and put it up for adoption or to have an abortion. After a few days and a discussion with the father of the child, their decision is to have an abortion.

Kelly returns to the campus health clinic for her test results so that she can take them to the abortion clinic. The nurse refuses to give Kelly the test results, saying, "You'll have to talk to the nurse practitioner. I don't believe in abortion." The nurse practitioner gives Kelly the laboratory results. Discuss.

As you read in the last chapter, licensure offers some benefits, but it also brings many regulations. The rules and regulations for physicians and some other providers can be found in the **medical practice acts** passed by each state. These are state statutes that define the practice of medicine, describe methods of licensure, and set guidelines for suspension or revocation of a license. All 50 states have such statutes to protect their citizens from harm by unqualified health-care professionals.

LICENSURE (MDs AND DOs)

Physicians (doctors of medicine [MDs] and doctors of osteopathic medicine [DOs]) must be licensed to practice medicine in the United States. States differ in their licensing requirements. The more common requirements include a 4-year undergraduate degree, graduation from an accredited medical school, completion of an internship, and successful completion of the United States Medical Licensing Examination (USMLE), which was implemented in 1994. Physicians must then meet the requirements for the state in which they wish to practice. This process usually involves completing an application, providing proof of required education and training, and paying an application fee.

Physicians who choose to practice in more than one state must satisfy the license requirements of each state. This process may require a physician to meet each state's reciprocity requirements. Not all states have reciprocity or endorsement, so rules for each individual state need to be researched. Each state also differs on its requirements for non–U.S.-trained and non–U.S.-educated providers. Most of the state regulations include additional education and/or internships. All states require the individual to pass the USMLE before being allowed to practice in the United States.

Many states require a complete and unrestricted license to provide medical services. The Department of Defense is encouraging states to require full licensure of its military personnel even when they are currently only serving in military medical services. Providers engaging strictly in research and not practicing medicine need not have a license in some states.

LICENSE RENEWAL

Physicians periodically renew their licenses to practice, usually every 2 years. Once a physician receives notice at the time of renewal, he or she is required to complete a renewal application form and pay a fee. Documentation of continuing medical education (CME) is a common requirement for license renewal in most states; however, some states require only payment of a fee. Specific state requirements differ, but CME credits may include (1) reading books, papers, and publications; (2) teaching health professionals; (3) attending approved courses, workshops, and seminars; and (4) self-instruction.

A clinic manager may be responsible for keeping records of the physician's CME activities and will want to have the state's requirements on file in order to verify the appropriate credits.

LICENSE REVOCATION AND SUSPENSION

A physician's license to practice may be revoked or suspended as a result of (1) conviction of a crime, (2) unprofessional conduct, and (3) personal or professional incapacity. Each of these conditions is defined by state statute.

Conviction of a crime is a more obvious reason for license revocation than is unprofessional conduct or personal or professional incapacity. Examples of crimes that would result in revocation would include conviction of child abuse or sexual assault against a client.

Unprofessional conduct of physicians and other licensed health-care professionals is defined by law. Although unprofessional conduct may not be considered a crime, such conduct is unacceptable according to state law and therefore is punishable. Examples of unprofessional conduct include falsifying any records regarding licensing, being dishonest, and impersonating another practitioner. Personal or professional incapacity includes chronic substance abuse, continuing to practice when severe physical limitations prevent adequate care, and practicing outside the scope of training.

Usually charges against physicians are made by the state's licensing board in all three conditions, necessitating the suspension or revocation of a provider's license. In all states, the basic procedure for disciplinary action is similar. Most boards are required to give the physician licensee sufficient notice of the charges and allow the physician legal counsel and a hearing. The board then investigates, prosecutes, makes a judgment, and sentences the physician. Some states have empowered their licensing boards to suspend a license to practice on a temporary basis without a hearing (i.e., due process) when the physician poses an immediate threat.

Case Study

On a cold, icy, winter day, Dr. Roberts was severely injured in a motor vehicle crash on his way to the hospital. He was listed in critical condition for several days, lapsing in and out of a coma. Dr. Roberts finally stabilized and was released home after 2 weeks. With lots of hard work and rehabilitation, Dr. Roberts went back to work after 5 months. Within 2 weeks, his support staff and the hospital personnel started noticing his forgetfulness. He forgot to document that he had ordered an x-ray. He argued with an MA regarding his request that a narcotic medication be called in for a client. The answering service called the hospital on a weekend when they could not find Dr. Roberts, who was on call. Instead, Dr. Roberts forgot he was on call and left town unexpectedly. The hospital's board of trustees is about to take action that rarely occurs. They feel the need to deem Dr. Roberts incompetent to practice medicine and have his license revoked.

If you are a member of Dr. Roberts' staff, what might you do in this situation?
Does this situation fall under ethics or law? Explain your response.
Is there any other action that might be taken by the hospital's board of trustees?

PRESCRIPTIONS

Note: *Throughout this section, the terms* non-narcotic *and* narcotic *are used because they are referenced in the Controlled Substances Act. However, the majority of medical practitioners now use the terms* nonopioid *and* opioid *to refer to medications.*

A prescription is an order for medication that is dispensed to or for a client. To order a non-narcotic prescription for a client, a provider must be licensed in the state in which he or she practices medicine and possess a National Provider Identification (NPI). An NPI is a 10-digit number that can be obtained from the Centers for Medicare and Medicaid Services (CMS) by any healthcare provider. This number is used for various reasons, including prescribing medications and submitting claims for services to insurance carriers.

TRANSMISSION OF PRESCRIPTIONS

Prescriptions can be supplied in a variety of ways. They may be handwritten, electronically printed, e-scripted (sent electronically directly to the pharmacy), phoned, or faxed to a pharmacy. For years, the usual transmission method has been the handwritten prescription. The handwritten method has proved to be problematic because of illegible handwriting of most providers causing many prescription medication errors.

In 2004, the first electronic-prescribing tools appeared in clinics and were offered first by insurance carriers. These tools were stand-alone devices, similar to a palm pilot, into which the insurance carriers input their drug formulary, hoping to coax the provider to prescribe only their approved medications. The provider created a database of clients on the device, making refills relatively simple. Once created, the electronic prescription was printed or sent electronically to the pharmacy.

E-prescribing can improve health care and hopefully reduce costs by increasing compliance with formularies and the use of generic medications. E-prescribing tools are also now available within electronic medical records (EMRs) software. Since the passage of the American Recovery and Reinvestment Act of 2009, there has been an increased push for providers to adopt EMRs. In 2011, the federal government began, through Medicare and Medicaid programs, to provide incentive payments to providers to encourage e-prescribing.

The following statement comes from the Department of Health and Human Services related to Medicare: "Although e-prescribing will be optional for physicians and pharmacies, Medicare Part D will require drug plans participating in the new prescription benefit to support electronic prescribing."

UNDERSTANDING NARCOTIC AND NON-NARCOTIC PRESCRIPTIONS

Medications fall into one of two categories—narcotics and non-narcotics. Prescriptions for non-narcotics are identified first.

NON-NARCOTIC PRESCRIPTIONS

A non-narcotic prescription can be transmitted to a pharmacy by any of the manners mentioned previously. Valid prescriptions can be filled anytime within a 6-month period. The provider may order up to a year's worth of refills for such medications as birth control and some chronic conditions. However, in order to ensure that the client is evaluated on a regular basis, the provider usually prescribes only five refills, requiring the client to be reevaluated before additional refills are given. Insurance carriers, who partially or totally pay for their subscriber's medications, usually limit the quantity dispensed to 1 month's worth at a time. The only exception is when the client mails a prescription to an insurance carrier's approved pharmacy, at which time they will allow a quantity of up to 3 months' worth to be sent to the client.

The practitioner is responsible for ensuring that the prescription conforms to all requirements of both federal and state laws and regulations. A non-narcotic prescription issued by a provider may be communicated to the pharmacist by health-care employees.

Drug Sample Closets

There are providers across the country that choose to maintain a closet of drug samples of the most commonly prescribed non-narcotic medications for the convenience of their clients. A provider may choose to do this for several reasons, among which is having medications on hand so that when starting a client on a new medication, the client can try samples before purchasing a whole prescription. This cost savings for clients is beneficial, especially if there is uncertainty about the medication's success for a client. Medication samples also help clients who do not have health insurance or cannot afford their medications.

MAs may be responsible, under the direction of the provider, for many of the requirements related to record keeping, inventory, and security of the drug sample closets. All distribution of samples must be logged on an inventory sheet with the following information:

- Date and time of dispensing
- Client's name and date of birth
- Name of medication
- Dosage
- Lot number
- Expiration date
- Prescriber (provider)

And, as always, documentation in the client's record is *vital*.

The drug sample closet records must be kept for 2 years and are subject to Drug Enforcement Administration (DEA) inspection. An inventory of the drug sample closet should be done every 8 to 12 weeks to ensure that any outdated medications are removed. Any added medications to the drug sample closet must be logged in as well. Security is necessary for any drug closet. The drugs must be kept in a locked closet or cabinet that is substantially constructed.

There are many providers who are opposed to drug sample closets. These providers believe that they are being encouraged to prescribe new, more expensive brand-name medications supplied by pharmaceutical company representatives. These providers also strive to help keep health-care costs down by prescribing generic drugs as often as possible.

Another method to acquire needed medications for a client is for the provider or the MA to contact the pharmaceutical company directly. Many pharmaceutical companies have what is known as an *indigent program*. Working with the provider, the client provides income verification so that the pharmaceutical company can determine his or her needs and if he or she qualifies for the medication free of charge. If the client is eligible, the drugs are mailed to and dispensed by the provider.

NARCOTICS

Drug Enforcement Administration Registration

Federal law requires that a provider must have a separate registration to prescribe narcotic drugs. Registration is made with the DEA, a subdivision of the Department of Justice. An application or renewal can be completed by paper or online (providing a credit card for the application fee) at the DEA Web site, www.justice.gov/dea. The current registration fee (for initial and renewal applications) is $551. Upon receipt of the application or renewal form and payment of the fee, a DEA registration number is assigned to each legitimate provider, and registration is renewed every 3 years. Updating a provider profile (i.e., address change), if needed, can also be accomplished through the Web site.

Providers must also know the narcotic-related laws of their particular state. The provider is required to follow the strictest regulations, whether federal or state. The renewal date of a provider's DEA certificate should be in a tickler file for the office clinic manager to ensure timely renewal and proper compliance.

 ## CONTROLLED SUBSTANCES ACT

The Comprehensive Drug Abuse Prevention and Control Act of 1970, more commonly known as the Controlled Substances Act, is administered by the DEA. These narcotics are controlled because of their potential for abuse and dependence. The DEA has divided these potentially abusive drugs into different categories.

DRUG SCHEDULES

The Controlled Substances Act lists controlled drugs in five schedules (I, II, III, IV, and V). This act and the *U.S. Code of Federal Regulations* are important to all providers but are especially pertinent to any who will administer a drug, prescribe a drug, or dispense a drug that is listed in the five schedules. See Figure 4-1 for definitions and examples of each of the five schedules.

The DEA mandates strict regulations on prescription writing for a narcotic. Prescriptions for a controlled substance must include the following information:

- Patient's full name, date of birth, and address
- The practitioner's full name, address, and DEA registration number
- Drug name
- Drug strength
- Dosage form (liquid, pill, or capsule)
- Directions for use
- Quantity prescribed
- Number of refills (if any) authorized
- Date and signature when issued

A prescription for a controlled substance must be written in ink, usually black, and must be manually signed by the practitioner.

Some states and many insurance carriers limit the quantity of a controlled substance dispensed to a 30-day supply, and most providers follow the same guidelines. However, there are no specific federal limits to quantities of drugs dispensed through a prescription.

Narcotics laws should be studied carefully by any provider who practices medicine or opens a medical office or clinic. The *U.S. Code of Federal Regulations* should be obtained either through

Controlled Substances Drug Schedules

Schedule I

Drugs on this list:

* Include drugs of high potential for abuse and that have no currently accepted medical use
* Can be used by physicians only for purposes of research, which must be approved by the Food and Drug Administration and the DEA, and only after a separate DEA registration as a researcher is obtained
* Are prohibited from manufacture, importation, and sale
* Include such examples as heroin, marijuana, and lysergic acid diethylamide (LSD)

Schedule II

Drugs on this list:

* Have current accepted medical use in the United States, but with severe restrictions; have a high potential of abuse that may lead to severe psychological or physical dependence
* Include such examples as morphine, codeine, and oxycodone with aspirin (Percodan)
* Include such nonnarcotic examples as amphetamines, methylphenidate (Ritalin), and pentobarbital (Nembutal)
* Require physicians to use a special order form that is:
  - Preprinted with the physician's name and address
  - Issued in triplicate
  - Kept in the physician's file (1 copy); remaining copies are forwarded to the supplier, who, after filling the order, keeps a copy and forwards the third copy to the nearest DEA office
* Must have prescription orders written and signed by the physician
  - Some states, by law, require special prescription blanks with more than one copy
  - Physician's registration number must appear on the prescription
  - Prescription may not be telephoned in to the pharmacy except in an emergency, as defined by the DEA
  - May not be refilled

Schedule III–V

* Require either a written or oral prescription by the prescribing physician
  - If authorized by the physician on the initial prescription, the client may have the prescription refilled up to the number of refills authorized, which may not exceed five times or beyond 6 months from the date that the prescription was issued

Schedule III

Drugs on this list:

* Have less potential for abuse than substances in schedules I and II
* Have accepted medical use for treatment in the United States, but abuse may lead to moderate or low physical dependence or high psychological dependence
* Include such examples as various drug combinations containing codeine and paregoric
* Include such nonnarcotic examples as amphetamine-like compounds and secobarbital

Schedule IV

Drugs on this list:

* Have a lower potential for abuse than those in schedule III and have accepted medical use in the United States, but their abuse still may lead to limited physical or psychological dependence
* Include such examples as chloral hydrate, meprobamate, chlordiazepoxide (Librium), diazepam (Valium), and propoxyphene (Darvon)

Schedule V

Drugs on this list:

* Have less potential for abuse than drugs in schedule IV and their abuse may be limited to physical or psychological dependence
* Include such examples as cough medications containing codeine and antidiarrheals such as diphenoxylate/atropine (Lomotil)

Figure 4-1. Controlled Substances Drug Schedules.

the Internet or from the nearest federal government bookstore and studied carefully before controlled substances are managed in the health-care setting.

The majority of providers do not keep narcotics or any medications in their clinics. The threat of theft and mandatory record keeping are the driving force for this decision. Also, the liability of keeping narcotics is high, so most providers refrain from keeping them on-site. However, any provider performing in-clinic surgical procedures may have narcotics in the clinic. Loss of any narcotic is to be reported to the regional DEA office and local law enforcement.

██ SUBSTANCE ABUSE

Substance abuse is found in every sector of society. No group is exempt. It is commonplace in schools, colleges, all professions, and industry. The most commonly abused substances are drugs and alcohol. The Controlled Substances Act is driven, in part, by the fear of drug abuse.

DRUG ABUSE

Providers must be particularly mindful of persons who abuse drugs and are seeking controlled substances for their personal use or for resale on the street. Pharmacists must also be mindful of fake prescription requests on the telephone and forged written prescriptions in their stores.

Health professionals themselves also are vulnerable to drug and alcohol abuse, perhaps more so to narcotics because of their availability in the workplace. However, providers and their employees have a public duty to be alert to all forms of substance abuse and to do everything possible to prevent its increase.

A common problem in the health-care setting is a person who abuses drugs and secures the same prescription drug from more than one provider and pharmacy in a geographic area. Often these individuals go from door to door at medical clinics with a convincing tale of woe or a set of symptoms they hope warrants a prescription for narcotics. A person who abuses narcotics may be a well-established, well-liked client who for medical reasons has developed a need for excessive drugs. The client may be seeing a specialist for the same complaint and receive several prescriptions. Quite often, the client also makes excuses for missing prescriptions, such as "they fell in the sink," "I left them in my hotel room on vacation," or "someone stole my purse." Providers and staff that are alert will start to notice patterns among clients that point to drug addiction.

Another problem occurs when a provider becomes known as a "script doctor," one who freely and excessively prescribes potentially dangerous drugs. People who abuse drugs quickly learn who these providers are and become their regular clients.

The abuse of prescription medications, especially by young adults, is rampant. Teens steal their parents' medications, take them to school, and sell them for more potent and illicit drugs, or take the medications themselves. Young adults have learned that street drugs may be laced with very dangerous and poisonous substances and are very costly, and they often consider stolen prescription medications as free and safe.

The market for prescription drugs on the street is a lucrative one. The street price of prescription drugs varies according to the drug and the location. A recent study showed the following values for three samplings of drugs, from the cheaper drugs to the higher-priced drugs:

- Tylenol #3 (street name, *T3s*), a pain medication, has a street value of approximately $1.50/pill.
- Talwin & Ritalin (street name, *Ts n Rs*), used to control hyperactivity, has a street value of approximately $30.00/pill.
- MS Contin (street name, *Red Peelers*), another pain medication, has a street value of approximately $75.00/pill.

Case Law

A Florida physician, David W. Webb, MD, was sentenced to life imprisonment for distribution of and conspiracy to distribute controlled substances resulting in death. He was convicted of 36 counts of health-care fraud, 90 counts of illegal distribution of controlled substances, 2 counts of conspiracy to commit those offenses, and 2 counts of identity theft. He was found also responsible for the deaths of three of his patients who overdosed on drugs that he had prescribed. Dr. Webb had been prescribing controlled narcotics, sedatives, and stimulants in quantities and dosages that caused patients to abuse, misuse, and become addicted to these drugs.

Even after his patients suffered overdoses, he continued to prescribe the same prescriptions to them. During the trial, the evidence showed that the defendant failed to monitor his patients' use of drugs and failed to document the patients' files with sufficient medical justification for prescribing the drugs. In the cases of more than 100 of the patients to whom the defendant prescribed controlled substances, agents were able to find no evidence that the defendant kept any patient file. Dr. Webb was found to be prescribing controlled substances over the Internet to patients he had never seen. Once Dr. Webb's DEA certificate had been suspended, he continued to prescribe controlled drugs under another physician's number.

U.S. Department of Justice, Northern District of Florida v David W. Webb, Pensacola, Florida. January 28, 2010

ALCOHOL ABUSE

Another substance that is greatly abused is alcohol. Much of the information related to drug abuse is the same for alcohol abuse. It knows no socioeconomic boundaries, afflicts both genders, and is rampant among today's youth. One major difference between drug abuse and alcohol abuse is that alcohol is more readily available to most anyone at any time. The World Health Organization estimates that about 76 million people throughout the world suffer from alcohol-related disorders. According to the Centers for Disease Control and Prevention, "alcohol is the most commonly used and abused drug among youth in the United States, more than tobacco and illicit drugs. Although drinking by persons under the age of 21 is illegal, people aged 12 to 20 years drink 11% of all alcohol consumed in the United States; 90% of this drinking is binge drinking."

Alcohol abuse can cause multiple problems at any age, but youths are more at risk because the alcohol can interrupt the progression of their normal development. Among the problems seen in alcohol abusing teens are:

- Disruption of normal growth and sexual development
- Memory problems
- Changes in brain development that may have life-long effects
- Social and school problems

PREVENTION OF SUBSTANCE ABUSE

Clinic policies can aid greatly in the control of narcotics abuse. The following stipulations should be part of every clinic's policy and procedure manual:

- When checking in for the first time, a client needs to produce picture identification to verify the correct name and match the name to the face.
- The provider will authorize no controlled substance prescriptions without first seeing the client.
- The provider needs to see the client on a regular basis before any refills will be authorized.
- A picture ID is needed to pick up a narcotic prescription.

Providers and clinic staff still using handwritten prescriptions must keep prescription pads in a secure place. They should be carried in the provider's pocket and should not be kept in the examination room, on counters, or in drawers, where clients have access to them while waiting for the provider. The increased use of e-prescribing will help to rid the clinic of the liability of stolen prescription pads.

Whether the drug of choice is alcohol, prescription medications, or illicit street drugs, the approach is the same. Substance abuse of any kind is injurious to the health and well-being of clients. Providers and health professionals must establish firm and clear procedures to curb the increase of substance abuse. Health-care professionals who have the most success with such clients are those who are able to honestly discuss the abuse issues and possible treatment plans without judgment or condemnation.

A frank, honest discussion must be conducted with all clients, especially young adults, that encourages saying "no" to alcohol and drugs; yet, health-care professionals must be careful to keep an open dialog so that their clients are comfortable in admitting any substance abuse problems. In the case of young adults, this kind of discussion is best held when parents or guardians are not present.

All health-care professionals should take a comprehensive substance abuse history from their clients. This history taking is often administered as a self-assessment questionnaire. Clients may present with a current substance abuse condition in addition to another disease or illness, so both must be addressed. It is imperative for health-care professionals to be knowledgeable of signs and symptoms of substance abuse and report them to the provider.

If health-care professionals abuse substances, their ability to function safely will be impaired, and the problem needs to be addressed in a quick and efficient manner to avoid errors. Such abuse and impairment are cause for loss of the health-care professional's license.

Case Law

An MA employed in a fairly large medical clinic, Emerald Providers, in Hyannis, Massachusetts, has been charged with three counts of conspiracy to violate drug laws, three counts of passing a false prescription, six counts of document forgery, larceny of a value less than $250, and receiving stolen property of a value less than $250. The medical director of the clinic contacted police after Lyndsay Thacher, 23, was caught allegedly using false identification to secure a fraudulent oxycodone prescription at a Hyannis pharmacy. Ms. Thacher pled not guilty. A pretrial hearing was set.

  April 8, 2010; Barnstable District Court.

HEALTH INSURANCE PORTABILITY AND ACCOUNTABILITY ACT

Another federal regulation, the Health Insurance Portability and Accountability Act (HIPAA), was passed by Congress in 1996 and became effective in April 2003. HIPAA requires (1) standardization of electronic client health data, administrative data, and financial data; (2) unique health identifiers for individuals, employees, health plans, and health-care providers (NPIs); and (3) security standards to protect the confidentiality and integrity of the individually identifiable health information, past, present, or future (Privacy Rule).

HIPAA established for the first time a set of national standards for the protection of health information. According to the U.S. Department of Health and Human Services, the major goal of the Privacy Rule is to "assure that individuals' health information is properly protected while allowing the flow of health information needed to provide and promote high quality health care and to protect the public's health and well-being." The Privacy Rule protects "all individually identifiable health information," which is called protected health information (PHI).

Under HIPAA, clients must grant written consent or permission to provide or disclose their PHI for any reason. Providers must provide clients with a notice of their privacy practices, which must include the right to:

1. Restrict use of PHI
2. Request confidential communication
3. Inspect and obtain a copy of the PHI
4. Request any amendment to the PHI
5. Receive an accounting of PHI disclosures

Clients should sign a form stating they have received the privacy statement.

This is just a brief introduction to HIPAA regulations. Criminal penalties can be levied for non-compliance of the security standards of $100 per violation up to $25,000 per person for all identified violations in a calendar year. Depending on the circumstances of a breach of confidentiality, fines that can reach up to $1.5 million and imprisonment of 1 year can be levied against offenders.

 ## CONFIDENTIALITY

As we have seen, one of the main purposes of HIPAA is to ensure and protect a client's privacy related to health-care issues.

 Unless otherwise required by law, providers must keep confidential any communication necessary to treatment of the client. ●

The client's privacy must be protected. Providers and their employees must be extremely careful that all information gained through the care of the client is kept confidential and given only to those health professionals who have a medical need to know. Care should also be taken that any information communicated about a client cannot be overheard by others (see Fig. 4-2).

In many cases, HIPAA regulations have meant that clinics reconsidered how clients are greeted, how basic personal information is viewed, how billing is discussed, and how clients are addressed in the reception area and any other areas when personal information may be seen or heard. For example, a clinic with a very open reception area created a cubicle at one side of the reception area for the exchange of private information. Another clinic chose to enclose the reception area in glass. Even this glass enclosure does not guarantee privacy. The receptionist needs to keep his or her voice lowered to maintain confidentiality. No telephone calls are made to remind clients of appointments or to discuss bills or laboratory results where any other party can hear. It is imperative that clients' charts or any personal information be out of view of others. Another area of concern within the physical setup of the clinic is the use and placement of computers. Placement should be where only

Figure 4-2. An example of a breach of confidentiality.

the employee can view the computer screen. Additionally the computer should have a screen protector that fits over the monitor so that any information is distorted to anyone except the employee who is looking straight at the monitor. Health-care professionals should be directed to log off any time they leave the computer. The confidentiality of the client is of utmost concern, and all physical areas and policies should be constantly monitored to ensure that privacy.

Case Study

In your podiatrist's office, there is a sign-in sheet at the reception desk requesting your name, phone number, insurance number, and Social Security number.

What do you do?

Can't I Tell My Friend?

To continue with the dilemma of Kelly's pregnancy in the vignette, "Who Has a Right To Know?" consider the following information.

Several days later in the MA's clinical class, another MA instructor overhears Nancy, a student who is receiving work experience in the campus health center, breach a confidence and tell other students in the class about Kelly's pregnancy and abortion.

The program's coordinator privately speaks with Nancy about the breach of confidentiality. Nancy responds, "I didn't tell the whole class. I only told my friend."

Is this situation HIPAA compliant? How would you respond if you were the coordinator?

HEALTHCARE REFORM ACT OF 2010

The intent of the national health-care reform bill is to make health care available to as many Americans as possible. The passage of this bill is considered one of the most historic domestic policy achievements since the creation of Medicare in 1965. Since the major changes related to health-care reform will not take place until 2014, continued adjustments, even reductions in health-care coverage, are likely in the interim.

The hope is that health-care reform will provide solutions to some of the major health issues in the United States. Medicare and Medicaid now pay less of the total bill for elderly and indigent clients than was originally planned, and managed care is instituting every cost-saving measure possible, thus dictating to providers what and how costs will be covered. For example, an uncomplicated hernia surgery formerly required 2 to 3 days of hospitalization following general anesthesia surgery. Today, the same surgery is performed on an outpatient or same-day surgery basis under local anesthesia, and the client is sent home later in the day. Another example is that, increasingly, hospitals find themselves in the "ambulatory care" business when uninsured clients come to their emergency rooms after being turned away from the care and attention that is normally available from providers in a clinic or medical office setting. As the burden of quality health-care costs shifts, states struggle to pass laws regarding the equitable distribution of health-care dollars and additional ethical concerns raised over that distribution.

The Healthcare Reform Bill is being implemented in stages that started in September 2010 and will be fully implemented by 2014. Since its passage, it has already undergone many changes and, perhaps by the time it is enacted, will look entirely different than it does today.

As part of the health-care reform taking place, President Obama signed into law the Affordable Care Act in March 2010. Its main goal is to "put American consumers back in charge of their health coverage and care." Under this Act, on June 22, 2010, the Department of Health and Human Services

(DHHS) issued new regulations to implement a new Patient Bill of Rights. (Not to be confused with the Hospital Patient Bill of Rights noted in Chapter 1.) The Affordable Care Act and the new Patient Bill of Rights offer the following protection for consumers:

- No preexisting condition exclusions for children under age 19 years (eventually this will include all Americans)
- No arbitrary rescissions (cancellations) of insurance coverage
- No lifetime limits on coverage
- Restricted annual dollar limits on coverage
- Protection of the client's choice of doctors
- Removal of insurance company barriers to emergency department services

The Healthcare Reform Act is a major area to watch in the next several years as this reform is put into place and changes are made to the health-care system in the United States. Keep up to date on this changing piece of legislation at the following Web site: www.healthcare.gov/.

SUMMARY

Providers must be aware of all state and federal rules and regulations to practice medicine. Among those regulations are licenses to practice and DEA certificates of registration. Another federal regulation is HIPAA, which helps to protect the confidentiality of the client. Health-care professionals have a responsibility, as public servants, to both prevent substance abuse and treat those who abuse either drugs or alcohol. Any health-care professional must also understand that there are numerous changes taking place not only with treatments and research but also with the organization and the methods of delivery of health care that may affect both federal and state regulations.

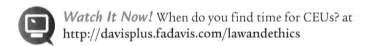 **Watch It Now!** When do you find time for CEUs? at
http://davisplus.fadavis.com/lawandethics

Questions for Review

SELECT THE BEST ANSWER

1. When a drug is introduced into a client's body, it is known as
   a. Dispensing a drug.
   b. Prescribing a drug.
   c. Administering a drug.
   d. All of the above.
   e. None of the above.

2. The controlled substances act divides narcotics into how many schedules?
   a. Two (2)
   b. Three (3)
   c. Four (4)
   d. Five (5)
   e. Six (6)

3. The Affordable Care Act and the Patient Bill of Rights provide which of the following benefits for clients?
   a. No rescinding of insurance coverage
   b. Limit on the amount of co-pay
   c. No preexisting condition exclusions for all clients
   d. Protects the client's choice of doctors
   e. Only a and d above

4. A provider's license may be revoked for which of the following reasons?
   a. Conviction of a crime
   b. Professional incapacity
   c. Personal incapacity
   d. All of the above
   e. Only a and b above

5. The acronym DEA stands for
   a. Department of Environmental Agency.
   b. Department of Drug Agency.
   c. Drug Enforcement Administration.
   d. Drug Education Agency.
   e. Drug Enforcement Agency.

TRUE OR FALSE

T F 1. A medical licensing board may revoke a provider's license without due process if the board feels that the provider is a threat to the community.

T F 2. A license to practice medicine in any U.S. state entitles a provider to practice medicine anywhere within the country.

T F 3. A medical assistant working within a medical clinic may take and use samples of drugs as long as they are for his or her own personal use.

T F 4. Health-care professionals are very cognizant of their health, so it is hard to find one who abuses drugs or alcohol.

T F 5. A janitor who cleans a medical clinic is not held to the same confidentiality rules as the medical professional.

CLASSROOM EXERCISES

1. Ben LaPaglia, your provider's client, who is a practicing attorney, is being weighed on the scale in the hallway. He looks up and sees the daily client's schedule posted by the provider's office door. He says to you, "Is that where you always post the schedule?" Discuss.

2. What might constitute license revocation?

3. In the vignette "Who Has a Right to Know?" could the program coordinator do anything more than speak with Nancy about her breach of confidentiality? Discuss.

4. Identify medical specialty clinics that might dispense as well as prescribe controlled substances and discuss their uses.

INTERNET ACTIVITIES

1. Assume that you are the clinic manager for a family practice. You are responsible for keeping track of your provider's license renewal and CMEs. Go to your particular state's board of registration in medicine. Research the requirements for provider license renewal and the regulations regarding CMEs and what activities constitute CMEs.

2. Research the *U.S. Code of Federal Regulations.* Who and what do they regulate? What topics do they cover when it comes to drugs and medications?

3. Research the Healthcare Reform Act of 2010 to see what changes have been made to the Act since its passage. What reforms have been put into place already?

4. Research the pros and cons of keeping a "drug sample closet" in a provider's clinic. Decide where you would stand with regard to this topic. Debate a fellow classmate who holds a different opinion than yours.

5. Explore your state's Board of Registration in Medicine. What helpful information can you find there that would aid you in your career as a medical assistant? Describe.

WEB RESOURCES

Drug Enforcement Administration
  www.justice.gov/dea

Governmental health-care site
  www.healthcare.gov/law/introduction/index.html

Governmental site on health-care reform
  www.healthreform.gov/newsroom/new_patients_bill_of_rights.html

Naturopathic Licensing Jurisdictions in the United States
  www.oregon.gov/OBNM/PopDocs/NaturopathicBoardsOfAmerica.pdf?ga=t

Physician Licensing Requirements by State
  www.visalaw.com/IMG/physicianchart.pdf

State Medical Licensing Boards
  www.circare.org/boards/statebrds.htm#ak

Underage Drinking
  www.cdc.gov/alcohol/fact-sheets/underage-drinking.htm

U.S. Code of Federal Regulations
  www.gpoaccess.gov/ecfr

U.S. Department of Health and Human Services
  www.hhs.gov/ocr/privacy/hipaa/understanding/summary/privacysummary.pdf

 DavisPlus | For additional resources please visit
http://davisplus.fadavis.com

CHAPTER 5

Professional Liability

"Character is much easier kept than recovered."—Thomas Paine (1737–1809); Controversial revolutionary propagandist

KEY TERMS

agent Person (the health-care employee) appointed by a principal party (the physician or provider) to perform authorized acts in the name and under the control and direction of the principal.

alternative dispute resolution (ADR) Methods outside the judicial system used to solve potential malpractice actions; methods include arbitration and mediation.

assault A threat to inflict injury with an apparent ability to do so.

battery The unlawful touching, beating, or laying hold of persons or their clothing without consent.

breach of contract Failure to comply with the terms of a valid contract.

civil liability Identifies conflicts between individuals, corporations, government bodies, and other organizations.

compliance plan Guidelines established to protect a clinic from fraud and litigation charges.

contract A voluntary agreement between parties.

criminal liability When an individual commits an act that is considered to be an offense against society as a whole.

defamation Spoken or written words concerning someone that tend to injure that person's reputation and for which damages can be recovered. Two types of defamation are:

  libel False, defamatory writing, such as published material, effigies, or pictures.

  slander False, malicious, or defamatory spoken words.

fiduciary Holding in confidence or trust.

malfeasance Commission of an unlawful act.

medical malpractice Professional negligence of physicians or providers.

misfeasance Improper performance of an act resulting in injury to another.

negligence (medical) Doing some act that a reasonable and prudent provider would not do or failing to do some act that a reasonable and prudent provider would do.

nonfeasance Failure to perform an act when there is a duty to do so.

res ipsa loquitur A Latin phrase meaning "the thing speaks for itself"; a doctrine of negligence law.

respondeat superior A Latin phrase meaning "let the master answer"; that is, the provider is responsible for employee acts.

tort Wrongful act committed by one person against another person or against property; distinguished from a breach of contract.

vicarious liability Legal doctrine assigns liability for injury to a person or institution who did not cause the injury but who has a particular legal relationship to the person who did act negligently.

LEARNING OUTCOMES

Upon successful completion of this chapter, you will be able to:

5.1   Define key terms.

5.2   List three elements necessary for a contract to be valid.

5.3   Describe how a contract may be breached.

5.4   Discuss the meaning of standard of care.

5.5   Explain professional liability for providers.

5.6   Identify the four Ds of medical negligence.

5.7   Compare and contrast intentional and unintentional torts.

5.8   Restate, in your own words, the importance of professional liability (malpractice) insurance.

5.9   Name two alternative methods to litigation.

5.10 Recall 10 guidelines for risk management.

COMPETENCIES

CAAHEP

- Describe liability, professional, personal injury, and third party insurance. (CAAHEP IX.C.6)
- Compare and contrast physician or provider and medical assistant roles in terms of the standard of care. (CAAHEP IX.C.7)
- Provide an example of tort law as it would apply to a medical assistant. (CAAHEP IX.C.9)
- Explain how the following impact the medical assistant's practice and give examples:
  - Negligence (CAAHEP IX.C.10.a)
  - Malpractice (CAAHEP IX.C.10.b)
- Describe the process to follow if an error is made in patient care. (CAAHEP IX.C.14)
- Practice within the standard of care for a medical assistant. (CAAHEP IX.P.4)

ABHES

- Follow established policies when initiating or terminating medical treatment. (ABHES 4.5)
- Understand the importance of maintaining liability coverage once employed in the industry. (ABHES 4.d)
- Perform risk management procedures. (ABHES 4.e)

Is There Professional Responsibility?

Nicole, an Arkansas resident, calls the office of the obstetrician who delivered her first child 2 years ago. She reports to the receptionist that she is having minor cramping and discomfort and believes she also may be pregnant due to a missed period. The receptionist tells Nicole "not to worry at this stage." She also informs Nicole that her obstetrician is not taking new patients. Later that night Nicole is admitted to the hospital as a result of shock due to blood loss from a ruptured ectopic pregnancy. As a result of the rupture and complications, Nicole required a hysterectomy.

Once physicians and certain providers become licensed, they become legally liable for their actions as physicians and providers. They are responsible, accountable, obligated, and legally bound by law; this is known as *professional liability.* ●

PROFESSIONAL LIABILITY

Professional liability can be criminal or civil, or both, but criminal liability is less common in health care than civil liability. Criminal liability results when an individual commits an act that is considered to be an offense against society as a whole. The legal term malfeasance reflects this liability. Malfeasance is the commission or performance of an unlawful act.

Examples of criminal liability for providers and their employees include fraud in insurance billing, client abuse, the evasion or breach of the Controlled Substances Act, or aiding in the death of a client in a state that does not allow physician-assisted death. Physicians or providers found to be grossly negligent or reckless in the injury or death of a client also may be held criminally responsible. The medical assistant (MA) who breaks the law or aids a provider in a criminal act becomes liable for a criminal act as well.

Civil liability identifies conflicts between individuals, corporations, government bodies, and other organizations. Most of the time, examples of civil liability for health professionals include a breach of contract or commission of a tort. A contract is a voluntary agreement between parties. A tort is a wrongful act or injury committed by one person against another person that is not dependent on a contract. Misfeasance is another term that is used in tort law to describe an act that is legal but performed improperly. Contract law and tort law related to medical care are identified here.

CONTRACTS

Health-care professionals are liable for professional negligence issues that often arise related to contract principles. A contract or a provider–client relationship is normally a prerequisite for any professional negligence on the part of the provider before any litigation can occur. This is known as *contract law*. Health-care employees and their providers are parties to contracts on a daily basis. When a provider accepts a client, a contract has been made. When the clinic assistant calls an office supply company to reorder office stationery, the assistant acts as the provider's agent in making a contract.

For a contract to be valid, it must be (1) an agreement between two or more competent people, (2) an agreement to do or not to do a certain task for payment or for the rendering of a benefit, and (3) a lawful agreement. An example of a contract in health care occurs when a client calls the clinic to make an appointment for an annual physical examination. Assuming that the provider is legally able and capable to practice medicine and the client is a competent adult, the first two parts of the contract exist and are valid. The performance of a physical examination is a lawful act, so part three of the contract exists and is valid. The client is given a statement of the charges, and the fee is paid. Hence, the contract is valid in all respects.

A contract can be expressed or implied. An *expressed contract* can be written or oral, but all facets of the contract must still be specifically stated and understood. (Fig. 5-1). An *oral contract* is as legally binding as a written one; however, it may be more difficult to prove. Providers' telephone contacts with clients are examples of oral contracts, especially when medical advice is given. A *written contract* requires that all necessary aspects of the agreement be in writing and signed by each party. Each state, in its statute of frauds, identifies those contracts that must be in writing. Usually included in this list are deeds and mortgages. Most states' statutes of frauds include a section that is pertinent to health care, that is, an agreement made by a third party to pay for the medical expenses of another. Such an agreement must be in writing to be valid. For example, if Joel tells the medical

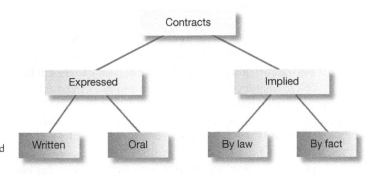

Figure 5-1. Contracts, either expressed or implied, can be legally binding.

receptionist that he will pay the medical expenses for his partner, Dwayne, the receptionist should have Joel fill out a form to that effect and affix his signature to it. If not properly executed, it may be impossible to collect payment for the bill.

Implied contracts are the most common form of contracts occurring in health care. Such contracts occur every time the provider and client discuss what course of treatment to take and an agreement is reached. An implied agreement does not require a specific expression of the parties involved but is still valid if all points of the contract exist. An implied contract may be implied from the facts or circumstances of the situation or by the law. For example, when a client complains of a sore throat and the provider does a throat culture to diagnose and treat the ailment, a contract is implied by the circumstances of the situation. Another example of an implied contract would be of a provider who administers epinephrine after a client goes into anaphylactic shock. In this example, the law will say that the provider did what the client would have requested had there been an expressed agreement.

Other contractual agreements determine obligations for providers. Providers who practice in institutions, such as hospitals or long-term care facilities, must provide health care to whomever comes into the facility within the limits of their employment contracts with the institution. Similarly, providers who are a part of a health maintenance organization (HMO) have a duty to treat plan members as a result of their written contractual obligation to the HMO.

Contracts made by the mentally incompetent, the legally insane, those under heavy influence of drugs or alcohol, infants, and some minors are not valid. Such persons are not considered by the law to be competent to enter into binding contracts.

Health-care employees are generally considered agents of their provider-employer. An agent is a person (the health-care employee) appointed by a principal party (the provider) to perform authorized acts in the name and under the control and direction of the principal. As agents, health-care employees must be careful of their actions, which could become binding to their providers. For example, an employee might promise a client a cure that in fact is not possible. ●

BREACH OF CONTRACT

A breach of contract arises when one of the parties involved fails to meet the contractual components. For example, the contract may be violated when the client does not pay the bill or refuses to follow medical advice. The contract can be breached when the provider fails to use the treatment promised, promises to perform a procedure and then allows someone else to do the procedure, or promises a cure and no cure results. Such breaches of contract are cause for litigation in which the court will attempt to reward reimbursement to the offended party. Usually this reimbursement is in the form of a monetary reward to offset any incurred losses.

ABANDONMENT

A provider's fiduciary or trusted obligation, posed by his or her professional ethics, causes the law to look outside the parameters of contract law when determining the provider's obligation to treat a client. Health-care professionals are constrained in their ability to withdraw from contractual relationships by judicial case law, which has set rules against abandonment.

Once the provider–client relationship has been established, providers can be found liable if they abandon their clients. Abandonment seems like a harsh term, but in this context, it refers to the provider's action or desire to no longer serve a client. To avoid charges of abandonment, it is recommended that a provider withdraw formally from a case or formally discharge a client. This withdrawal or discharge requires giving reasonable notice to the client with the recommendation for the client to seek further medical care. The written notice should be sent so that the client has ample time to secure another provider.

A point to remember is that some managed care contracts limit a provider's ability to terminate a provider-client relationship. A provider should carefully read the contract to determine whether termination is possible and how to give notice to the managed care plan. If a provider leaves a managed care plan for some reason, even though the managed care plan will give notice to its clients, it is a good idea for the provider to send his or her own written communication (i.e., letter) advising clients what arrangements have been made for the continuation of their care.

Additionally, a provider may wish to withdraw from a case if a client fails to follow instructions, take the prescribed medications, disclose information pertinent to the care, or return for recommended appointments. Almost any nondiscriminatory reason is valid as long as proper written notice is given. To withdraw formally from a case, a provider should notify the client in writing, state the reasons for the dismissal, and indicate a future date when the provider is no longer responsible. Such a letter should be sent by certified mail with restricted delivery only to the person specified and a return receipt requested providing that individual's signature. Figure 5-2 shows an example of a letter of withdrawal. A copy of the letter and the returned receipt are kept in the

---

RECOMMENDED TERMINATION LETTER

Letter of Withdrawal to a Client

Dear_____:

You may recall from your most recent visit that we discussed the possibility that it may be better for you to seek medical attention from a different provider.

After further consideration of that discussion, I find it necessary to withdraw my professional services as your primary care provider. This action is necessary because you have not followed the instructions in my personal treatment plan for you. Please place yourself in the care of another provider as soon as possible, but no later than 14 days from the time you receive this letter.

Upon receipt of a written request from your chosen provider, your case history with my diagnostic and treatment recommendations will be promptly supplied. Since your condition requires medical attention, please do not delay in finding another provider among the many competent providers in this area.

I regret the need to take this action, but believe it is best for your continuing medical care. Thank you for your cooperation in making this change as quickly as possible.

Sincerely yours,

Provider's Name and Credentials

SEND BY CERTIFIED MAIL WITH RESTRICTED DELIVERY AND RETURN RECEIPT

Figure 5-2. Recommended withdrawal letter.

client's record. To further protect a provider from abandonment charges, any canceled or missed appointments should be noted in the client's record.

Clients, too, may wish to terminate the contractual relationship with a provider at any time and for any reason. Most of the time clients simply stop making appointments rather than officially withdrawing from the provider's care. It is important, however, for the provider to acknowledge in writing even this kind of termination, when known, if the client still needs medical care. Knowledge of such a termination may happen when clients request that their records be sent to another provider. The clinic staff should never respond to such a request without their provider-employer's knowledge and instructions.

 ## STANDARD OF CARE

One cannot fully understand professional liability without some knowledge of "standard of care" principles. Acceptable *standard of care* requires that providers use the ordinary and reasonable skill that would be commonly used by other reputable practitioners when caring for individuals. They are expected to perform those acts that a reasonable and prudent provider would perform. Failure to perform an act when there is a duty to do so is known as nonfeasance. Standard of care also dictates that providers must not perform any acts that a reasonable and prudent provider would not perform. Providers should always practice in the realm of safety and obtain all necessary data on which to base a sound judgment. This practice includes obtaining a thorough medical history, a complete physical examination, and necessary laboratory tests. Providers are expected to know what new therapeutic developments might benefit those in their care and still not subject them to undue risk.

Employees in health care also must adhere to a standard of care. The standard a health-care employee will be measured against depends on the task the employee is undertaking; the education, training, credentialing, and experience of the employee; and the responsibility the provider has given to the employee. For example, if an MA makes a diagnosis or treats a client, the MA can be held to the same standard of care as the provider. If the MA is acting outside his or her level of competency and if the client is injured as a result, the MA is negligent. An MA will be expected to use the same standard skill and reasonable judgment that would be commonly used by other reputable MAs in the same area when assisting with clients. Health-care employees often act in a variety of roles, and they must understand the standard to which they can be held. If, on the other hand, the health-care employee is mopping the floor, he or she will be held to the reasonable standard of a custodial person rather than the standard of a specific health-care professional.

Unfortunately, errors can be made. By the very nature of today's ambulatory health-care environment, where clients with multiple illnesses are being cared for, providers are seeing more clients for shorter periods of time and may be processing as many as 900 laboratory results in any given week; serious but preventable errors can be made. A study in the *Journal of the American Medical Association* reports that diagnostic errors are implicated in about 46% of malpractice claims, followed by errors in treatment at 30%.

Errors made by MAs require immediate reporting to the provider or supervisor, admitting the error, making corrections when possible, and helping to plan procedures to prevent a recurrence.

PROFESSIONAL NEGLIGENCE OR MALPRACTICE

Failure to perform professional duties according to the accepted standard of care is called negligence. More specifically, negligence occurs when a reasonable and prudent provider performs an act that he or she would not perform or fails to perform an act that he or she would perform according to acceptable guidelines in the standard of care. Professional negligence has the same meaning as malpractice, and malpractice may be referred to as professional negligence.

Professional negligence is more easily prevented than defended. Obviously, providers and their employees do not wish to be found negligent or become involved in a malpractice suit of any kind. However, consumers are quite aware of their rights in today's society. Therefore, all health professionals must protect the provider–client relationship at all times and be above reproach in the performance of their duties.

THE FOUR Ds OF MEDICAL NEGLIGENCE

To more clearly understand professional negligence, the four Ds of medical negligence are often used as guidelines. They include duty, derelict, direct cause, and damages:

1. *Duty* exists when the provider–client relationship has been established. For example, the client calls the office to make an appointment, keeps the appointment, and makes another to return for further treatment.
2. *Derelict* is more difficult to define. The client must prove that the provider failed to comply with the standards required and dictated by the profession.
3. *Direct cause* implies that any damage or injuries that resulted from the provider's breach of duty were directly related to that breach and that no intermittent circumstances or intervening acts could have caused the damages.
4. *Damages* refer to the compensation provided for injuries suffered by the client. The most common in medical professional liability cases is monetary compensation, which may be actual, or compensatory damages and exemplary or punitive damages. *Actual damages* are those that compensate the client for injuries sustained and nothing more. These include past medical care, loss of wages, and future medical care. *Exemplary* or *punitive* damages are compensation that punishes the defendant and awards the client for pain, suffering, and mental anguish. Punitive damages may be limited by law in some states.

▍ TORTS

Tort law is an area of law that health-care professionals are most likely to be involved in because the law identifies negligence and medical malpractice. Health-care employees or providers may commit a tort that can result in litigation.

A tort is a wrongful act committed by one person against another person or property that causes harm to that person or property. A tort results if there is damage or injury to the client directly or indirectly caused by the conduct of the provider or the health-care employee that does not meet the standard of care governing either the provider or the health-care employee (see the Four Ds of Medical Negligence). If a provider commits a wrongful act against a client with no resultant client harm, a tort has not been committed.

The two main classifications of torts are *intentional* and *unintentional/negligent* acts. Intentional torts or wrongs involve the intentional commission or a violation of another person's rights. Unintentional or negligent wrongs may be the result of the omission or the commission of an act. Malpractice is an unintentional tort (Fig. 5-3). It is a specific type of negligence that occurs when the standard of care commonly expected from a health-care professional is not met. It is also known as *professional negligence.*

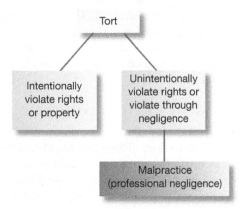

Figure 5-3. Torts are violations, either intentional or unintentional.

INTENTIONAL TORTS

Intentional torts are intentional acts that violate another person's rights or property. The ethical obligation to "do no harm" to a client *(nonfeasance)* is the basis for any intentional tort action. If the principle of nonfeasance was never violated and there was no harm to the client, there could be no grounds for litigation based on intentional tort.

Some of the more common intentional torts that may occur in ambulatory health care are assault and battery, defamation, and invasion of privacy. Assault and battery are terms often used together; however, assault rarely occurs in the medical setting. Assault refers to a threat to inflict injury with an apparent ability to do so. Battery, in the medical context, occurs when a client receives treatment without having given consent to do so; it is the unlawful touching, beating, or laying hold of persons or their clothing without consent. Some intentional torts such as assault and battery may also violate criminal laws and can become complaints in both criminal court and civil court. In this situation, separate trials will be held, one criminal and one civil. In a civil case the plaintiff must show, by a preponderance of evidence, that a tort has been committed, whereas in a criminal case the prosecution must prove its case beyond a reasonable doubt.

When battery occurs, an individual's right has been invaded. Individuals have the right to be free from invasion of their persons. Regardless of whether the procedure constituting the battery improves the client's health, the client must consent to the treatment.

Defamation is spoken or written words that tend to injure a person's reputation and for which damages can be recovered. One type of defamation is libel, which is false, malicious, defamatory writing, such as published material, effigies, and pictures. Another type of defamation is slander, which is the false and malicious defamatory spoken word. For defamation to be a tort, a third person must hear or see the slander or libel and understand it.

Invasion of privacy is the unauthorized publicity of client information. Medical records and treatments cannot be released without the client's knowledge and permission. Clients have the right to be left alone and the right to be free from unwanted publicity and exposure to public view (i.e., Health Insurance Portability and Accountability Act [HIPAA]).

UNINTENTIONAL TORTS OR MALPRACTICE

An example of an unintentional tort occurs in the medical profession when a provider prescribes a pain medication over the phone for a client with a migraine-like headache, not recalling that this client is recovering from hepatitis. Because the pain medication is contraindicated in hepatitis, the client becomes violently ill and suffers liver damage. Although the provider did not intentionally prescribe an inappropriate medication, negligence did cause injury to the client for which the provider is liable.

Unintentional torts are the basis for the majority of civil lawsuits against health-care professionals. When the standard of care is not very carefully adhered to, errors can be made, and the client suffers the consequences.

Torts are best prevented by practicing legally and ethically. The standard of care in the health-care setting needs to be excellent. The privacy of clients must be guarded, their bodies and possessions are to be respected, and their reputations are to be protected. The rights of clients must be protected by all who come in contact with them. All health professionals must perform only within their scope of training, education, credentialing, and recognize the standard of care required for each action taken.

DOCTRINE OF *RES IPSA LOQUITUR*

Another rule of the law of negligence is the doctrine of *res ipsa loquitur,* "the thing speaks for itself." It relates chiefly to cases of foreign bodies being left in clients, instruments slipping during surgical procedures, burns from heating modalities, and injury to a portion of the client's body outside the field of treatment. In other words, the negligence is obvious; the result was such that it could not have occurred without someone being negligent.

Case Law

Mrs. Farley had a tubal ligation. She was informed of the risks and signed consent forms before surgery. Five months later she returned to the same provider, who determined that she was pregnant. After the birth of Mrs. Farley's baby, the attending provider examined both of her fallopian tubes and found that one was ligated, but the other appeared normal. Mrs. Farley sued the provider who performed the tubal ligation on the basis of *res ipsa loquitur.*

Outcome: The court held that Mrs. Farley could not rely on the doctrine of *res ipsa loquitur* to establish the medical malpractice claim against the provider. The court held that "the doctrine of *res ipsa loquitur* cannot be invoked where the existence of negligence is wholly a matter of conjecture and the circumstances are not proved, but must themselves be presumed, or when it may be inferred that there was no negligence on the part of the defendant." The doctrine only holds in cases in which the defendant's negligence is the only inference that can reasonably and legitimately be drawn from the circumstances. This was not the case here. The court stated that this was probably one of those cases in which the sterilization procedure failed; the ligation was performed, but the ligation band came off soon thereafter.

Farley v Meadows, 404 SE2D 537 (1991)

DOCTRINE OF *RESPONDEAT SUPERIOR*

As stated earlier, professional liability exists for both employer and employee. Physicians and providers are responsible not only for their own actions of negligence but also for the negligent actions of their employees under the doctrine of *respondeat superior.* This Latin phrase means "let the master answer." For example, consider an MA who administers an allergy shot, dismisses the client, and hastens on to the next task without keeping the client under observation for 20 minutes. The client collapses in the parking lot a few minutes later as a result of anaphylactic shock from the injection. The provider-employer is responsible for the negligence of the MA; however, the MA is also liable for not following the proper standard of care.

The doctrine of *respondeat superior* may extend to a hospital or HMO that employs providers and their assistants, thus making the institution liable for negligent acts of their employees or agents when they are performing within the scope of their employment, even if the organization was not at fault in any way. The legal term used in this situation is vicarious liability. You learned in Chapter 2, Medical Practice Management, that increasing numbers of providers are becoming employees of hospitals and HMOs; therefore, it becomes important for many reasons to be able to identify the legal relationship between the organization and the provider.

Case Study

A woman in her 80s, recovering from hip surgery, returns to her surgeon's clinic for a checkup. The MA is cautious to make certain the woman's walker is carefully placed over the scale. With chart and pen in hand, the MA stands to the right of the client on the scale. While the MA is recording the weight, the woman steps back and falls backward off the scale. Her hip is reinjured, and there are other injuries as well. The instant the MA turned to enter data in the chart, the fall occurred. The client and her family are suing both the surgeon and the MA.

The provider-employer is responsible for ensuring that all employees perform only those tasks within the scope of their knowledge and training. However, the employer's responsibility does not diminish employees' responsibility to perform any acts within the scope of their knowledge and training. In the situation in the previous case study, both the provider and the employee can be found liable when injury occurs to the client as a result of the employee's actions.

The provider's employee also has a responsibility to question an order if there is good reason, and a prudent employee in such a position would do so. If the order is not questioned and negligence occurs as a result, both the provider and the employee may be liable. For example, an MA tells the provider that the client he saw 2 days ago for a cold now is coughing up yellow sputum. The provider orders penicillin to be added to the treatment regimen. Before calling the pharmacy, the MA notices that the patient is allergic to penicillin and so questions the provider.

Professional liability is a concern of all health professionals, but providers are most concerned because they are in a position of higher authority and responsibility.

PROFESSIONAL LIABILITY/MALPRACTICE INSURANCE

The need for providers to carry professional liability insurance is obvious for numerous reasons. The most important, perhaps, is financial protection. Some states mandate the minimum amount of professional liability insurance that a provider must carry.

Providers need liability insurance protection whether they are employees or employers. For example, employment in a corporation, an HMO, or a hospital does not guarantee professional liability coverage. Many employers or institutions carry professional liability insurance merely on themselves or the institution, not on their employees. Some hospitals require a minimum amount of professional liability insurance before hospital privileges are granted. In some cases, clients sue both the employer and the employee.

One of the reasons employers will carry professional liability insurance is the doctrine of *respondeat superior*. Providers may not be directly negligent, but they are liable for the acts of their employees, even while the employees are liable for their own actions.

Employees will want to remember that the only way in which they can be covered under an employer's liability insurance policy is by being specifically named in that policy—something that is very rare. Employees are advised to carry their own professional liability insurance. For example, MAs who are members of the American Association of Medical Assistants may purchase professional and personal liability insurance through the organization.

Many providers carry professional liability insurance because they are often asked for medical advice or assistance from friends or neighbors in a "casual setting." For example, at an outdoor barbecue, a neighbor asks the provider, "My back is killing me. What can I do?" In the case of strangers when medical care may be emergent and the provider is the only one available to provide the care, an employer's or institution's policy probably will not extend coverage in this situation. The Good Samaritan Law, which may be applied in such an emergency, is discussed in Chapter 7, Public Duties.

COST OF PROFESSIONAL LIABILITY INSURANCE

The kind and amount of liability coverage to carry vary according to the type of practice, the community economic level, the level of risk of the specialty, and the claims-consciousness of the clients. Most professional liability policies, however, should address (1) what the insurer will pay, (2) effective policy dates, (3) the power of the insurer in obtaining legal counsel, (4) the power of the insurer in seeking settlement, (5) what costs are covered, and (6) how payment is to be made. The professional liability insurance policy will specify monetary limits for each claim. For example, a policy may have professional medical liability of $1 million for each claim and $3 million aggregate as a total amount.

Some providers are limiting their practice and their professional liability insurance coverage because of the high cost of premiums. This can be seen when a family practitioner chooses not to perform surgeries or deliver babies, thus reducing the cost of professional liability insurance.

States have been diligent in writing legislation that would limit or control the monetary amounts awarded to plaintiffs (i.e., clients) in malpractice claims, but have not been fully successful. Even in states that have been successful in tort reform legislation, the cost of professional liability insurance has decreased only a little. Therefore, insurance costs will vary by state and by specialty. Insurance premiums for an internist, for example, may range from $6000 a year in states with a "low-end" rate to as much as $56,000 per year in states with a "high-end" insurance rate. An obstetrics/gynecology specialist may pay as much as $55,000 per year in a state with low-end insurance premiums and as much as $100,000 in a state with high-end insurance rates. Why is there a difference? Providers say the high cost of malpractice insurance is not about lawsuits, but rather is about insurance companies making up for investment losses. Insurance companies generally decline to reveal how premiums are established but insist that skyrocketing rates are related to the increasing costs of health care and clients' litigious nature to sue.

ALTERNATIVES TO LITIGATION

Some providers and institutions have tried solving the malpractice dilemma with alternative dispute resolution (ADR) methods, such as arbitration and mediation. These methods eliminate the use of the court system. The client voluntarily agrees, sometimes in advance, with the provider or institution to permit a neutral person or persons to arbitrate the dispute. The parties involved generally select the impartial third party, who is an expert in the area of controversy. In most instances, the decision of the arbitrator is binding, and there is limited judicial review of the process. In mediation, there is no third party; rather, the mediator is selected by both parties and attempts to facilitate negotiation between them.

A number of states have statutes addressing the use of arbitration and mediation. Some states have established ADR centers, often with the state bar association, for such alternatives to litigation. Generally, the cost of arbitration and mediation is less than a court-litigated solution and saves time for both parties. Such arbitration and mediation cases also may remain more private.

RISK MANAGEMENT AND COMPLIANCE PLANS

Generally, if a healthy provider–client relationship exists, litigation is less likely to occur. Also, the clinic that has taken the time to develop a compliance plan is further protected because steps have been taken to ensure that precautions are in place.

The Office of the Inspector General (OIG) suggests that a medical practice's focus on quality client care is enhanced with the adoption of a voluntary compliance program. Compliance plans are an aid to avoid litigation, to help prevent problems from arising in the delivery of health care, and to remind employees of the importance of every aspect of the practice. A fully effective compliance plan has seven basic components as identified by the OIG:

- Establishes written policies, procedures, and standards for major areas of the clinic/practice
- Names a compliance officer (often the clinic manager or supervisor) to monitor and enforce the compliance plan
- Educates all employees so that the compliance plan is well understood
- Develops open lines of communication so that employees feel comfortable reporting any unsafe activities or potentially fraudulent areas and to continually update employees on the status of the plan
- Audits and monitors all aspects of the plan on a regular basis
- Enforces disciplinary standards through well-publicized guidelines
- Corrects action for detected offenses appropriately and promptly

There is not just one compliance plan for a medical practice; there are several. High-risk areas that will benefit from a compliance plan include confidentiality, documentation, coding and billing, and employee and client safety. When a compliance plan is in place and appropriately followed, areas of concern can be noted and corrected before they become major problems. Fraud cases are determined on "intentional fraud." A clinic with a plan in place can show that compliance is strived for, helping to refute any fraud charges.

RISK MANAGEMENT WITHIN THE AMBULATORY HEALTH-CARE SETTING

All employees can help to manage risks. This can be accomplished in their work habits and in their dealings with clients.

Risk Management with Good Work Habits

1. Perform within the scope of training, education, and credentialing.
2. Comply with all state and federal regulations and statutes, including HIPAA.
3. Keep the clinic safe and equipment in readiness.
4. Diligently practice standard precautions.
5. Log telephone calls. Return all calls to clients within a reasonable time.
6. Have all diagnostic test results viewed and initialed by the provider before filing.
7. Select employees carefully, and encourage a team approach.
8. Keep all matters related to client care confidential.
9. Follow up on missed or canceled appointments and incomplete documents.
10. Continue to grow professionally.
11. Formally document (a) withdrawing from a case and/or (b) discharging clients.
12. Keep accurate and meticulous records.
13. Limit practice to scope of training and to a manageable number of clients.
14. Document when clients are called with test results.
15. Document all canceled appointments and no-shows.
16. Always retain original records or radiographs.
17. Pay meticulous attention to coding and billing.
18. Have provider review accounts before sending any to a collection agency.
19. Consider turning the reception area into an education area.
20. Continue to build on your knowledge base in all areas of the practice.
21. Maintain professional certification, registration, and/or licensure.
22. Document, document, document.

Risk Management with Clients

1. Practice uninterrupted listening during the critical first 60 seconds of any conversation with a client.
2. Provide an opportunity for clients to ask questions.
3. Provide time- and action-specific instructions at the close of client contact and indicate the expected time for follow-up or recovery.
4. Put verbal instructions in writing, and give a copy to the client.
5. Do not criticize other practitioners.
6. Explain any appointment delays. Do not keep clients waiting more than 20 minutes. Offer another appointment if feasible.
7. Discuss fees before treatment.
8. Treat all persons equally.
9. Never guarantee a cure.
10. Secure informed consent.
11. Listen to clients, and always tell your provider-employer when a complaint occurs.
12. Call clients at home the day after outpatient surgery to check on their progress. Document the follow-up in the client's chart.
13. Tell clients how to get care on nights and weekends.
14. Regularly survey clients for satisfaction and follow suggestions for improvement.

In addition to the risk management guidelines discussed previously, the Bayer Institute for Health Care recommends the four Es of client interaction to help health professionals prevent malpractice. They are: (1) engage, (2) empathize, (3) educate, and (4) enlist clients in management of their health care. These suggestions can further help in risk management.

Case Study

As clinic manager, you want to find ways to improve your clients' satisfaction in your large clinic. You know of a company that 'infiltrates' your clinic and actually 'pretends' to be some of your clients. The company's 'clients' call to make appointments, come in to see your providers, use your laboratories, and other ancillary services. A report is made to the employers. It becomes an ongoing practice to help you identify areas for improvement. You use the report to educate your staff.

If you are a staff person, what do you think of this practice?
Should the results regarding a particular individual be used in the employee evaluations?

SUMMARY

Once physicians and certain providers become licensed, they become professionally liable for themselves and their employees. Well-established compliance plans and employees who are conscientious with regard to risk management will aid the provider in managing the clinic's risks. If litigation becomes a reality, however, it is advisable to seek professional legal advice promptly.

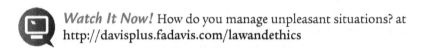

Watch It Now! How do you manage unpleasant situations? at
http://davisplus.fadavis.com/lawandethics

Questions for Review

SELECT THE BEST ANSWER

1. Professional negligence
   a. Is more easily prevented than defended.
   b. May be described as malpractice.
   c. Can be the result of either a provider or an employee error.
   d. All of the above.
   e. Only a and b above.

2. *Res ipsa loquitur* means
   a. Let the master answer.
   b. Let the buyer beware.
   c. The thing speaks for itself.
   d. Defamation has occurred.
   e. A name has been slandered.

3. A contract may be
   a. Expressed or implied.
   b. Written or oral.
   c. Invalid if the agreement is unlawful.
   d. All of the above.
   e. Only a and b above.

4. Tort
   a. Is a French dessert.
   b. Identifies negligence and medical malpractice.
   c. Is a lawful act committed by one person against another.
   d. Is a wrongful act against another with no resultant harm.
   e. Is an action not covered in professional liability insurance.

5. Alternatives to litigation may include
   a. Alternative dispute resolution.
   b. Arbitration and mediation.
   c. An impartial third party.
   d. A heavy fee for the service.
   e. Only a, b, and c above.

TRUE OR FALSE

T   F   1. Some providers limit their practice because of the high cost of malpractice insurance.

T   F   2. One type of defamation is battery.

T   F   3. Libel is false and malicious defamatory spoken words.

T   F   4. The four Ds of medical negligence are duty, derelict, direct cause, and damages.

T   F   5. Two classifications of torts are intentional and unintentional acts.

CLASSROOM EXERCISES

1. It has been reported that because providers fear litigation, they often order testing on clients that is not actually necessary just to be certain that no "stone is left unturned." Discuss the implications of this practice for the provider, the client, and health care in general.

2. List and describe medical practices that are deemed "higher risk" and are apt to require larger fees for malpractice insurance. Justify your choices.

3. Describe the standard of care for the MA in the ambulatory care setting.

4. Identify steps to be taken if you make an error while attending to a client's needs.

5. If you do all the coding for insurance in the clinic in which you are employed, but you are not a professional coder, is it possible you could be held to the same standard as a professional coder? Explain your answer.

6. In the *vignette* at the beginning of the chapter, identify the errors that were made by the obstetrician's office. What action might have prevented this scenario? Do you think Nicole might have basis for a lawsuit? Justify your response.

INTERNET ACTIVITIES

1. Search the Internet for recent legal cases in your area's district court related to medical malpractice. Describe your findings.

2. Research tort reform in your state. Describe your findings.

REFERENCES

Furrow, B. R., Greaney, T. L., Johnson, S. H., Jost, T. S., & Schwartz, R. L.: *Health Law Cases, Materials and Problems, Abridged 6th Edition*. St. Paul, MN: Thomson West, 2008.

Harris, D. M.: *Contemporary Issues in Healthcare Law and Ethics, 3rd Edition*. Chicago: Health Administration Press, 2008.

"Managing Your Practice," Medical Insurance Exchange of California. Advisory Number 2. 2000.

WEB RESOURCE

U.S. Department of Justice, Office of Public Affairs
www.usdoj.gov/opa/pr/2009/March/09-crm-244-html

DavisPlus | For additional resources please visit
http://davisplus.fadavis.com

CHAPTER 6

Law for Health Professionals

"The virtue of a man ought to be measured, not by his extraordinary exertions, but by his everyday conduct."—Pascal (1623–1662); French mathematician, physicist, inventor, and writer

KEY TERMS

appellant One who appeals a court decision to a higher court.

arraignment The procedure of calling someone before a court to answer a charge.

civil case Court action between private parties, corporations, government bodies, or other organizations. Compensation is usually monetary. Recovery of private rights is sought.

closing arguments Summary and last statements made by opposing attorneys at a hearing or trial.

Congress The law-making body of the federal government. It is made up of two separate groups, the House of Representatives and the Senate.

court of appeals Court that reviews decisions made by a lower court; may reverse, remand, modify, or affirm lower court decision.

court order An order issued only by a judge to appear or to request certain records. The release of any records requested in a court order does not require the client's permission.

criminal case Court action brought by the state against individuals or groups of people accused of committing a crime; punishment is usually imprisonment and/or a fine; includes recovery of rights of society.

cross-examination Examination of a witness by an opposing attorney at a hearing or trial.

defendant The person or group accused in a court action.

deliberation The process whereby a jury considers the evidence presented in a case.

deposition A written record of oral testimony made before a public officer and/or both attorneys. It is for use in either a criminal or a civil case and is completed outside of court before the trial begins.

direct examination Examination of a witness by the attorney calling the witness at a hearing or trial.

examination of witness Questioning of a witness by attorneys during a court action.

expert witness (medical) Person trained in medicine who can testify in a court of law as to what the professional standard of care is in the same or similar circumstances.

felony A serious crime, such as murder, larceny, assault, or rape. The punishment is usually severe.

higher (superior) court The court to which appeals of trial court decisions can be made; a court with broader judicial authority than a lower or inferior court.

judge A public official who directs court proceedings, instructs the jury on the law governing the case, and pronounces sentence.

jurisdiction The limits or territory within which authority may be exercised.

jury Six to twelve individuals, usually randomly selected, who are administered an oath and serve in court proceedings to reach a fair verdict on the basis of the evidence presented.

law Rule or regulation that is advisable or obligatory to observe.

litigation A lawsuit; a contest in court.

lower (inferior) court Usually, the court in which a case is first presented to the trial court; a court with limited judicial authority.

misdemeanor Type of crime less serious than a felony; examples include property theft, and certain cases of intimate partner violence and elder abuse.

opening statements Statements made by opposing attorneys at the beginning of a court action to outline what they hope to establish in the trial.

plaintiff The person or group initiating the action in litigation.

probate (estate) court State court that manages wills and settles estates.

sentencing Imposition of punishment in a criminal proceeding.

small claims court Special court intended to simplify and expedite the handling of small claims or debts.

subpoena An order to appear in court under penalty for failure to do so.

subpoena duces tecum A court order requiring a witness to appear and bring certain records or tangible items to a trial or deposition.

summons An order, in a civil case, from the court directing the sheriff or other appropriate official to notify the defendant where and when to appear to answer charges against him or her.

verdict Findings or decision of a jury.

LEARNING OUTCOMES

Upon successful completion of this chapter, you will be able to:

6.1   Define key terms.

6.2   Explain in a brief paragraph why knowledge of the law is necessary for health professionals.

6.3   Describe the source of law.

6.4   List the three branches of government in the United States.

6.5   Give an example of each of the following terms: (a) constitutional law, (b) common law, (c) statutory law, (d) administrative law, (e) plaintiff, (f) defendant, (g) felony, and (h) misdemeanor.

6.6   List two similarities and two dissimilarities between criminal and civil law.

6.7   Review, in diagram form, the process for a (a) civil case, (b) misdemeanor case, and (c) felony case.

6.8   Diagram the federal court system and state court system.

6.9   List two factors that determine in which court a case is heard.

6.10   Discuss the use of probate and small claims courts.

6.11   List two similarities and two dissimilarities among a subpoena, *subpoena duces tecum,* and court order.

6.12   Explain, in your own words, the trial process.

6.13   Name two circumstances that might require the services of an expert witness.

COMPETENCIES

CAAHEP
- Compare criminal and civil law as it applies to the practicing medical assistant. (CAAHEP IX.C.8)
- Explain how the following impacts the medical assistant's practice and give examples:
  - Statute of limitations (CAAHEP IX.C.10.c)

ABHES
- Comply with federal, state, and local health laws and regulations. (ABHES 4.f)

VIGNETTE

Can She Be an Expert Witness?

As a medical assistant educator with several years of experience in the administrative area and a recognized authority on medical records, you have been asked to testify as an expert witness regarding protocol for making corrections in a medical record. You agree.

When you are interviewed by the attorney and given the records to review, you recognize that the person responsible for the data entered in the record is a former student and a practicing certified medical assistant. It appears obvious that the records have been altered after the fact.

The U.S. legal system is complex and multifaceted. It can baffle even the most astute citizen. Basically, there is one federal legal system and 50 different and unique state legal systems, all created by federal and state constitutions. Most legal actions pertinent to health care occur within the state and local systems.

SOURCES OF LAW

Law encompasses rules derived from several sources. The Constitution of the United States provides the highest judicial authority. Adopted in 1787, it provides the framework for our government. The Constitution, federal law, and treaties take precedence over the constitutional law of the states. The Constitution of the United States is a legal document that defines the structure and function of federal, state, and local government.

The federal government has three branches: (1) the legislative branch is the lawmaking body, called the Congress; (2) the executive branch is the administrator of the law and includes the president; and (3) the judicial branch is the judges and courts, including the Supreme Court. Each branch provides a system of checks and balances for the other two. For example, the power of lawmaking belongs to Congress, but the president can veto its legislation, and the judiciary is empowered to review legislation. Congress, in turn, can investigate the president and control the appellate jurisdiction of the federal courts. No one branch has absolute authority. In addition to the federal government, each state has a constitution defining its own specific governing bodies. All powers not conferred specifically on the federal government are retained by the state, yet states vary widely in their assumption of that power.

TYPES OF LAW

The two basic types of law are common law and statutory law. *Common law* was developed by judges in England and France over many centuries. It emerged from customs, the ways things were done over time in England and in France. Common law was brought to the United States with the early settlers. Common law, views decided by judges, is always evolving as established principles are tested and adapted in new case situations. Common law is also called *judge-made law* or *case law.*

Many of the legal doctrines applied by the courts in the United States are products of the common law developed in England (or in the case of Louisiana, from France). Common law is a body of law based on judicial decisions that attempts to apply general principles to specific situations that arise. It has the force of statutory law, although common law is not enacted by the legislature.

Congressional and state legislative bodies enact rules (laws) known as legislative or *statutory law.* These laws make up the bulk of our laws as they exist today. Publications containing these statutes are known as *codes.* An example of a statute pertaining to health care is a medical practice act, which defines and outlines the practice of medicine in a given state. (See Chapter 4, State and Federal

Regulations.) A federal law will be uniformly applied throughout the country. A state law applies only in that given state. If there is a conflict between a federal and state law, the Constitution mandates that the federal law governs.

Legislative bodies, however, do not have the time or knowledge to enact all laws necessary for the smooth functioning of the government. Thus administrative agencies are given the power to enact regulations that also have the force of law. This type of law is called *administrative law*. The Internal Revenue Service and Federal Trade Commission are examples of administrative agencies. Both implement extensive rules in their areas of concern.

Administrative law, an extension of statutory law, affects the health-care employee. The state health department, the state board of medical examiners, and the state board of nurse examiners are administrative agencies that dictate rules and regulations for health care. Further, licensing and accrediting bodies, as well as such federal government programs as Medicare and Medicaid, directly influence many policies, procedures, and functions of health care and fall under the category of administrative law. The Drug Enforcement Agency, an administrative agency of the Department of Justice, enforces the Controlled Substances Act.

CIVIL AND CRIMINAL LAW

Law may also be classified as civil, criminal, international, and military. International and military law are not considered here. This book concentrates on civil and criminal law because of their importance in the health-care setting. Figure 6-1 provides a brief overview of the trial process.

CIVIL LAW

Civil law affects relations between individuals, corporations, government bodies, and other organizations. Restitution for a civil wrong is usually monetary in nature. The bulk of law dealt with in health care is civil in nature.

In a civil case, the party bringing the action (plaintiff) must prove the case by presenting evidence that is more convincing to the judge or jury than the opposing evidence, a preponderance of evidence. The procedure for a civil case is shown in Figure 6-2. The plaintiff's complaint is filed in the proper court, usually by an attorney for the plaintiff. The defendant is formally summoned, prepares an answer, and files it in the court. If the defendant fails to answer the summons within the prescribed time, the plaintiff will win the case by default, and judgment will be entered against the defendant.

The case may be disposed of without a trial. For example, the complaint may be dismissed because of some technical error, the summons may have been improperly served, or the complaint may not have set forth a claim recognized by law. The parties also may decide to settle out of court.

Case Study

Consider, for example, a "slip, trip, and fall" case. Fran enters her provider's office and slips and falls as she approaches the reception desk. She suffers a simple fracture of the left femur. When the receptionist comes to her aid, they discover that a snag from the rug caught the heel of Fran's shoe. Fran later takes civil action and sues her provider for medical fees and loss of employment wages for the time she was unable to work as a result of her injuries. As the plaintiff, she must prove that her provider (the defendant) was negligent.

How might this case be settled in a civil suit?

The Trial Process

```
        ┌─────────────────┐
        │ Jury selection  │
        └────────┬────────┘
                 │
                 ▼
        ┌─────────────────┐
        │Opening statements│
        └────────┬────────┘
                 │
                 ▼
        ┌─────────────────┐
        │  Examination    │
        └────────┬────────┘
                 │
                 ▼
        ┌─────────────────┐
        │Cross examination│
        └────────┬────────┘
                 │
                 ▼
        ┌─────────────────┐
        │Closing arguments│
        └────────┬────────┘
                 │
                 ▼
        ┌─────────────────┐
        │Jury deliberation│
        └────────┬────────┘
                 │
                 ▼
        ┌─────────────────┐
        │    Verdict      │
        └──┬───────────┬──┘
           │           │
           ▼           ▼
    ┌──────────┐  ┌──────────┐
    │Not guilty│  │  Guilty  │
    └────┬─────┘  │Sentencing or│
         │        │settlement│
         ▼        └──────────┘
    ┌──────────┐
    │Dismissed │
    └──────────┘
```

Figure 6-1. A general example of the trial process.

CRIMINAL LAW

Criminal law pertains to crimes and punishment of persons violating the law. Criminal law affects relations between individuals and government. Criminal wrongs are acts against the welfare and safety of the public or society as a whole. Criminal acts usually result in a punishment of imprisonment and/or a fine.

A criminal case is brought by the state against individuals or groups of people accused of committing a crime. The prosecuting, district, or state attorney prosecutes the charge against the accused person (defendant) on behalf of the state (plaintiff). The prosecution must prove that the defendant is guilty beyond a reasonable doubt. In other words, the prosecution must be able to prove to the satisfaction of the court that a criminal act was, beyond reasonable doubt, committed by the accused.

A crime is a felony or misdemeanor that is statutorily defined. Felonies are more serious crimes and include murder, larceny (thefts of large amounts of money), assault, and rape. Misdemeanors

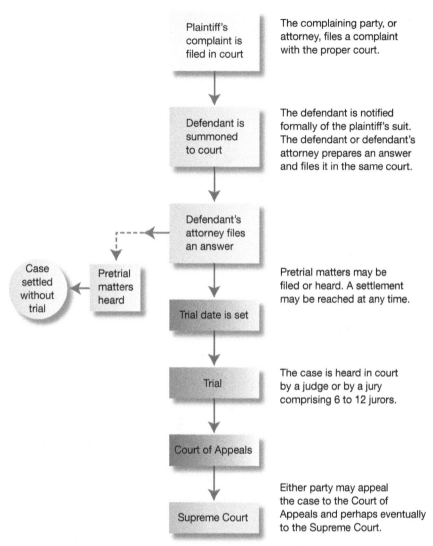

Figure 6-2. Chart explaining the procedure for a civil trial. Each state has a similar process. Compare with your state's civil trial process.

are considered lesser offenses. These include disorderly conduct, thefts of small amounts of property, and breaking into an automobile.

In a misdemeanor case (Fig. 6-3), the prosecuting attorney is made aware of violations of the law either by traffic or police citations, by police arrest, or by citizen information. When the prosecutor determines that enough evidence is present, the court arraigns the person on the prosecutor's charge. The charged person may plead guilty and consequently face sentencing. The guilty person may be put on probation, may serve a jail term and/or pay a fine, or may go through the appeal or appellate process. If the charged person pleads not guilty, a trial date is set. At the end of the trial, a verdict is given of either guilty or not guilty. If the person is found not guilty, the charge is dismissed. If found guilty, the person faces a jail term, probation, and/or must pay a fine. The guilty person (appellant) may also use the appeal process.

The felony case process is shown in Figure 6-4. When evidence exists that a crime may have been committed, the police begin their investigation. Then the information is either filed by the

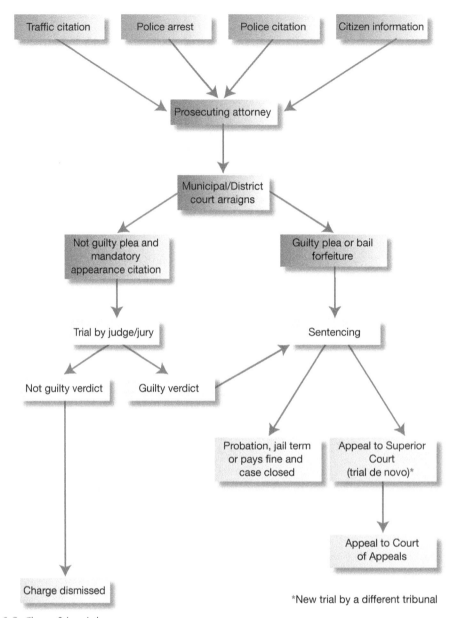

Figure 6-3. Chart of the misdemeanor case process.

prosecuting attorney or given to a grand jury, depending on the practice of the particular jurisdiction and severity of the charge. If the evidence is sufficient, the individual is charged. Pretrial proceedings, to plan the manner in which cases will proceed, are generally informal in nature, and many cases are settled at this point.

If the accused pleads guilty, he or she is sentenced to imprisonment, probation, and/or a fine. The appellate process then may be available. If the person pleads not guilty, the trial is set, the facts of the case are determined, the principles of law relating to those facts are applied, and a conclusion as to guilt or innocence is reached. If the verdict and judgment are guilty, the individual goes through the same sentencing process as in the guilty plea. If the verdict is not guilty, the person is acquitted, and the charges are dismissed.

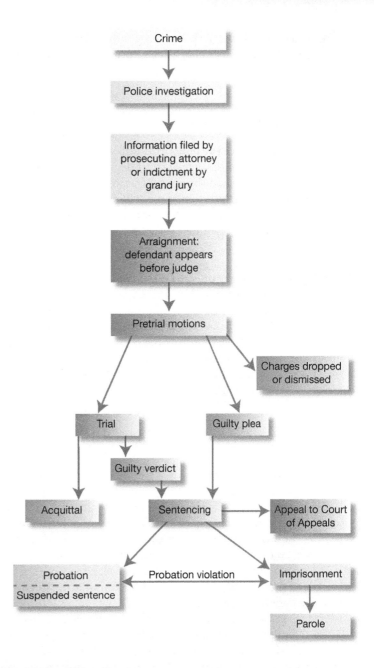

Figure 6-4. Chart of the felony case process.

Case Study

To illustrate both civil and criminal law, consider the following situation. Drunk driver Earle is involved in an automobile crash that causes the death of a homemaker who has two children. Earle is charged by law enforcement officials with involuntary manslaughter and reckless driving while speeding and intoxicated. The courts later find Earle guilty. This is criminal law protecting society. Taking this situation a step further, the husband of the homemaker then sues Earle for a substantial monetary amount to care for the two children, who are now without a mother. On the basis of the facts of the case, the court grants a monetary award. This is civil law.

Identify similar actions that you are aware of in your locale.

In a criminal case the proof is beyond a reasonable doubt. In a civil case there only needs to be a preponderance of evidence. So, a person can be found not guilty in a criminal case but then found guilty in a civil case. ●

TYPES OF COURT

As indicated earlier, the type of court that hears a particular case depends on the offense or complaint. In criminal cases, the type of court depends on the nature of the offense and where it occurs. In civil cases, it depends on the amount of money involved and where the parties reside. The jury and judge are neutral arbitrators of the evidence.

Courts also are classified as lower or higher, inferior or superior. A lower or inferior court has less authority than a higher or superior court.

FEDERAL COURT

Three jurisdictions belong only to federal courts: federal crimes, such as racketeering and bank robbery; constitutional issues; and civil action involving parties not living in the same state.

The U.S. Supreme Court is the highest court in the federal court system. Directly under the jurisdiction of the U.S. Supreme Court are the U.S. Court of Claims, the U.S. Court of Customs and Patent Office, and the U.S. Court of Appeals. The U.S. Supreme Court directs the actions of all courts: federal, state, trial, and appellate.

The circuit courts are below the Supreme Court, and they direct the actions of the U.S. Federal District Courts and Tax Courts.

Case Law

In August 2009, a group of Florida medical professionals who filed $11 million in false Medicare claims for HIV infusion therapy were sentenced to prison.

The case involved two clinics in Miami, two physicians (Dr. Keith Russell and Dr. David Rothman), two physician assistants, a medical assistant, additional staff members, a pharmaceutical wholesale supplier, and clients of the clinic. Testimony at the trial proved that the clinics were established for the sole purpose of defrauding Medicare.

The state of Florida, in its suit, claimed that clients of the clinic would visit and then have their blood drawn. The medical assistant manipulated the client's blood samples to indicate that they were HIV positive.

A bogus prescription would be written by one of the providers and sent to a pharmaceutical wholesale supplier who would send a minimal amount of medication but provide invoices for large quantities. The clients would then return for the purpose of the intravenous (IV) therapy (which they did not receive) and the services and medications would be billed using the client's Medicare numbers. The owner of the clinic testified that the clients were paid $200 in kickbacks for their part in the scheme.

The participants in this Medicare fraud scheme received various sentences ranging from 5 to 8 years in federal prison, and all were ordered to pay back millions of dollars to the Medicare system.

Miami Federal Court, Criminal Division, 09-244

Federal law enforcement officials from several agencies continue to investigate Medicare fraud throughout the country and are making great strides in detecting and punishing offenders.

STATE COURT

The pattern for state courts is similar to the pattern for federal courts. There are inferior or lower courts and a process of appeals. Figure 6-5 illustrates the state court system. The lower courts (district or municipal court) hear cases involving civil matters, small claims, housing, traffic, and some misdemeanors. The State Superior Court has general jurisdiction in all types of civil and criminal cases. The court of appeals has power to review decisions of this court. The court of appeals may reverse, remand, modify, or affirm a decision of a lower court. The final route of appeal is to the State Supreme Court, the determination of which becomes the law of the state.

Each state defines by statute the types of cases a particular court will hear and the maximum money value of the cases over which it has jurisdiction. In the event litigation does arise in a civil matter, providers and their health-care employees will most likely find themselves in a state court. Other civil matters may also take place in probate court and small claims court.

PROBATE COURT

Probate law oversees the distribution of a person's estate upon death. In probate court (sometimes called estate court), a provider may decide to initiate action on the collection of a bill owed by a deceased client if all other options have been unsuccessful. Generally, a health-care employee represents the interests of the provider and attempts to locate the responsible person or party for the debt,

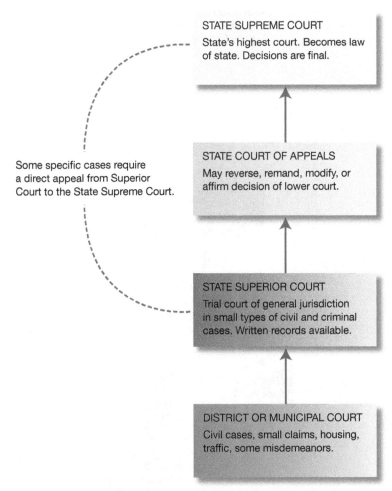

STATE SUPREME COURT
State's highest court. Becomes law of state. Decisions are final.

STATE COURT OF APPEALS
May reverse, remand, modify, or affirm decision of lower court.

Some specific cases require a direct appeal from Superior Court to the State Supreme Court.

STATE SUPERIOR COURT
Trial court of general jurisdiction in small types of civil and criminal cases. Written records available.

DISTRICT OR MUNICIPAL COURT
Civil cases, small claims, housing, traffic, some misdemeanors.

Figure 6-5. Titles of courts vary from state to state, but this diagram illustrates the overall structure of the court system in most states.

whose name can be obtained from the deceased client's family or lawyer, or from the mortuary. If unable to obtain a name from these sources, the health-care employee must write or call the county seat in which the estate is being settled. The county probate court recorder will provide information concerning the filing of the claim (in court, to the executor of the estate, or elsewhere), the proper forms to file, and when the claim must be submitted (see Fig. 6-6). Quick action is required because most states have a file period from 4 to 12 months after the publication of notice in a newspaper by the administrator or executor.

Once the probate forms are ready to be mailed, the health-care employee sends them by certified mail, return receipt requested. This step establishes that the documents were received and by whom. The administrator will either accept or reject the claim. If it is accepted, payment will follow, but it may be delayed for months in the courts. If it is rejected and the provider believes the bill is justified, a lawsuit may be filed against the administrator within a designated amount of time, depending on the state. Health-care employees should be aware of their particular state's time limits.

 Keep in mind that even though you may be hesitant to collect a deceased client's bill, the provider rendered services for the client and deserves payment. Failure to file a claim may be construed by others as an admission of poor medical care on the part of the provider. ●

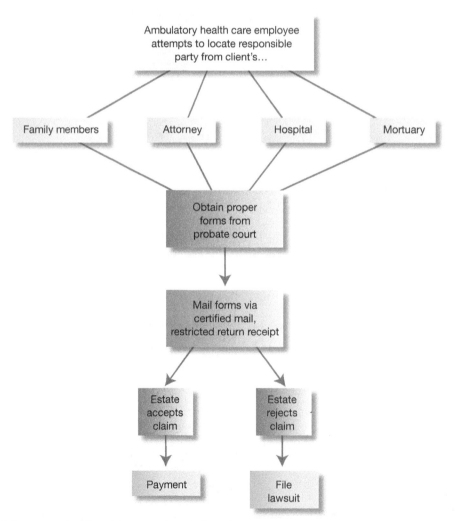

Figure 6-6. An example of financial recovery through the probate process.

SMALL CLAIMS COURT

Small claims court allows the provider or the provider's representative to file action against a client for an unpaid or delinquent account. In the state of Virginia, for example, small claims court has jurisdiction over cases when the plaintiff seeks monetary judgment up to $2000. In addition to the judgment of the amount owed, the provider plaintiff may also recover the costs of the litigation. There is no representation by attorney. The plaintiff bringing the action files a preprinted form identifying facts in the account to be collected. A summons is issued on the complaint requesting the appearance of the defendant before the judge.

The defendant is given time to file a cross-complaint against the plaintiff for any possible grievance the defendant may have. A date is set for delivery and decision.

The plaintiff presents the facts in the case, and the defendant responds to the allegations or charges. Both parties may subpoena witnesses to testify on their behalf. After all information is heard, the matter goes to the judge for a decision. If judgment is in favor of the defendant, there is no right to appeal. However, if judgment is in favor of the plaintiff, the defendant may appeal the decision to a higher court.

The prudent health-care employee will contact the clerk of the small claims court for instructions and information regarding the procedures to follow. This is in direct contrast to lawsuits in higher courts, where court clerks cannot assist the parties in completing forms.

 ## SUBPOENAS

Providers may find themselves in court even though they and their employees have practiced good preventive measures. No matter what the dispute or reason for litigation, providers need to be adequately prepared. The reasons for court appearances are numerous, but most commonly the provider will be a defendant, a witness, or an expert witness (medical) in civil or criminal trials; in sanity and probate contests; in personal injury actions; or in cases arising under insurance policies including life, health, or accident.

In any of these cases, providers may appear with or without a subpoena. A subpoena is an order commanding attendance in a specific court or office, at a specific time, under penalty for failure to do so unless a protective order from the court invalidates the requirement. The subpoena may be signed by the clerk of the court, a notary public, or an attorney. The subpoena may require a deposition to be taken rather than an actual appearance in court.

The attendance requested in a subpoena may be of a person (provider or health-care employee) or of data (medical record). The summons is referred to as a *subpoena duces tecum,* which requires the witness to appear and to bring certain records. The provider most likely would not need to appear to identify a record; proper identification usually can be done by an employee. The provider would be required to appear, however, if the record needed to be interpreted. The health-care employee should verify with the court magistrate whether his or her appearance is necessary or if just a copy of the medical records would suffice. In most cases, it is a copy of the medical record that is needed.

A court order is an order issued only by a judge to appear or to request certain records. The release of any records requested in a court order does not require the client's permission. However, out of courtesy to clients, the provider will notify them of the request. Any records related to substance abuse, mental health, or dangerous communicable diseases also require a court order. State laws differ on rules related to court orders, but generally these orders have stronger force of the law than a summons, a subpoena, or a *subpoena duces tecum.*

Whether a subpoena or a court order, it should authorize witness fees, photocopying fees, or mileage fees. If fees are not authorized, they are to be requested when the subpoena is served. If the provider is being subpoenaed, the subpoena must be hand-delivered to the provider. However, because so many subpoenas are served and there are so few officers to serve them, some subpoenas may be served to the provider's employee instead of to the provider. In such cases, the provider, out of courtesy, appears in court as though the subpoena was served by an officer to him or her. If the medical record is subpoenaed, the subpoena may be served to an employee. Legal advice should be sought for any questions about a subpoena or its circumstances. Any questions can be answered by the provider's malpractice insurance company or by the risk management department at the affiliated hospital.

 ## THE TRIAL PROCESS

A case may be tried before a judge or a judge and jury. Usually, trial courts have a jury, but the parties to a trial may waive (voluntarily give up) their right to a jury trial.

First, the jury, consisting of 6 to 12 people, must be selected. A pool of potential jurors is chosen at random from voter registration lists and auto license records in the area. How the actual jurors are picked from this pool depends on the level of court, the type of case being tried, and local court rules. Once the jurors are selected, they are given the oath by a clerk or judge.

The trial procedure (arraignment) then begins. Opening statements usually are made by each attorney, first for the plaintiff and then for the defendant. Such statements outline the facts each party hopes to establish during the trial. The plaintiff's attorney calls the first witness and asks questions (examination of witness). This part of the process is called direct examination. The defendant's attorney then questions the witness (cross-examination). This procedure continues until the plaintiff's entire case has been presented. The case for the defense is presented in the same manner. The direct examinations and cross-examinations recur. In a criminal case, the state must prove guilt "beyond a reasonable doubt," whereas in a civil case it is by "a preponderance of evidence." Then both attorneys rest their cases, that is, indicate that no further evidence or testimony is to be given.

If it is a jury trial, the judge then instructs the jury on the law governing the case. The attorney for each party is allowed closing arguments, after which the judge charges the jury to reach a fair verdict based on the evidence presented. Then the jury is ushered from the courtroom to consider the case (deliberation) and reach a verdict.

In civil court, the judge or jury finds for the plaintiff or for the defendant. If the verdict is found in favor of the defendant, the case is dismissed. If the plaintiff wins the case, a monetary settlement usually is awarded, the amount determined by the judge or jury.

In a criminal trial, if the defendant is found guilty, the judge imposes sentence. At sentencing, the court can commit the defendant to an institution or allow probation. At the end of the trial, the judge informs the defendant of all rights to appeal. If the defendant is found not guilty, the case is dismissed.

 ## EXPERT WITNESS

In medical cases, an expert witness is a person specifically qualified in medicine who can testify in court as to what the professional standard of care is in the same or a similar community. An expert witness is necessary if the subject of the court action is beyond the general understanding of the average layperson or if the knowledge of the expert witness will aid in discovering the truth.

As expert witnesses, providers testify as to what they see, hear, know to be fact, and is the recognized standard of care. Opinions not based on their experience or expertise, certain out-of-court statements, and conclusions are not admissible in most cases. Expert witnesses in medical cases are usually skilled in the art, science, or profession of medicine and may be practicing medicine or teaching in a school of medicine. In litigation, attorneys may have difficulty obtaining an expert witness who is geographically close because experts are often hesitant to testify about a situation that may appear to contradict their own peers.

Expert witnesses are expected to be reputable, honest, and impartial. The attorney who has called the witness will try to establish the witness's training, experience, intelligence, and accuracy. Witnesses should talk in lay terms rather than medical language and bear in mind that their dress and appearance may influence the judge and jury. Attorneys cannot prompt or cue witnesses.

Expert witnesses may wish to illustrate or clarify their testimony by employing such visual aids as electronic media, photographs, diagrams, charts, radiographs, skeletons, and human-type models.

In some instances, sketch artists or illustrators may be employed. During cross-examination, witnesses may face difficulties. The cross-examining attorney may try to intimidate the witness or create confusion. Witnesses should take their time and answer truthfully. They should not be afraid to say, "I don't know," if that is the case.

Expert witnesses are entitled to a fee commensurate with their time away from their practice or teaching for the case, their preparation for the case, and their participation in the case. If questioned during cross-examination regarding a fee for witnessing, they should answer truthfully. A fee should be established before serving as an expert witness rather than on a contingency basis.

If a health-care employee or a provider is subpoenaed to be an expert witness, legal counsel should be sought. Ethically such testimony should not be seen as adversarial to peers. An attorney will guide, advise, and take whatever legal action is indicated.

STATUTE OF LIMITATIONS

State legislatures have established statutes of limitations that restrict the time allowed for individuals to initiate any type of legal action. The length of time allowed for starting a lawsuit varies greatly from state to state. For example, in the case of injury to an individual, the statutes of limitations range from 1 year in Louisiana, to 6 years in Maine, and up to 10 years in Oregon.

The statute of limitations most commonly begins at the time when the negligent act was allegedly committed; when the client discovered or should have discovered the alleged negligence; or when the care, treatment, or provider–client relationship ended. However, states have differing statutes of limitations. Health-care professionals should understand their state's law on the subject as well as how the law has been interpreted in case law. Tort actions and contracts usually have separate statutes of limitations. The statute of limitations is typically longer for contracts than for torts.

Circumstances that may alter the statute of limitations occur with a person who is legally insane or when an individual has not yet reached the age of maturity. Therefore, a person declared legally insane will not come under the statute of limitations until the period of insanity has ended. In the case of minors, the statute of limitations may not apply until the child has reached the age of maturity, usually 18 years. Thus, it does not matter what age a child was when a situation occurred, the statute of limitations does not begin until the 18th birthday. This fact is of special concern to pediatricians and obstetricians.

Providers and their employees must concern themselves with the statute of limitations when considering the retention of their medical records as well as when they could be involved in a malpractice suit (refer to Chapter 9, Medical Records). Legal counsel should be sought for interpretations and advice.

Case Study

On a winter morning in Oklahoma, Lisa Boudreau, a 40-year-old mother of two, started to sweat profusely even though she was outdoors building snowmen with her children. She also was dizzy. Lisa was frightened and extremely concerned because her mother had suffered from the same symptoms 4 years earlier and died from unknown causes. Lisa called her neighbor, Barb, who rushed over. Barb called 911. By the time Lisa reached the hospital, she was in a coma. Tests determined that Lisa was diabetic. With aggressive treatment, Lisa recovered and was released from the hospital. In discussing the situation with her neighbor, Lisa realized that her mother probably had diabetes also and just was not diagnosed. Lisa ponders on whether to sue the doctor and the hospital where her mother died for not diagnosing her condition properly.

What additional information would Lisa need before approaching an attorney?
What is the statute of limitations in Oklahoma?
Do you think Lisa's case went to court? Justify your response.

It cannot be overstressed enough how important legal counsel is in the case of any questions or doubts. Providers often seek consultation on difficult medical problems and should do no less for themselves and their employees if faced with litigation.

SUMMARY

This introduction to law does not attempt to provide all the necessary information the health-care employee may need. It provides basic information, not legal advice. However, ambulatory health-care employees must be knowledgeable of the law and aware of their professional responsibilities so that they can act responsibly. Many activities in health care require this knowledge of the law to prevent illegal acts; however, when in doubt always seek legal counsel.

Watch It Now! Why is law important in health care? at
http://davisplus.fadavis.com/lawandethics

Questions for Review

SELECT THE BEST ANSWER

1. A court order calling someone to court to answer a charge is a
   a. Subpoena.
   b. Summons.
   c. *Subpoena duces tecum.*
   d. Misdemeanor.
   e. Felony.

2. A court that manages wills and settles estates is a
   a. Probate court.
   b. District court.
   c. Superior court.
   d. Supreme court.
   e. Appellate court.

3. A public official who directs court proceedings is a
   a. Plaintiff.
   b. Jury.
   c. District attorney.
   d. Judge.
   e. Defense lawyer.

4. A person who brings a claim against another individual is a
   a. Plaintiff.
   b. Jury.
   c. District attorney.
   d. Defendant.
   e. Judge.

5. A person who must appear in court to answer charges against them is a
   a. Plaintiff.
   b. Jury.
   c. District attorney.
   d. Defendant.
   e. Judge.

TRUE OR FALSE

T   F   1. Congress is the law-making body of the federal government.

T   F   2. Another name for a probate court is an estate court.

T   F   3. A felony is less serious than a misdemeanor.

T   F   4. A civil case is when a state brings court action against an individual for committing a crime.

T   F   5. A court of appeals reviews decisions made by a lower court.

CLASSROOM EXERCISES

1. State laws cannot override federal laws, yet states may enact a statute that does just that (i.e., numerous states' action to allow provider-assisted death). What happens when that occurs? Discuss the "checks and balances" that exist in the United States.

2. Describe a situation in which an understanding of the law is important to a medical receptionist.

3. If you were involved in a civil case, describe the process the case would follow and identify the factors that would determine the appropriate court.

4. Compare and contrast a summons, a subpoena, and court order. Give an example of the use of each.

5. In the vignette at the beginning of the chapter, "Can She Be an Expert Witness?" what issues does the medical assistant educator consider?

6. Although probate court and small claims court are avenues to collect a client's account, discuss the disadvantages of doing so.

INTERNET ACTIVITIES

1. Research and identify the statute of limitations for malpractice in your state.

2. Go to the Web site for your state judicial system and describe how your states' court system is organized.

WEB RESOURCE

Statutes of Limitations by state.
   http://public.findlaw.com/library/legal-system/state-statutes-of-limitations.html

 For additional resources please visit
http://davisplus.fadavis.com

CHAPTER 7

Public Duties

"The return from your work must be the satisfaction which that work brings you and the world's need of that work. With this, life is heaven, or as near heaven as you can get. Without this—with work which you despise, which bores you, and which the world does not need—this life is hell."—William Edward Burghardt Du Bois

(1868–1963); Sociologist, author, and civil rights leader

KEY TERMS

autopsy Examination by specially trained medical personnel of a body after death to determine cause of death or pathological conditions.

coroner An official, usually elected, who investigates death from sudden, unknown, or violent causes; may or may not be a physician.

intimate partner violence (IPV) Intimate partner violence refers to violence/abuse between a spouse or former spouse; boyfriend, girlfriend, or former boyfriend/girlfriend; same-sex or heterosexual intimate partner, or former same-sex or heterosexual intimate partner.

mandatory reporter A person mandated by law to report abuse or neglect to the proper authorities.

notifiable or reportable disease A disease that concerns the public welfare and requires reporting to the proper authority; a potentially pathological condition that may be transmitted directly or indirectly from one individual to another.

notifiable or reportable injury An injury that concerns the public welfare and requires reporting to the proper authority; for example, injuries resulting from gun or knife wounds.

LEARNING OUTCOMES

Upon successful completion of this chapter, you will be able to:

7.1 Define key terms.

7.2 List at least five areas of public duties for physicians and providers.

7.3 Discuss the importance of completing birth and death certificates.

7.4 Identify three circumstances in which a county coroner or medical examiner would be called to investigate a death.

7.5 Discuss the importance of prompt reporting of the death of a client.

7.6 Describe the process necessary for reporting communicable and notifiable diseases.

7.7 Restate the protocol to use for reporting adverse events of vaccines and toxoids.

7.8 List at least four injuries that are reportable.

7.9 Discuss child and elder abuse laws.
7.10 Identify professionals who are required to report suspected child abuse.
7.11 Summarize the five main types of intimate partner violence.
7.12 Describe the process used in gathering and securing evidence in the health-care setting.
7.13 Discuss Good Samaritan laws.

COMPETENCIES

CAAHEP

- Recognize the role of patient advocacy in the practice of medical assisting. (CAAHEP IV.C.14)
- Explain how the following impacts the medical assistant's practice and give examples:
  - Good Samaritan Act (CAAHEP IX.C.10.d)
- Identify where to report illegal and/or unsafe activities and behaviors that affect health, safety, and welfare of others. (CAAHEP X.C.4)
- Report illegal and/or unsafe activities and behaviors that affect health, safety, and welfare of others to proper authorities. (CAAHEP X.P.1)

ABHES

- Comply with federal, state, and local health laws and regulations. (ABHES 4.f)
- Advocate on behalf of family/patients, having ability to deal and communicate with family. (ABHES 5.e)

VIGNETTE

What Would You Do?

Jose Gonzalez, a long-time client who owns a popular Mexican restaurant where you have often eaten, comes into the clinic not feeling well and looking sick. He is seen by the provider and tests are ordered. A day later the tests results reveal hepatitis A. Jose is called and asked to return to the clinic immediately. The provider informs Jose of the diagnosis and the need to rest and take medication to cure this illness. The provider also informs Jose of the fact that he cannot return to his restaurant until he is cured and that he must inform the county health department of his diagnosis. Jose is devastated. When he leaves, he tells you there is no way he can stay away from the restaurant; it cannot run without him.

What is your responsibility in this situation?

REPORTING REQUIREMENTS

Physicians, as licensed professionals, and many other health-care professionals have a duty to protect the health of their clients but also have a responsibility to protect the health of the community as a whole. They must follow certain statutory and regulatory requirements. Reports of births, communicable diseases, and abuse are a just a few examples. Reporting requirements vary among states, but there are a number of similarities. Health-care employees will want to be familiar with the statutes, regulations, and reporting requirements for the state in which they are employed.

Good Samaritan laws are discussed in this chapter so that health-care professionals realize when their professional responsibility goes beyond the health-care setting.

Reporting statistical data and information gathered by health professionals may become an impersonal task, but it is important to remember that these data represent individuals. Therefore the task is a personal matter. Deaths, rapes, and abuse are sensitive issues. Individuals involved need special care.

BIRTHS AND DEATHS

The recording of births and deaths is an important function of the provider. These certificates are legal documents and require truthfulness and prompt and proper completion. In some states, a criminal penalty will result if birth or death certificates are not properly completed. Some states refuse to accept certificates completed in inks other than black; others refuse to accept a certificate with any blanks.

BIRTH CERTIFICATES

A birth certificate will be used throughout a person's life to prove age, parentage, and citizenship. A child will need a birth certificate when entering school. Adults will need a birth certificate to register to vote or to obtain a driver's license, a marriage license, a passport, veteran's benefits, welfare aid, and Social Security benefits.

Birth certificate requirements vary from state to state. A stillbirth or fetal death, in which the fetus has not reached the 20th week of gestation, may require neither a birth nor a death certificate. In some states, however, a special stillbirth form is used; in others, it is necessary to file both a birth and death certificate. If the birth is considered a live birth and then the infant dies, both a standard birth and death certificate are to be completed. In the event of a nonhospital birth, the person in attendance is responsible for initiating the birth certificate. In such a delivery, a parent should verify that the process is completed according to state regulations.

Check with your state's public health or vital statistics department, which offers information regarding reporting of birth and death certificates. This agency provides detailed information for completing the standard forms.

DEATH CERTIFICATES

Generally speaking, physicians (MDs and DOs) sign a certificate giving the cause of death of the deceased upon whom they have been in professional attendance. Some states allow nurse practitioners and physician assistants to sign if they, too, were providing care to the deceased. In some circumstances, someone of greater authority, such as the county health officer or coroner, will assume the responsibility. A death may need to be reported to the coroner in the following instances: a death occurring within 24 hours after a client is admitted to a hospital or licensed health-care facility, nonattendance by a physician during the 3 days before death, or death of an individual outside a hospital or licensed health-care facility. The rules vary by state. For example, in Massachusetts, any death needs to be reported to the coroner unless the client is in hospice. In that case, the hospice nurse calls the physician to discuss the death and then completes a pronouncement form. Within 24 hours the physician will complete a death certificate.

The top two thirds of the death certificate is completed by the funeral home, and the bottom one third is completed by the physician. It is then turned in to the city or town hall for recording.

In some states, a physician is forbidden by law to sign certain death certificates. Examples include, but are not limited to, a death caused by criminal activity, a death from an undetermined cause, and a death that is the result of an accident or an occupational or environmental hazard. In these cases, the police, who are likely the first responders, immediately call the coroner, medical examiner, or equivalent official for investigation. The police will ensure that the bodily remains are not disturbed, and evidence will be collected by both the police and the coroner and his or her team. This is particularly significant if an investigation or autopsy is to be performed. An investigation may result in prosecution of criminals and alteration of survivors' rights or other benefits. The client's provider may also be consulted with regard to the deceased client's medical record and his or her most recent condition.

Once the cause of death has been determined, a death certificate is issued. At this time a consultation with the next of kin or person financially responsible for the burial will take place, and the body can then be released to a mortician.

As a courtesy to the deceased's family, it is imperative that the death certificate be completed and signed as quickly as possible so that funeral and financial arrangements can begin. Many states have a requirement that the death certificate be filed within 24 to 72 hours.

Health-care professionals should understand the rules for completion of death certificates, and some blank certificates may be kept on hand for quick completion. They should realize that no arrangements can be made until the death certificate is signed. As a courtesy, many morticians will complete the death certificate for a physician and bring it to the clinic where the physician will review and sign the certificate.

The death certificate proves a person has died. A certified copy of a death certificate is generally necessary in obtaining access to insurance policy monies, bank accounts, safe-deposit boxes, dispersal of estates, real estate transactions, tax base information, Internal Revenue Service information, and Social Security and veteran's benefits.

NOTIFIABLE DISEASES

A notifiable or reportable disease concerns the public welfare and is a potentially pathological condition that may be transmitted directly or indirectly from one individual to another. In Georgia, the Department of Health succinctly states that the purpose of reportable disease surveillance is to:

1. Identify in a timely way any diseases or conditions that may require immediate public health intervention and follow-up;
2. Detect changing trends or patterns in disease occurrence;
3. Identify areas or communities that require special public health response as a result of changes in disease patterns; and
4. Assess and evaluate control and prevention interventions.

Statistics and records on reportable diseases began in the 19th century, but in 1961, the Centers for Disease Control and Prevention (CDC) assumed responsibility for the collection and publication of data concerning nationally notifiable diseases.

 According to the CDC Web site: "The list of nationally notifiable infectious diseases is revised periodically. For example, a disease may be added to the list as a new pathogen emerges, or a disease may be deleted as its incidence declines. Public health officials in state health departments and the CDC continue to collaborate in determining which diseases should be notifiable at the national level; however, reporting of nationally notifiable diseases to the CDC by the states is voluntary. Reporting is currently mandated (i.e., by state legislation or regulation) only at the state level. The list of diseases that are considered notifiable, therefore, varies slightly by state. All states generally report the internationally quarantinable diseases (i.e., cholera, plague, and yellow fever) in compliance with the World Health Organization's International Health Regulations." ●

The current list of notifiable diseases is available at the CDC Web site, listed by years: **www.cdc.gov/ncphi/disss/nndss/phs/infdis.htm.** Each state publishes a list of 30 or more notifiable diseases and their required reporting format.

Providers have a duty to report notifiable diseases according to the state's requirements. Reports are usually made by the medical assistant, who telephones the local health department and furnishes the following information that may require a written follow-up:

1. Disease (or suspected disease)
2. Name, address, age, and occupation of person with suspected disease
3. Date of onset of disease
4. Name of person reporting

To report by mail, the appropriate forms furnished by the health department are used. A check with the local health department may reveal 20 or more specific forms for diseases. Some states encourage reporting by phone, with the statistical data being collected by the health department. Other states require that the initial paperwork be completed at the time the notifiable disease is detected. Whatever method of reporting is used, it should be prompt, consistent, factual, and complete. A copy of the report is kept for the files. The health department's responsibility is to determine the source of infection and mode of transmission so that public health will be protected. The list in Figure 7-1 is not exhaustive; however, it identifies those communicable diseases that most threaten public safety.

CHILDHOOD AND ADOLESCENT VACCINATIONS

For more than two centuries humans have benefited from vaccines. Vaccine discovery started with Edward Jenner, who in 1790 developed a vaccine for smallpox. Until Jenner's time, such contagious diseases as smallpox, measles, diphtheria, and pertussis topped the list for childhood killers. Since Jenner's discovery, many more vaccines have been identified for diseases. Through widespread distribution of effective, safe, and affordable vaccines, industrialized nations have been able to contain these devastating diseases.

Health-care providers have a duty to the public to immunize children. The CDC publishes a schedule each year listing at what age the immunizations should be administered. The American Academy of Family Physicians and the American Academy of Pediatrics follow these same recommendations (see Fig. 7-2).

Before any immunizations are given, the parent or guardian is to receive a Vaccine Information Statement (VIS). The VIS is given before each vaccination, regardless of whether it is the first or third in a series. The VIS is a pamphlet published by the CDC that contains the following topics:

• Why the child should be vaccinated
• Description of the specific vaccine

Anthrax	Botulism (foodborne and wound)
Brucellosis	Cholera
Chickenpox	Guillain-Barré syndrome
Diphtheria	Encephalitis
Haemophilus influenzae (invasive)	Hantavirus pulmonary syndrome
Hepatitis A, B	Measles (Rubeola)
Meningococcal diseases	Pertussis
Plague	Poliomyelitis
Rabies (human)	Ricin poisoning
Rubella	Severe acute respiratory syndrome (SARS)
Smallpox	*Staphylococcus aureus* (VRSA/VISA)
Tuberculosis	Tularemia
Typhoid fever	Viral hemorrhagic fevers
Yellow fever	

Many states also add: animal bites, coccidioidomycosis, giardiasis, paralytic shellfish poisoning, mumps, syphilis, West Nile virus.

*See Web site for each state's particular requirements; e.g., Rhode Island
http://www.health.ri.gov/disease/communicable/providers.php

Figure 7-1. Communicable and infectious conditions commonly reported immediately by telephone.

According to the American Academy of Pediatrics (AAP) and the American Academy of Family Physicians (AAFP), the recommended childhood immunizations as of 2011 are as follows:

Diphtheria, tetanus, and pertussis

Hepatitis A

Hepatitis B

Haemophilus influenzae type b (Hib)

Influenza

Measles, mumps, and rubella

Meningococcal

Pneumococcal

Poliovirus, inactivated

Rotavirus

Varicella

For more detailed information visit the Centers for Disease Control and Prevention (CDC), AAFP, or AAP Web sites.

Figure 7-2. Recommended childhood immunizations.

- Who should get the vaccine
- Who should not get the vaccine
- Identified risks
- What to do if there is a severe reaction
- The National Vaccine Injury Compensation Program phone number and website address
- How to learn more

 After the parent or guardian has read the pertinent VIS, the health-care professional should have a consent form signed stating that they have received the VIS, have had their questions answered, and have agreed to the vaccination for the child. ●

Providers who administer certain childhood vaccines and toxoids are required by law to record the following information in each person's medical or health record:

- Type of vaccine
- Date of the vaccine's administration
- Dose
- Route
- Site
- Manufacturer and lot number of the vaccine
- Date on the VIS and date given
- Vaccine administrator's initials.

This information aids the clinic if an adverse reaction or a vaccine recall occurs.

The path of vaccine administration has not been straight or easy. There have been many bumps in the road, including adverse reactions, supply shortages, and litigation. Providers must also report any adverse events following administration. In 1986, Congress passed the National Childhood Vaccine Injury Act (NCVIA) to address concerns about vaccine supply, safety, and liability. The primary purpose of NCVIA was to create the National Vaccine Injury Compensation Program (NVICP) to compensate those injured by vaccine on a no-fault basis. The program covers all routinely recommended childhood vaccinations.

A Vaccine Injury table was created to identify those injured by vaccines and due compensation. The table is updated as information becomes available from research on vaccine adverse effects. Qualification for compensation occurs in three ways: (1) by showing that an injury found on the Vaccine Injury table occurred in the appropriate time interval following immunization; (2) by proving that the vaccine caused the condition; or (3) by proving that the vaccine aggravated a preexisting condition. Initially awards were paid from taxpayer funds, but since October 1, 1988, awards are paid from the Vaccine Injury Compensation Trust Fund. The funds come from an excise tax on every dose of covered vaccine that is purchased.

The Vaccine Adverse Event Reporting System (VAERS) was created in 1990 to provide a computerized database management system for the collection and analysis of these reports. It is operated jointly by the CDC and the U.S. Food and Drug Administration (FDA). These agencies monitor VAERS data to detect previously unknown adverse events or increases in known adverse events.

Not only do health-care providers have a responsibility for appropriate immunizations, but also school districts in all states have immunization requirements for children before they can be admitted to school. Individuals (regardless of age) must produce a record of vaccination dates or blood work proving the establishment of antibodies to the diseases. Most states follow the recommendations of the CDC. The fear of adverse effects of several of the vaccines has caused many individuals to oppose immunizations for themselves and their children. Most schools will grant exemptions for individuals with medical or religious reasons.

The CDC constantly monitors vaccines and any adverse reactions. The CDC makes recommendations regarding what vaccines should be given, on what schedule, and when any recalls of vaccines occur. Local Boards of Health will alert clinics in their area of any changes. Vaccine package inserts will assist a medical assistant on the proper storage of the vaccine. Health-care professionals must understand the rules, regulations, and schedules for vaccines and immunizations.

NOTIFIABLE OR REPORTABLE INJURY

A notifiable or reportable injury is identified when it concerns the public welfare and reporting is required to the proper authority; for example, injuries resulting from gun or knife wounds. Most states have detailed requirements for reporting injuries. Check with the local or state medical associations and law enforcement agencies for specific requirements.

Generally, however, injuries caused by lethal weapons, such as guns and knives, are treated in emergency or hospital facilities and are always reported. When persons who have been raped or battered seek and receive treatment from ambulatory health-care providers, they can be treated in the clinic or may be referred to the emergency room of a local hospital.

Questions may surface concerning reporting requirements. For example, if an adult survivor reports for medical care in an ambulatory health-care facility after a spousal rape, must it be reported? What if the client begs the provider not to report the incident? If the physician suspects abuse, must it be reported? To whom and how? At least 50 state variances govern the reporting of such incidents. In some states, marital rape laws may mandate reporting of spousal abuse; others do not. In the states where reporting is required, failure to report child, elder, and spousal abuse may be specifically considered a misdemeanor. Information that follows is important for the health professional in identifying and recognizing abuse and violence.

ABUSE

The responsibilities and tasks performed in the health-care setting can sometimes be very stressful. Abuse is one of the most serious of those stressors. Emotions are especially charged when there is evidence of child or elder abuse but are equally as difficult to hold in check when there is abuse in family or close personal relationships. The most difficult task may not be in treating the individual abused but rather in remaining calm and nonjudgmental about the circumstances that bring the abused and/or the abuser to the health-care setting.

CHILD ABUSE

Culturally, the issue is complex because there is the belief in a majority of cultures that parents are best able to provide for the care and discipline of their children. There may be the belief that parents have a moral obligation to correct a child's misbehavior. The idea of "spare the rod, spoil the child" is a paraphrase from a Bible scripture. The Mother Goose rhymes some learned as children express the frustration of the old woman in a shoe who did not know what to do with all her children, so she "whipped them all soundly and put them to bed."

Incidents of child abuse and neglect may be seen in a hospital or a clinic when a child displays fractures, burns, severe bruises, and questionable injuries. Not so obvious injuries may include dislocations, cerebrospinal trauma, and internal injuries resulting from blows to the abdomen. Malnutrition, lower than expected growth rate, poor hygiene, gross dental problems, and unattended medical needs also may indicate neglect or abuse.

Definitions of child abuse are essential for understanding what is to be reported.

- *Neglect:* Failure to provide for basic care, including food, clothing, shelter, or medical attention that endangers the health of the child.
- *Physical injury:* Burns, severe bruising, lacerations, fractures, injuries to internal organs, or serious bodily injury. Injury is often obvious, but many abusers will harm a child in places that are not obvious so that the casual observer will not notice.
- *Mental injury:* Harm to a child's well-being that damages his or her psychological or intellectual development. The child may be emotionally withdrawn, depressed, anxious, or aggressive, but injury is not obvious.
- *Sexual abuse:* Using a child to engage in sexual activity of any sort, including rape, molestation, incest, prostitution, or sexual exploitation. Physical evidence may be present.
- *Sexually explicit conduct:* Actual or simulated sexual intercourse with a child (same sex or opposite sex), masturbation, exhibition of genitalia, or sadistic or masochistic abuse; likely is not obvious to health-care professionals.
- *Child molestation:* Oral-genital contact or viewing and fondling of genitals; likely is not obvious to health-care professionals.
- *Sexual exploitation:* Child pornography, child prostitution, or sexual explicit use of child's image in electronic media; likely is not obvious to health-care professionals.
- *Incest:* Sexual relations between children or parents or siblings in the same family; may be recognized by health-care professionals.

All 50 states and the District of Columbia have laws that mandate the reporting of child abuse and neglect. The report is made to an agency named in the state statute. Certain individuals are required to report suspected abuse and neglect. These mandatory reporters include health professionals, social service personnel, law enforcement personnel, educators, and any professional person working with children. Some states also allow a hospital administrator or a physician to detain a child legally without a guardian's consent in such instances. Individuals making the report are protected from civil and criminal liability if the report is found to be false. Failure to report is a misdemeanor in some states. The function of reporting is to identify incidents of suspected abuse and neglect, not to prove abuse or neglect. The report may be oral, written, or both. Immediate reporting is paramount so that a proper investigation can be initiated. Information required in the report may include the following:

1. Name, address, and age of child
2. Name and address of child's parents (or guardians)
3. Nature and extent of the injury, neglect, or abuse
4. Any evidence of previous incidents of abuse or neglect, including their nature and extent
5. Any other information that may be helpful in establishing the cause of the child's injuries, neglect, or death and the identity of the perpetrator

If a crime has been committed, law enforcement must be notified.

Case Study ▬▬▬▬

Jacqueline was new to the Girl Scout Brownie troop. The leader, Mrs. Linnette, noticed that when Jacqueline sat down, she was very hesitant and did so gently. Being busy with twelve 8-year-old girls, the leader didn't think twice about it. The next week Jacqueline appeared with a broken finger that she injured when she "ran into a door." Mrs. Linnette filed the information in the back of her mind but again got busy helping the girls complete a project. When taking attendance at the next troop meeting, however, the leader noticed that Jacqueline was not at the meeting. One of the Brownie members mentioned that Jacqueline had broken her leg when she "fell down the stairs" at home.

Should Mrs. Linnette be concerned? What are her options? Discuss and decide what you would do if you were Mrs. Linnette.

INTIMATE PARTNER VIOLENCE

For many years, the terms spousal abuse and domestic violence have been used. Today intimate partner violence (IPV) more accurately describes the problem. IPV refers to violence or abuse between a spouse or former spouse; boyfriend, girlfriend, or former boyfriend or girlfriend; same-sex or heterosexual intimate partner, or former same-sex or heterosexual intimate partner. The phrase *teen date violence* also falls into this category. IPV refers to actual or threatened physical, sexual, or psychological harm to another individual. The term *survivor* rather than *victim* is used because survivor is believed to be a more appropriate and empowering term.

Four main types of IPV are identified:

1. Physical violence is the intent to do harm or cause disability, injury, or death. Some examples include hitting, pushing, grabbing, biting, punching, slapping, restraining, burning, or using a weapon and one's strength to hurt another person.
2. Sexual violence is forcing another to commit a sex act against his or her will; having sex with someone who is unable to understand, decline participation, or say "no" because he or she is disabled or under the influence of alcohol or drugs; or having abusive sexual contact. Date rape falls under this category.
3. Threats of physical or sexual violence occur when gestures, words, or weapons are used to cause harm, injury, disability, or death.
4. Psychological or emotional violence refers to trauma that includes humiliation, control, and any acts to embarrass or diminish a partner; isolating a partner from family and friends; and denying access to monetary funds or basic resources.

Another form of IPV has been added, called *stalking*. Stalking is the act of following, spying on, making repeated calls or contacts after being asked not to, appearing at one's home or place of employment, and making threats, with or without a weapon.

No one knows for certain how much IPV occurs because not all incidences are reported. Men as well as women may be abusers; however, more women than men are abused. IPV is a criminal offense in some states. Not all states require IPV to be reported; often it depends on whether a weapon is used. In many states, there is no criminal action unless the abused individual wishes to file a claim. Any form of IPV that is acknowledged in the health-care setting will have to be reported when required to do so. All attempts should be made to keep the survivor as safe as possible. Referral and resources should be made available to survivors who seek protection.

RAPE

Rape, a crime of violence, is forced sexual intercourse or penetration of a bodily orifice by a penis or some other object. If a weapon is used, aggravated criminal assault has occurred. One or more persons may commit rape against an individual, and gang rape can involve several individuals. Rape is a reportable criminal act.

Rape is a serious crisis for survivors, who are likely to react to the experience in four phases.

1. *Disorganization:* phase of fear, shock, denial, and a feeling of loss of control
2. *Denial:* phase when the survivor outwardly appears normal, but inwardly has suppressed the incident; gradually begins to gain control
3. *Reorganization:* phase when the survivor is no longer in denial, but often becomes depressed; may feel a need to talk about the rape
4. *Recovery:* phase when survivors realize they are not to blame for the rape

It helps if survivors are able to vent their feelings of anger, guilt, and shame during the recovery process. Women and girls are more often raped than men. Men and boys, however, are more likely to be gang-raped.

ELDER ABUSE

Intentional or unintentional harm, physical or psychological, to someone 60 years of age or older is termed *elder abuse*. Elderly persons may be more vulnerable than others because of their social isolation and mental impairment. Their abusers may include professional caregivers, family members, partners, doctors, lawyers, bankers, accountants, or strangers. Elder abuse may occur anywhere but is more commonly found in the home, a nursing home, or other institution.

The types of elder abuse are as follows:

- *Physical abuse:* Violence that results in bodily harm or severe mental stress. Assault, beating, whipping, hitting, punching, pushing, shoving, pinching, force-feeding, shaking, or rough handling during caregiving are some of the examples of physical abuse.
- *Financial abuse:* Financial or material exploitation of an elder's resources. The improper use of money, assets, or property is financial abuse. Examples include withdrawing cash from accounts without permission, cashing checks received (e.g., pension and Social Security) and denying those funds to the elder person, forcing an elderly person to alter a will, and forging a senior's signature.
- *Emotional/psychological abuse:* Actions that dehumanize an elderly person, including social isolation, name-calling, harassment, humiliating, insulting, threatening to punish, treating an elderly person like a child, and yelling or screaming. This form of abuse usually accompanies one of the other forms.
- *Sexual abuse:* Any sexual contact with an elderly person without his or her permission, including fondling, touching, kissing; forcing the elder to observe sexual acts, rape, or sodomy; spying on the elder in the bathroom or bedroom; and coerced nudity.
- *Neglect:* Careless lack of attention that results in harm. Neglect may be emotional or physical. Examples include withholding medication or necessary medical attention, personal care, food and water, or any basic necessities of life. Abandonment, lack of assistance with mobility, failure to provide adequate diaper changes, and insufficient help with hygiene or bathing also constitute neglect.

Case Law

Chiyeko Tanouye was 80 years old at the time of her death. She had lived in an adult care home operated by Raquel Bermisa for only a few months, but her condition had worsened dramatically and quickly.

Ms. Tanouye was taken to her doctor's office for treatment of a urinary tract infection. She was found to also have a decubitus ulcer that needed treatment. A week later on a follow-up visit, the ulcer had not cleared up. She was referred to a specialist. Ms. Tanouye was seen by the specialist just 2 days later, but her condition had worsened markedly. He saw two decubitus

Continued

ulcers; both had areas of dead tissue. He treated the ulcers and instructed Ms. Bermisa to change the dressing 2 to 3 times each day. He scheduled a follow-up visit for a week later, but Ms. Bermisa and Ms. Tanouye did not return.

Instead, Ms. Bermisa arrived at the Pali Momi emergency room a month later with Ms. Tanouye in the front seat of her car. She told nurses at the emergency room that something was wrong with Ms. Tanouye.

Upon examination, Ms. Tanouye's decubitus ulcers had grown much larger and showed no signs of treatment. The smell from the ulcers was overpowering to the nurses. Despite aggressive treatment, Ms. Tanouye died the next day.

Ms. Bermisa was charged with manslaughter for her apparent failure to provide adequate care. Ms. Bermisa appealed the decision, but the Hawaii Court of Appeals affirmed Ms. Bermisa's conviction.

State v Bermisa, May 7, 2004

The majority of states have enacted legislation addressing elder abuse or abuse of vulnerable adults. The laws generally name a health-care professional as one who reports the abuse, and in some states, it is a requirement to report the suspected abuse. States may protect the reporter of suspected elder abuse from civil and criminal liability. The reporting agency varies in each state but generally is a social or welfare agency, a long-term care facility, or police. Risk factors for elder abuse include advanced age, female gender, dependence on a caregiver, social isolation, behavior problems, and increased physical and mental impairment.

ETHICS CHECK

Basic considerations when dealing with the abused survivor include the following:

1. Consider the vulnerability to future assault. Providers may feel an ethical obligation and choose to intervene. Such intervention might include questioning the possibility of abuse, discussing safety options, providing a list of community referrals and resources, giving therapeutic support, and documenting the situation for future reference.
2. Respect the survivor's right not to report abuse if this is permissible by law.
3. Remember that both the survivor and the abuser need professional care and have rights protected by law.

Caring for individuals who have been abused is emotionally difficult; requirements for reporting abuse will vary by state. Urban areas have community service agencies, such as rape relief and sexual assault centers. The provider may refer the survivor to such an agency for additional, specialized services. However, if these services are unavailable or the survivor chooses to be treated by the provider alone, information is needed from law enforcement agencies regarding reporting the incident and obtaining, securing, and handling medicolegal evidence.

The survivor should be treated as soon as possible after the injury or assault, not only for the survivor's welfare but also to preserve evidence of possible criminal acts. Rape survivors need to feel supported and cared for and to feel that the violent act will make no difference in how they are treated by people.

 ## EVIDENCE

Gathering of evidence is more likely to occur in the emergency room or hospital setting. Situations will arise in the ambulatory health-care setting, however, in which employees and providers need to be knowledgeable about the methods of proper collection and preservation of evidence. (See Chapter 6, Law for Health Professionals, for an explanation of the trial process.) When in doubt, seek professional guidance from attorneys and the proper authorities.

In the ambulatory health-care setting, providers may gather legal evidence knowingly or unknowingly. Later they may be asked to offer the evidence or may be subpoenaed to give the evidence. Office and clinic situations in which evidence will be collected include the female child's urinalysis showing sperm, the young boy receiving medical treatment who reveals he has been gang raped, or a client entering with a superficial knife wound. The circumstances just described may involve providers as witnesses in litigation; therefore, proper examination and documentation are essential.

One of the first sources of evidence is documentation in medical records. Malpractice lawsuits are commonly lost because of improper documentation. Specifically, providers must record the time of client arrival; a complete explanation of the client's condition, both physical and emotional; and what was done for the client. Obviously, treatment and care of the client is primary, but documentation in the client's medical record must follow. The written documentation must be clear, concise, complete, and in order.

Evidence may be in the form of a complete written description, x-rays, photographs, clothing, samples for laboratory testing, or samples of foreign objects. Photographs and x-rays need to be dated and labeled with the client's name. Photographs may need a brief description relaying what is pictured. Both x-rays and photographs should be stored in envelopes to protect them. Any objects and clothing must be properly and carefully removed, labeled, and stored. Clothing should not be cut unless necessary and then along seams. Clothing should not be rinsed or washed. In fact, wearing gloves and not handling clothing any more than necessary will avoid changing or damaging evidence. Any body fluids, such as vomitus or gastric washing, should be saved, especially in poisoning cases, for future analysis.

You may be requested by law enforcement to take such client samples as blood; semen; vaginal, oral, or rectal smears; or skin, fingernail, or hair clippings. Samples must be properly labeled and preserved. Every piece of evidence needs to be preserved as much as possible and securely stored in a locked place to avoid tampering or loss.

Having only one employee handle all evidence can prevent it from becoming inadmissible because it cannot be properly traced or verified. When giving evidence to the proper authorities, providers should ask for a receipt for their files. They should know to whom they are giving the evidence.

Providers should cooperate with law enforcement authorities who need to talk to the client. The provider and clinic staff should not be overprotective of the client, nor should the client be jeopardized. The authorities need to receive information on the client so that they can begin their investigation immediately.

If a client dies in the ambulatory care facility or arrives deceased, the medical examiner or coroner should be called immediately, and the bodily remains should not be touched or removed. Health-care employees should not touch, tamper, or remove any tubes or paraphernalia from the client. The deceased client should be left as is; otherwise, evidence may be useless to authorities.

Good Samaritan laws are laws or acts protecting from liability those who choose to aid others who are injured or ill. Good Samaritan statutes exist in all 50 states, yet their content varies widely with regard to who is protected, the standard of care required, and the circumstances under which protection is provided. The statute itself is a legal doctrine meant to encourage physicians and health-care professionals to render emergency first-aid treatment to accident victims without liability for negligence. In some states it does not apply to an emergency arising in a clinic, hospital, or office where the client–physician relationship exists. However, the scene of an emergency may include the emergency room of the hospital in the event of a medical disaster. Most Good Samaritan laws state that the person administering the aid cannot benefit financially or receive any rewards.

The Good Samaritan statutes mainly apply to physicians, but many also address other health-care professionals. A few statutes include laypersons. In most states, no one, including physicians and health-care professionals, has the legal obligation to render first aid in a life-threatening situation.

Most Good Samaritan statutes merely attempt to protect the physician or health-care professional who gives first aid and acts "in good faith" and "without gross negligence." In some states you must be a Good Samaritan or face a penalty, whereas in others legislation states that physicians must administer emergency treatment to the best of their ability. In most states a professional should not leave an individual during an emergency (1) unless it is to call for assistance, (2) until an equally competent professional is available, or (3) unless it is unsafe to continue.

The majority of Good Samaritan statutes are poorly written and leave many unanswered questions. Not many define the following: What is an emergency? What is care rendered gratuitously? Where and to what extent can care be given and be covered by the statute? ●

Many health-care professionals are reluctant to render aid in an emergency. Reasons for this attitude may include the laws that are vague, the legal and professional advice to be cautious, and the fear that the situation may require skills outside of one's training and education. The health professional may be as anxious to avoid getting involved as the layperson. The risk for liability, however, has been grossly exaggerated. In some states such as Vermont there is a fine for those who fail to offer such assistance.

Case Law

A patient underwent elective surgery for a total hip replacement. Early during the surgery, the assistant surgeon became so ill he had to lie down on the operating room floor. The hospital called another physician (Dr. Howard), who had his office across the street from the hospital. He canceled his office appointments, came to the hospital, and completed the surgery with the surgeon. After the surgery, the patient suffered complications and sued Dr. Howard.

Outcome: Under the Good Samaritan law in California, the court ruled that Dr. Howard "did not commit any willful act or omission" while assisting the surgeon. Dr. Howard was rendering emergency care in "good faith," which addresses the quality of the intentions and not the quality of the care delivered. Also, Dr. Howard had no preexisting duty of professional care to this patient; the patient was not an established patient of his. This is another requirement of the Good Samaritan law. Further, the court stated that, as a matter of public policy, the Good Samaritan law encourages physicians to respond to emergency requests.

Perkins v Howard, 283 Cal Rptr 764 (1991)

Note: Although this case involves physicians working in a hospital, the legal implications are strong for ambulatory care professionals as well.

All health-care professionals and their employees ought to know their Good Samaritan laws and specifically what and whom they address. Certainly, the legal and ethical ramifications of rendering aid in an emergency should be considered before an emergency presents itself. Although the health-care professional may feel inadequate and unprotected in an emergency, the general public considers such a professional to be far more qualified than any layperson appearing on the scene.

Health-care professionals who do render aid in an emergency must remember to treat within the scope of their training and to give adequate care in light of the circumstances. They also should take comfort in the fact that the chance of a lawsuit is slim.

For protection from possible liability for performing under the Good Samaritan law, always act on behalf of the victim. Continue to update cardiopulmonary resuscitation (CPR) and first aid classes. Follow your scope of practice (see Chapter 3, The Health-Care Team in the Ambulatory Setting) and use common sense. Do not do anything you are not trained, educated, or credentialed to do. Do not, under any circumstances, accept gifts or rewards. ●

SUMMARY

The health-care climate of today indicates that hospitals are often full, and emergency rooms are overcrowded and understaffed. The result is that many clients turn toward their primary care provider in the ambulatory health-care setting for treatment that might otherwise be given in the hospital or emergency room. Many births take place in the home or birthing center, placing emphasis on the attending physician or midwife to file the information for the birth certificate. Clients with communicable and reportable diseases are likely first seen in ambulatory care settings. Increasingly, some individuals who are abused or harmed in an abusive situation are less comfortable in the hospital emergency environment than they are with their personal primary care provider. Health-care professionals must be prepared and have the appropriate knowledge and education to provide the best medical care. They must function within legal and ethical guidelines.

Establish policies regarding public duties including the inquiry and reporting process in your clinic. Each employee should know what kind of inquiry to make, how reporting is done, who is responsible, what information is required, and when and where the report is filed. A copy should always be kept for the facility. Be knowledgeable of any community agencies that are available to provide information for the clinic and to provide valuable services for the clients.

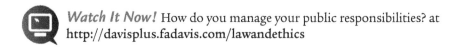

Watch It Now! How do you manage your public responsibilities? at http://davisplus.fadavis.com/lawandethics

Questions for Review

SELECT THE BEST ANSWER

1. An individual who is required by law to report child abuse is a
   a. Medical reporter.
   b. Good Samaritan.
   c. Mandatory reporter.
   d. Only a and b above.
   e. None of the above.

2. Child abuse includes which of the following?
   a. Physical injury
   b. Sexual exploitation
   c. Psychological harm
   d. Neglect
   e. All of the above

3. All of the following are phases that a rape survivor may experience except
   a. Denial.
   b. Disorganization.
   c. Neglect.
   d. Reorganization.
   e. Recovery.

4. The list of notifiable diseases comes from
   a. The CDC.
   b. Hospitals and medical providers.
   c. VAERS.
   d. American Medical Association.
   e. Only a and b above.

5. Death certificates are
   a. Mandated by law.
   b. Signed by provider in attendance at time of death.
   c. Required before release of body to mortician.
   d. Filed within 24 to 72 hours of death.
   e. All the above.

TRUE OR FALSE

T   F   1. Most elder abuse occurs in the home.

T   F   2. The majority of Good Samaritan statutes protect only MDs.

T   F   3. IPV stands for Intimate Patient Violence.

T   F   4. Stalking is a form of IPV.

T   F   5. Medical assistants are rarely involved in any reporting process.

CLASSROOM EXERCISES

1. What problems occur when a death certificate remains unsigned?

2. What are the future implications if a birth is not reported?

3. Discuss the premise that global/world vaccinations help to stop the spread of disease into industrialized nations. Are any difficulties associated with global/world vaccinations? With vaccinations in the United States? Explain.

4. Explore agencies in your community for the referral of abused persons and share your findings.

5. The provider gives you an envelope of x-rays and a sealed bag of clothing items and asks you to keep them safe until law enforcement officials arrive. How do you keep them safe? Why is this important?

6. Identify cultures in which abuse (child, intimate partner, adult, elder) is defined differently. For example, consider the following:
   - The use of a belt to spank a child
   - A cultural attitude that recommends circumcision of young girls (removal of clitoris and suturing of the vaginal opening)
   - A culture that severely punishes a rapist but financially and emotionally supports the female survivor or a child born of that rape
   - A culture that kills its infants if they are infirm and there is not enough food and shelter available

7. Under what circumstances might a provider decide not to render emergency aid?

8. Intimate partner violence is a relatively new term. Discuss its relevance with a close friend.

9. Identify advantages and disadvantages of using the term survivor rather than victim. Which would you use? Justify your response.

INTERNET ACTIVITIES

1. Visit the Web site for your state's public health department and find the list of notifiable diseases. Print it for your future reference.

2. Visit the website for two additional states in different regions of the country. Find the list of notifiable diseases. Compare these lists to the list found for your own state. How are they the same or how do they differ?

3. Go to the CDC Web site and find the VIS for the current year's influenza vaccine.

4. Find the school entry requirements for vaccinations for your state:
   www.immunizationinfo.org/vaccines/state-requirements

5. Explore the Internet for the Good Samaritan statutes for your state. What do they provide for? Would you as a medical assistant be covered under this statute?

WEB RESOURCES

American Academy of Family Physicians. Various topics on immunizations.
http://search.aafp.org/search?q=immunizations&site=a&client=aafp&proxystylesheet=aafp&filter=0&output=xml_no_dtd&getfields=*&hl=en&lr=lang_en

American Academy of Pediatrics: Immunizations and vaccines
www.aap.org/healthtopics/immunizations.cfm

Centers for Disease Control and Prevention (CDC). Intimate Partner Violence Overview.
www.cdc.gov/violenceprevention/pdf/IPV_factsheet-a.pdf

Centers for Disease Control and Prevention (CDC). Teen Dating Violence Overview.
www.cdc.gov/violenceprevention/pdf/TeenDatingViolence_2010-a.pdf

Centers for Disease Control and Prevention (CDC): Vaccine schedules for various ages.
www.cdc.gov/vaccines/recs/schedules/default.htm

Georgia Department of Public Health, "Notifiable Disease Reporting."
http://health.state.ga.us/epi/disease/report.asp

National Center for Victims of Crime
www.ncvc.org/ncvc/Main.aspx

DavisPlus | For additional resources please visit
http://davisplus.fadavis.com

CHAPTER 8

Consent

"Realize that you always have choices. It's up to you." —Leo Buscaglia (1924–1998); Author, lecturer

KEY TERMS

consent Permission by a client to allow touching, examination, or treatment by medically authorized personnel.

expressed consent Written consent that is signed by the client, provider, and a witness; it is usually for invasive procedures.

implied consent An expression of consent to something through conduct; usually used for routine services.

informed consent Specific guidelines for consent; usually identified by medical practice acts at the state level.

minor A person who has not reached the age of maturity—18 years in most jurisdictions.

    emancipated minor A person younger than 18 years of age who is free of parental care and is financially responsible for himself or herself.

    mature minor A person, usually younger than 18 years of age, who possesses sufficient understanding and appreciation of the nature and consequences of treatment despite chronological age.

uninformed consent Client gives permission to allow touching, examination, or treatment by medically authorized personnel but does not understand what has been consented to.

LEARNING OUTCOMES

Upon successful completion of this chapter, you will be able to:

8.1 Define key terms.

8.2 Explain the legalities of consent.

8.3 Give an example of verbal consent, nonverbal consent, and written consent.

8.4 Compare informed and uninformed consent.

8.5 List the four elements of the doctrine of informed consent.

8.6 Identify the following special situations in consent: minors, spouses and domestic partners, language barriers, clinical research, and when consent is not necessary.

8.7 Discuss the role of the health-care employee in the consent process.

COMPETENCIES

CAAHEP

- Recognize the elements of oral communication using a sender-receiver process. (CAAHEP IV.C.5)
- Discuss applications of electronic technology in effective communication. (CAAHEP IV.C.9)

ABHES
• Perform risk management procedures. (ABHES 4.e)
• Recognize and understand various treatment protocols. (ABHES 9.d)

When Is Informed Consent Really Informed?

A client comes in for a consultation with his surgeon regarding a complicated surgical procedure. After the consultation, the medical assistant asks the client to read and sign the lengthy informed consent. The client states, "Here, just give me that thing to sign. I am NOT going to read all of this."

What are the implications of this action?

In the health-care field, a client has the right to be in charge of his or her care and treatment. To make the best decisions, the client should be thoroughly informed. Once informed, the client can consent or refuse the treatment or choose other treatment options.

Consent is the voluntary affirmation by clients to allow touching, examination, or treatment by medically authorized personnel. Consent allows clients to determine what will be done with their bodies.

All health-care employees are involved in the consent process with the clients they serve. Although the health-care provider has the primary responsibility to inform clients of proposed treatment and to obtain consent for a procedure, employees are often responsible for having the consent form signed, and clients commonly ask questions of those health-care employees. Consequently, everyone must understand all aspects of consent.

 ## IMPLIED AND EXPRESSED CONSENT

There are two types of consent: implied consent and expressed consent.

Implied consent usually occurs at the time of routine treatment but can also cover emergency circumstances. Consider the following examples:

1. A client calls complaining of a persistent, productive cough. When the receptionist makes the appointment with the provider, the client has given implied consent for examination, which may include throat examination and culture.
2. When a provider requires a blood test for diagnosis and the client comes to the laboratory and rolls up his or her shirt sleeve, implied consent is being given.
3. If a client who comes to the office suddenly stops breathing during the provider's examination, the provider will take immediate action to restore breathing and preserve life. Consent is implied by law in an emergency situation when a client is unable to give consent. An emergency is said to exist when the client is in immediate danger and action is necessary to save a life or prevent further damage.

Expressed consent is made in writing and usually is for surgical or invasive treatments. Consider the following examples:

1. A client is scheduled for an office surgical procedure and signs an informed consent form. This action constitutes a medical contract between the client and the provider.
2. A mother signs the consent form to authorize a vaccination for her son.

Expressed consent has been obtained in both circumstances. See Figure 8-1.

CONSENT

By word	By action	Informed	Uninformed
• oral • written	• nonverbal behavior	• client understands • often is written	• client does not understand

Figure 8-1. The four forms of consent.

INFORMED AND UNINFORMED CONSENT

Because of the many occasions arising in the ambulatory health-care setting involving complicated medical procedures that are often difficult for clients to understand, informed consent is important to give the provider permission to act. To ensure that proper consent is obtained, it usually is put in writing (known as expressed consent).

Informed consent is the communication process between a client and a provider that results in the client's agreement to undergo a particular medical procedure or treatment.

Two underlying reasons for obtaining informed consent are to ensure individual autonomy (the right to be left alone or the right to privacy) and to encourage rational decision making. Written consent also aids in protecting the provider in cases of malpractice.

Regardless of the type of consent, the ideal is that all consents should be informed where the client understands all facets of the consent including risks and expected outcomes of the medical treatment and/or procedures.

Uninformed consent occurs when clients give permission but do not understand or comprehend what they have consented to.

 Consent is a process, not a mere piece of paper or form to sign. The process implies a two-way communication between client and health-care provider that will maximize the client's participation and ensure full knowledge of any procedure. Without consent, intentional touching can be considered a criminal offense, such as battery. ●

Integral to consent is the client's belief that the health-care professional to whom consent is given has the knowledge, skill, and ability to perform such tasks. The client has a right to expect that the provider has the ability to determine the need for a throat culture, perform the required surgery, or administer emergency treatment. Likewise, the client can expect the laboratory technician to know proper venipuncture technique.

Case Law

Donna Johnson saw her primary care provider because of headaches. Following a computed tomography scan, she was referred to Dr. Richard Kokemoor, a neurosurgeon, who diagnosed an enlarging aneurysm at the rear of Donna's brain and recommended surgery to clip the aneurysm. Following surgery, Donna, who had no neurologic impairments before surgery, was rendered an incomplete quadriplegic. The patient sued Dr. Kokemoor, alleging his failure to obtain her informed consent according to Wisconsin law. When obtaining Donna's informed consent, Dr. Kokemoor failed to reveal that he had rather limited experience with aneurysm surgery and had never performed the surgery that Donna required. Dr. Kokemoor also misrepresented the risk associated with the surgery. The Circuit Court found in favor of Donna Johnson. The Supreme Court agreed with the Circuit Court decision.

Johnson v Kokemoor, Supreme Court of Wisconsin, 1996; 199 Wis.2d 615, 545 N.W.2d 495

THE DOCTRINE OF INFORMED CONSENT

Informed consent is a client's right to know and understand, before agreeing to, a procedure. It is the provider's sole responsibility to obtain consent from the client, even if other staff members assist in the process. Consent should be obtained in writing because written consent implies an intentional and deliberate decision. Health-care employees must understand their state's doctrine of informed consent laws.

States vary in their consent laws. The American Medical Association recommends the following topics to be included and discussed for informed consent:

1. The client's diagnosis, if known
2. The nature and purpose of a proposed treatment or procedure
3. The risks and benefits of a proposed treatment or procedure
4. Alternatives (regardless of their cost or the extent to which the treatment options are covered by health insurance)
5. The risks and benefits of the alternative treatment or procedure
6. The risks and benefits of not receiving or undergoing a treatment or procedure

Case Study

To further illustrate the necessary elements of informed consent, consider Phil, aged 65 years, who has been diagnosed by the oncologist with an adenocarcinoma. Phil's oncologist is careful to explain the nature of this particular disease to him as well as its possible progression in his body. Possible forms of treatment are outlined, including surgery, chemotherapy, and/or radiation, and a careful explanation of the risks and possible outcomes of each are outlined.

Sometimes a provider encourages a particular form of treatment even before the client asks for a recommendation. Here the oncologist has knowledge of Phil's particular case and may be expected to give credence to such a recommendation. However, the oncologist should be careful also to explain the possible risks of no treatment at all. Although the client often looks to the specialist for medical information and recommendations, the decision is the client's alone.

Phil states he wants to discuss all his options with his family before making a final decision.

Have all the points of informed consent been satisfied? Explain your response.

In Phil's situation (see the previous Case Study), as with most others, all health-care professionals must be sensitive to the impact of such a decision. For consent to be meaningful, Phil may need time to comprehend the essential elements of the consent. This may include talking with family members, seeking a second opinion, considering financial implications, or just being alone. Staff members also need to be prepared to clarify, further explain, or direct additional questions to the provider if the client so indicates. Not until a later time will written consent be obtained and the provider able to proceed. The written consent must reflect each of the elements previously described and should also contain the client's signature, the provider's signature, and the signature of a witness. The provider may ask Phil to explain in his own words what he believes is happening.

Case Law

Cindy Werth was expecting twins. Because she was a Jehovah's Witness and had a firm belief in the religion's teaching "that it is a sin to receive blood transfusions," Cindy signed a "Refusal to Permit Blood Transfusion" form as part of her hospital preregistration.

After delivery, Cindy had complications and was experiencing uterine bleeding. She was advised to undergo a dilatation and curettage and agreed. Again, she discussed her refusal to allow a blood transfusion with her obstetrician/gynecologist. After being placed under anesthesia and despite the specialist's efforts during surgery, Cindy continued to bleed and was experiencing, among other things, premature ventricular activity and a significant decrease in blood pressure. The anesthesiologist (Dr. Michael Taylor) determined that Cindy needed a blood transfusion to sustain her life. Cindy's obstetrician/gynecologist (OB/GYN) expressed Cindy's refusal of blood transfusions, but the anesthesiologist proceeded anyway stating that it was medically necessary.

The Werths filed a malpractice action, alleging that Dr. Taylor committed battery by performing the transfusion without Cindy's consent. Dr. Taylor moved for summary disposition "because Cindy's refusal was not conscious, competent, contemporaneous, and fully informed."

The trial court found that Cindy's refusals of a transfusion were made when she contemplated "merely routine elective surgery" and not life-threatening circumstances, and that "it could not be said that she made the decision to refuse a blood transfusion while in a competent state and while fully aware that death would result from such refusal." The record apparently reflected "the unexpected development of a medical emergency requiring blood transfusion to prevent death or serious compromise of the patient's well-being." The trial court therefore granted summary disposition in favor of Dr. Taylor.

The Michigan Court of Appeals affirmed the trial court's decision.

Werth v Taylor, 475 N.W.2d 426, 427 (Mich. Ct. App. 1991).

PROBLEMS IN CONSENT

Consent may be difficult to obtain in the treatment of a minor, a person who has not reached the age of maturity, which is 18 years old in most states. In some states, courts recognize two types of minors as being capable of informed consent. Mature minors are considered to possess sufficient understanding of treatment they are to receive and its consequences despite their chronological age. Emancipated minors have the legal capacity of an adult as indicated by age, maturity, intelligence, training, experience, economic independence, and/or freedom from parental control. In some states, someone who is married or in the military is an emancipated minor. Legal questions of capacity to consent related to both the mature minor and the emancipated minor are considered on a case-by-case basis because not all states recognize mature or emancipated minors.

In most states, minors are unable to give consent for medical care except as described previously or in special cases when minors are pregnant, request birth control or an abortion, have suspected sexually transmitted diseases, have possible problems with substance abuse, or are in need of psychiatric care. In all other situations, the provider or staff should attempt to reach the parents or legal guardians for consent.

Legal implications to consider when treating a minor are as follows:

1. A minor has the right to confidentiality. A 16-year-old who seeks a prescription for birth control pills has the right for that information to be kept confidential.
2. A minor who may legally consent to treatment may not be financially responsible. If the 16-year-old in the first example does not pay when services are given, collecting from parents who have not given their consent may be difficult and breaches confidentiality.
3. A minor's legal guardian may have to be determined—a special problem in the case of divorce and remarriage. If the father of a child is financially responsible, but the child resides with the mother, who may properly give consent for treatment?

Knowledge regarding your particular state's laws regarding minors is important. Also, seek an attorney's recommendations when questions occur regarding minor's rights.

The law that governs consent is not well defined for minors, and it may be vague or even non-existent with respect to spouses and/or domestic partners. Increased awareness of the rights of women and domestic partners has had a significant impact on the legal system. More advances can be expected in the future. A spouse has the legal right to consent to and receive medical care and treatment without a spouse's approval. Domestic partners also may consent without the other partner's approval.

Case Study

A 17-year-old ward of the court is pregnant and gives birth to a son. She identifies the father on the birth certificate. Social services garnish the father's wages for child support.

Discuss.
Should the father of an unborn child have any say if the mother seeks an abortion instead of giving birth? Discuss.

Other problems in consent may arise in the case of foster children, stroke clients who cannot communicate, persons who are mentally incompetent (including those in shock and trauma), demented clients, and those temporarily or permanently under the influence of drugs or alcohol. A legal guardian who can give consent may have to be appointed by the courts. The health-care staff must determine who is legally responsible in each case. When there is immediate danger to life and limb, however, the law implies consent for treatment for these individuals without consent from the responsible party.

Language can become a barrier to informed consent. An interpreter may be necessary so that information for consent can be given in a client's native tongue to ensure comprehension. If an interpreter is used, this should be documented on the consent form, and there should be a place for the interpreter's signature.

A number of exceptions to informed consent are particular to each state. Examples include the following:

1. The provider may not need to disclose commonly known risks.
2. The provider may not be responsible for failing to disclose risks when the knowledge might be detrimental to the client's best interest.
3. A provider may not need to disclose risks if the client requests to remain ignorant.

A client has the right to refuse treatment. In some situations, the court appoints a guardian, who then may give consent for the client. This is especially true in the case of minors. Check your state's doctrine of informed consent for specific exceptions and information. Local medical associations also may offer information.

A unique problem surfaces for consent when the client is going to be part of any clinical trial, experimental treatment, or human research. The federal Office for Human Research Protections (OHRP), a branch of the National Institutes of Health, oversees the safety of participants in federally funded research. Each major institution that conducts research also must perform its own audit of client safety and report its results. Audits of "human subject laws," however, reveal a number of problems:

1. Serious adverse reactions to experimental drugs often are not recorded or reported to clients.
2. Clients are coerced into waiving their rights to sue in case of malpractice or serious problems.
3. Clients are placed in trials that are medically inappropriate but that needed research subjects.
4. Informed consent is rushed because of the "desperate" nature of a participant's condition.

5. Researchers are allowed to have financial interests in the procedures or drugs that are used, which is in direct violation of federal regulations.
6. Not all benefits, risks, and possible alternatives are adequately explained.

OHRP records and the U.S. Food and Drug Administration (FDA) sources say the biggest problems surface at high-volume institutions where the pressure to do research is intense. Both agencies have the power to shut down clinical trials and do so; however, both agencies have limited budgets. Participation in any research places a burden on clients and their families to conduct their own investigation of the research in which they are involved.

 ## IMPLEMENTING CONSENT

Consent forms are prepared for the client's signature. The staff may be responsible for the preparation of specifically designed forms or the procurement of preprinted consent forms. In either case, the form must be understandable, protect the rights of the client, and be broad enough to cover anything contemplated but specific enough to create informed consent. A so-called blanket consent form, which seeks to cover all aspects of client care and is not specific, must be avoided.

Care should be given to be certain that all elements of informed consent have been understood by the client before a signature is affixed. The consent form should include an expiration date. In some states, 90 days is the maximum. Another consideration may be allowing a waiting period between consent and administration of the procedure or treatment.

The consent process ought to be concisely documented in the medical record. Some providers tape-record the informed consent process and save the tapes or have a staff member present who signs the consent form also. Others have a checklist for the informed consent interview. Whatever procedures are followed, informed consent should be sought as soon as possible after the need is identified (Fig. 8-2).

A health-care employee may be asked to witness a signature in order to verify that the signature is indeed that of the client. The provider is responsible for the explanation of medical treatment to the client, even though the employee may provide reinforcement through clarification. If the client has any further questions about the treatment or difficulties with the consent form, let the provider know. If the client signs with an X, two witnesses are required. Younger staff members should witness consent forms; this helps ensure the longevity of the witnesses should there be any problems in later years. At least three copies of the signed consent form are necessary—one for the client, one for the medical record, and one for the hospital, if necessary.

INADEQUACY OF CONVENTIONAL CONSENT FORMS

The typical preprinted consent form is often incomplete in that it does not contain all of the topics required. Most of these preprinted forms are fairly generic and vague in order to cover all situations. This inadequacy makes the provider liable for litigation.

Also, these forms often are missing some of the required signatures and are easily misplaced or lost.

 ## IMPROVING THE CONSENT PROCESS

With the growing number of lawsuits due to miscommunications, providers and hospitals are doing more to ensure that the client has been fully informed regarding the proposed procedure. They are now presenting the client with videos and diagrams to ensure that the client is well informed. Providers and hospitals are also turning to electronic consent forms in the hope that these hi-tech forms will fully meet the requirements for clear, informed consent forms.

These electronic consent forms can be tailored individually for each client. These software programs offer the following options:

1. A comprehensive library of education materials that describe different medical conditions and treatments so that the provider can choose which options meet the diagnosis of each client.

BOTULINUM TOXIN TYPE A
(Botox Cosmetic)

Botox is made from the Botulinum Toxin Type A, a protein produced by the bacteria Clostridium botulinum. For the purpose of improving the appearance of wrinkles, small doses of the toxin are injected into the affected muscles blocking the release of a chemical that would otherwise signal the muscle to contract. The toxin thus paralyzes or weakens the injected muscle. The treatment usually begins to work within 24 to 48 hours and can last up to four months. The Food and Drug Administration (FDA) approved the cosmetic use of Botulinum Toxin Type A for the temporary relief of moderate to severe frown lines between the brow and recommends that the procedure be performed no more frequently than once every three months.

It is not known whether Botulinum Toxin Type A can cause fetal harm when administered to pregnant women or can affect reproduction capabilities. It is also not known if Botulinum Toxin Type A is excreted in human milk. For these reasons, Botulinum Toxin Type A should not be used on pregnant or lactating women for cosmetic purposes.

Patient's
Initials

_____ The details of the procedure have been explained to me in terms I understand.
_____ Alternative methods and their benefits and disadvantages have been explained to me.
_____ I understand that the FDA has only approved the cosmetic use of Botulinum Toxin Type A for frown lines between the brow. Any other cosmetic use is considered "off-label".
_____ I understand and accept the most likely risks and complications of Botulunum Toxin Type A injection(s) that include but are not limited to:

- abnormal and/or lack of facial expression
- allergic reaction/violent allergic reaction
- disorientation, double vision, and/or past pointing
- facial pain
- headache, nausea, and/or flu-like symptoms
- inability to smile when injected in the lower face
- local numbness

- paralysis of a nearby muscle, which could interfere with opening the eye(s)
- product ineffective
- temporary asymmetrical appearance
- swallowing, speech, and/or respiratory disorders
- swelling, bruising, and/or redness at injection site

_____ I understand and accept that the long-term effects of repeated use of Botox Cosmetic are as yet unknown. Possible risk and complications that have been identified include but are not limited to:

- muscle atrophy
- nerve irritability

- production of antibodies with unknown effect to general health

_____ I understand and accept that there are complications, including the remote risk of death or serious disability, that exist with this procedure.
_____ I have informed the doctor of all my known allergies.
_____ I have informed the doctor of all medications I am currently taking, including prescriptions, over-the-counter remedies, herbal therapies and supplements, aspirin, and any other recreational drug or alcohol use.
_____ I have been advised whether I should take any or all of these medications on the days surrounding the procedure.
_____ I am aware and accept that no guarantees about the results of the procedure have been made or implied.
_____ I have been informed of what to expect post treatment, including but not limited to: estimated recovery time, anticipated activity level, and the necessity of additional procedures if I wish to maintain the appearance this procedure provides me.
_____ I am not currently pregnant or nursing, and I understand that should I become pregnant while using this drug, there are potential risks, including fetal malformation.
_____ If pre- and postoperative photos and/or videos are taken of the treatment for record purposes, I understand that these photos will be the property of the attending physician.
_____ I understand that these photos may only be used for scientific or record keeping purposes.
_____ I have been advised to seek immediate medical attention if swallowing, speech, or respiratory disorders arise.
_____ The doctor has answered all of my questions regarding this procedure.

I certify that I have read and understand this treatment agreement and that all blanks were filled in prior to my signature.

I authorize and direct _____ , M.D., with associates or assistants of his or her choice, to perform the following procedure of Botulinum Toxin Type A injection(s) on _____
for the treatment of_____ .   (patient name)
                              (i.e., brow, forehead, "crow's feet," etc.)

_____   _____
Patient or Legal Representative Signature/Date   Relationship to Patient

_____   _____
Print Patient or Legal Representative Name   Witness Signature/Date

I certify that I have explained the nature, purpose, benefits, risks, complications, and alternatives to the proposed procedure to the patient. I have answered all questions fully, and I believe that the patient fully understands what I have explained.

                              _____
_____ copy given to patient   Physician Signature/ Date   _____ original placed in chart
initial   initial

Figure 8-2. Informed consent forms: (A) for a botulinum toxin type A (Botox cosmetic) procedure.

Continued

FLEXIBLE SIGMOIDOSCOPY

Flexible sigmoidoscopy involves passing a lighted flexible tube (sigmoidoscope) through the anus into the lower intestinal tract (colon). This procedure allows the practitioner to examine the inside of the lower two feet of the colon. Sometimes small tissue growths (polyps) are removed during the sigmoidoscopy (polypectomy), as polyps can grow inside the colon and become cancerous. Occasionally biopsies (sampling of small pieces of colon) are performed during the sigmoidoscopy. Bleeding sites may be treated during the sigmoidoscopy by injection of sclerosing material or use of electrocautery. On rare occasions a narrowing or obstruction may be encountered during the sigmoidoscopy. The narrowing may be stretched (dilated) at the time of sigmoidoscopy.

Patient's
Initials

_____ The details of the procedure have been explained to me in terms I understand.
_____ Alternative methods and their benefits and disadvantages have been explained
to me.
_____ I understand and accept possible risks and complications include but are not
limited to:

- *bleeding*   • *need for surgery*
- *gassy discomfort/bloating*   • *pain*
- *infection*   • *perforation*

_____ I have informed the doctor of all my known allergies.
_____ I have informed the doctor of all medications I am currently taking, including
prescriptions, over-the-counter remedies, herbal therapies and supplements,
aspirin, and any other recreational drug or alcohol use.
_____ I have been advised whether I should avoid taking any or all of these medications
on the days surrounding the procedure.
_____ I am aware and accept that no guarantees about the results of the procedure have
been made.
_____ I have been informed of what to expect postoperatively, including but not limited to:
estimated recovery time, anticipated activity level, and the possibility of additional
procedures.
_____ I understand that any tissue/specimen removed during the surgery may be sent to
pathology for evaluation.
_____ The doctor has answered all of my questions regarding this procedure.

I certify that I have read and understand this treatment agreement and that all blanks
were filled in prior to my signature.

I authorize and direct _____ , with associates or
                                      (practitioner's name and title, i.e., M.D., N.P., P.A.)
assistants of his or her choice, to perform a flexible sigmoidoscopy on _____ .
                                                                                                    (patient name)
I further authorize the physician(s) and assistants to do any other procedure that in
their judgment may be necessary or advisable should unforeseen circumstances
arise during the procedure.

_____   _____
Patient or Legal Representative Signature/Date   Relationship to Patient

_____   _____
Print Patient or Legal Representative Name   Witness Signature/Date

I certify that I have explained the nature, purpose, benefits, risks, complications, and
alternatives to the proposed procedure to the patient or the patient's legal
representative. I have answered all questions fully, and I believe that the
patient/legal representative (circle one) fully understands what I have explained.

_____
Physician Signature/ Date

_____ copy given to patient   _____ original placed in chart
initial   initial

Figure 8-2. —cont'd (B) For a flexible sigmoidoscopy surgical procedure.

Refusal to Consent to Treatment

I have been advised by Dr. _____ that the following treatment _____ should be given to me/the below-named patient (please type or print): _____

Dr. _____ has fully explained to me the nature and purposes of the proposed treatment, the possible alternatives thereto and the risks and consequences of not proceeding.

I nonetheless refuse to consent to the proposed treatment.

I have been given an opportunity to ask questions, and all my questions have been answered to my satisfaction.

I hereby release Dr. _____ and _____ Hospital and their employees, students and medical staff from any liability for any ill effects that I may suffer from failure to perform the proposed treatment.

I confirm that I have read and fully understand the above and that all the blank spaces have been completed prior to my signing.

_____   _____
Patient or Legal Guardian Signature   Date

_____   _____
Witness   Relationship

I hereby certify I have explained the nature, purpose, benefits, and alternatives to, the proposed treatment and the risks and consequences of not proceeding, have offered to answer any questions and have fully answered all such questions. I believe that the patient/relative/guardian fully understands what I have explained and answered.

_____   _____
Physician Signature   Date

Note: This document must be made part of the patient's medical records.

Figure 8-2. —cont'd (C) For refusal to consent to treatment.

2. Detailed informed consent materials that facilitate a discussion of the given procedure or treatment, including:
   a. Description of the procedure for that particular client and their unique condition. These include risks, benefits, treatments, and likely outcomes if there is no treatment.
   b. An expansive collection of anatomical diagrams and images that facilitate the provider's ability to describe the nuances associated with a given condition or procedure.
   c. A wide range of postprocedural care instructions.
   d. A comprehensive library of drug information documents.

Therefore, an individualized consent form tailored directly to that client and his or her specific diagnosis and treatment plan will be developed by the provider and presented to the client. Once discussed and totally understood, the client signs the consent form on a digital pad, and this comprehensive, signed document is printed and saved electronically and automatically noted in the client's electronic medical record.

The Veterans Health Administration has been using these electronic consent forms for several years. When initiating them, Secretary of Veterans Affairs Anthony J. Principi said, "We owe it to our veterans to do all we can to ensure that they understand the care they receive and to make sure that the informed consent process is as patient-friendly as possible. This new program is a great complement to the success of VA's electronic patient records systems."

SUMMARY

Consent may be quite formal, requiring the signature of the client on a form that includes all the necessary components for informed consent. It may be very informal and implied, requiring no formal signature, and occurs in the routine activities of health care. What is most important, however, is that any consent be informed. Clients must understand and give permission for any procedures or tests to be performed. Any confusion or lack of understanding on the part of the client is an "open door" for difficulties later. Health-care employees must be particularly sensitive to making certain clients comprehend what is happening.

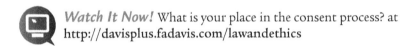

Watch It Now! What is your place in the consent process? at
http://davisplus.fadavis.com/lawandethics

Questions for Review

SELECT THE BEST ANSWER

1. When a client understands all aspects of a consent and signs a consent form, it is considered
   a. Informed consent.
   b. Uninformed consent.
   c. Informed express consent.
   d. Informed implied consent.
   e. None of the above.

2. An emancipated minor is
   a. Someone who lives at home with his parents but is older than 18 years.
   b. Someone who lives at home that is younger than 18 years.
   c. Someone who is younger than 18 years but is married.
   d. Someone who is living at college but is still under their parent's health insurance and the parents pay for their room and board.
   e. Only c and d above.

3. When creating a consent form, most states require which of the following?
   a. Name of the procedure
   b. The possible risks involved
   c. Any alternative procedures or treatments
   d. All of the above
   e. None of the above

4. In an uninformed consent, the client has done the following:
   a. Read the consent form
   b. Read, understood, and signed the consent form
   c. Read, not understood, but signed the consent form
   d. Only a and c above
   e. Only b and c above

5. With regard to clinical trials or human research, which of the following often occur?
   a. Clients are often desperate to get into a clinical trial and so will consent to anything.
   b. Clients are placed into inappropriate trials where there is a need for more subjects.
   c. Clients are usually coerced into waiving their rights to sue for any damages during the trial.
   d. All of the above.
   e. None of the above.

TRUE OR FALSE

T   F   1. A provider who does not obtain consent from a client is at risk for being accused of battery.

T   F   2. As long as a provider has the client's signature on a consent form, the client is considered to be informed.

T   F   3. Doctrine of informed consent laws are the same from state to state.

T   F   4. The Office for Human Research Protections oversees the safety of participants in federally funded research trials.

T   F   5. Consent for treatment is implied consent when a client makes an appointment and comes to the clinic as scheduled.

CLASSROOM EXERCISES

1. Jerod Hilton has just been informed that he has prostate cancer. His provider says that the only recommended course of treatment is surgery. Jerod has no hesitation in his response and immediately says, "No way doc, you aren't cutting me down there." After further discussion, Jerod's decision is unchanged. What steps, if any, should the doctor take?

2. In emergency situations, what type of consent exists? Explain and give an example.

3. The parents of a 6-year-old child consented to allow her to undergo "routine cardiac tests." One of the tests performed was a catheter arteriogram in which complications occurred. Questioning of the parents revealed that they did not fully understand the risks involved. What are the legal implications of this consent? Identify potential problems in this situation.

4. A 15-year-old boy enters your clinic requesting treatment for scalds received on his hand while emptying the dishwasher at his place of employment. Although his family receives medical treatment at the clinic, you are uncertain about seeing him without his parents' knowledge. Can he consent to treatment? What are the legal ramifications?

5. How specific should a consent form be? How general? Explain.

6. When you are asked to witness a signature, what does it legally mean?

7. An unmarried pregnant client requests an abortion. Assuming the abortion is legal, what rights, if any, does the father have in consent? Do you agree? Justify your reasoning.

8. After a client signed a consent form and you have witnessed it, she states, "I think this is the right decision." What would you reply? What would you do?

9. Detail what role medical assistants may assume in the consent process.

INTERNET ACTIVITIES

1. Search the Web site of the American Medical Association (AMA) regarding informed consent.

2. Go to the governmental Web site of your own state and find the rules and regulations regarding informed consent.

3. Visit the Web site for "iMedConsent" and explore a sample of electronic informed consent.

REFERENCE

Landro, L.: Consent forms that patients can understand, *Wall Street Journal*, Feb. 6, 2008. **http://online.wsj.com/article/SB120224055435844931.html#articleTabs%3Darticle.**

WEB RESOURCE

U.S. Department of Health and Human Services, Office for Human Research Protections (OHRP)
http://grants.nih.gov/grants/policy/hs/

DavisPlus | For additional resources please visit http://davisplus.fadavis.com

Workplace Issues

CHAPTER 9

Medical Records

"Do not put your faith in what statistics say until you have carefully considered what they do not say."—William W. Watt; Writer and author

KEY TERMS

Certification Commission for Health Information Technology (CCHIT) A group whose task is to set standards for electronic medical record (EMR) software.

Consolidated Health Informatics (CHI) An initiative to standardize computer applications so that they can communicate back and forth.

continuous positive airway pressure (CPAP) Small electrical pump that delivers pressurized air through a nasal mask. Used to prevent airway from closing while sleeping, leading to sleep apnea.

degauss To demagnetize. A computer reads stored information magnetically. If information is demagnetized (degaussed), the information is scrambled beyond recognition and cannot be read or reconstructed.

electronic health record (EHR) Combination of a client's care from multiple sources (in electronic format).

electronic medical record (EMR) Computerized version of a client's medical chart in a single clinic or facility.

Evaluation and Management (E&M) A set of codes used to identify a clinic visit rendered by a provider.

Health Information Technology for Economic and Clinical Health (HITECH) Act This law extends the Health Insurance Portability and Accountability Act (HIPAA) data privacy and security regulations to support business associates, such as billing companies, accounting firms, and others.

Holter monitor A device worn by a client to monitor the electrical activity or rhythm of the heart over a certain period of time.

Institute of Medicine (IOM) An organization that gives advice regarding government policies that affect public health.

microfiche Method of filing data on film using minute images.

problem-oriented medical record (POMR) A charting system, developed by Lawrence L. Weed, MD, that is based on client problems.

protected health information (PHI) Individually identifiable health information that is transmitted or maintained in any medium including oral statements.

purge A cleansing or clearing away; refers to the clearing away of old medical records that are no longer being used.

SOAP/SOAPER A charting method using subjective and objective data for client assessment and planning, education, and response.

telemonitoring An electronic observance of activity; in medicine, the monitoring of a client's health status.

LEARNING OUTCOMES

Upon successful completion of this chapter, you will be able to:

9.1 Define the key terms.

9.2 List six purposes of medical records in the ambulatory health-care setting.

9.3 Name and describe two types of charting.

9.4 Describe *SOAP/SOAPER* and its use in medical records.

9.5 Compare/contrast electronic medical records and electronic health records.

9.6 Demonstrate by example how and when to correct an error in medical records.

9.7 Discuss the impact of the Healthcare Insurance Portability and Accountability Act (HIPAA) on medical records.

9.8 Describe at least five guidelines for keeping client information private in electronic medical records and paper medical records.

9.9 Outline the process to follow when a subpoena or court order is received for records.

9.10 Explain the ownership of medical records.

9.11 Discuss retention and storage of medical records.

9.12 Discuss purging of medical records.

9.13 List the required information needed on a release of information form.

COMPETENCIES

CAAHEP

• Discuss applications of electronic technology in effective communication. (CAAHEP IV.C.9)

• Discuss principles of using EMRs. (CAAHEP V.C.11)

• Document accurately in the patient record. (CAAHEP IX.P.7)

ABHES

• Institute federal and state guidelines when releasing medical records or information. (ABHES 4.b)

• Prepare and maintain medical records. (ABHES 8.b)

The creation and care of medical records require careful attention from the health-care staff. Both employees and providers collect and enter data into clients' medical records. Medical records are a part of every person's life, beginning with the birth certificate and ending with the death certificate.

With increased health awareness, clients are more concerned about what goes into their medical records. Clients also care who has access to their records. Are the records legal documents? Are they confidential? What authorization is required to release clients' medical records? Who owns them? HIPAA regulations (see Chapter 4, State and Federal Regulations) mandate that health-care facilities address these questions. These are concerns health-care employees face daily.

Medical records can be in either a paper or electronic format. Regardless of the format, the primary goal of any medical record is the proper care and identification of the client. A client's medical record that is accurate, complete, and concise encourages quality medical care.

This chapter considers medical records specifically in the ambulatory care setting and discusses the various state statutes that apply to medical records, including access, retention, and destruction.

 ## PURPOSE

The medical record in the ambulatory health-care setting serves many purposes. Among them are:

1. Providing a base for managing client care that includes initiating, diagnosing, implementing, and evaluating.
2. Providing interoffice and intraoffice communication of client-related data.
3. Documenting total and complete health care from birth to death.

4. Allowing patterns to surface that will alert providers of clients' needs.
5. Serving as a legal basis for evidence in litigation and to protect the legal interests of clients and providers.
6. Providing clinical data for education and research.

MEDICAL RECORD CREATION AND CONTENT

A medical record is established at the first encounter between a provider and a client. It chronicles each interaction thereafter between the client and any member of the clinic's staff. The organization of the medical record will vary depending on the policies of the clinic, whether paper or electronic, but all medical records usually contain the same information (Fig. 9-1).

DOCUMENTATION

Documentation in the medical record facilitates the diagnosis and treatment of clients, ensures client safety and reduces medical errors, promotes health-care management, and serves as legal documents in risk management issues.

Documentation within the medical record should include the date, time, details of each encounter (in a nonjudgmental manner), and signature of the health-care professional who took part in the encounter. In paper charts, legible writing is a necessity.

The type of charting and medical record used in health-care settings varies. Specialists who see the client only once may have an abbreviated form of the medical record. By contrast, a provider who has had the same client for 30 years may have the equivalent of three file folders with several hundred sheets of medical data on that client. Documentation within the chart can be accomplished in a variety of ways. A few of the most popular documentation styles are explained here and work equally well with either the paper or electronic chart.

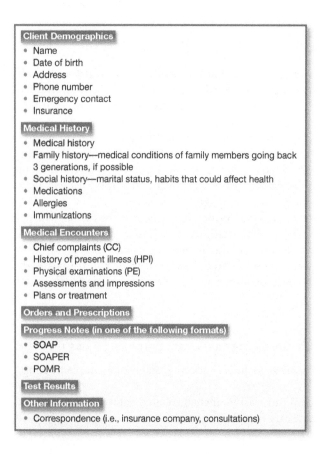

Client Demographics
- Name
- Date of birth
- Address
- Phone number
- Emergency contact
- Insurance

Medical History
- Medical history
- Family history—medical conditions of family members going back 3 generations, if possible
- Social history—marital status, habits that could affect health
- Medications
- Allergies
- Immunizations

Medical Encounters
- Chief complaints (CC)
- History of present illness (HPI)
- Physical examinations (PE)
- Assessments and impressions
- Plans or treatment

Orders and Prescriptions

Progress Notes (in one of the following formats)
- SOAP
- SOAPER
- POMR

Test Results

Other Information
- Correspondence (i.e., insurance company, consultations)

Figure 9-1. Contents of a medical record.

PROBLEM-ORIENTED MEDICAL RECORDS

The problem-oriented medical record (POMR) was developed by Dr. Lawrence L. Weed. The POMR is based on the client's problems, and every health-care employee, including the provider, adds to the chart in a particular place in the same manner. The POMR identifies the client's problems, not simply diagnoses that are based on defined data. A problem can be a condition or a behavior that results in physical or emotional distress or interferes with the client's functioning. Examples include pain in the knees and ankles, fear of falling, decreased appetite, and even an inability to pay medical bills. The problem list is usually numbered, appears early in the record usually on the chart face sheet, and serves as a checklist to ascertain the client's progress.

To identify clients' problems, the provider explores the client's problem and performs services that may include a physical examination, history, laboratory tests, and obtaining subjective data from the client. Every problem has a plan, and its progress is recorded in the medical record.

Weed also developed a computerized medical record that permits the healthcare provider to build a computer-based POMR while accessing data pertinent to the problem from current literature.

SOAP/SOAPER

Many ambulatory health-care settings use SOAP/SOAPER—subjective, objective, assessment, and plan, education, and response—as a method of charting. The format is as follows.

> _Subjective_ includes what the subject or client says, family comments, and hearsay; the client's exact words are recorded.
> _Objective_ includes events that are directly observed or measurable, including laboratory tests, radiograph results, and physical examination findings.
> _Assessment_ includes the provider's evaluation based on the subjective and objective data (S + O = A).
> _Plan_ includes the treatment plan and the actions taken.

Some providers may add two additional letters to the SOAP note, thus producing a SOAPER note. The additional letters are:

> _Education_ includes any education given to the client.
> _Response_ includes the client's understanding of the education and care given.

An example POMR charting in the SOAP/SOAPER format is shown in Figure 9-2.

Each time the client is seen by the provider, an entry (regardless of its style) is created by the provider, who either keys the information into the record at the time of the encounter or dictates the information to be transcribed by an employee. Whatever method of charting is used in medical records, it must be concise, complete, clear, and in chronological order.

Case Study

Candace works for Dr. Robert Ford, who has been in practice for 20 years. This provider has used paper medical records his entire career. Candace and her coworkers struggle to keep up with the large amount of paperwork within the clinic. The health-care employees know that electronic medical records, though time-consuming to establish, would solve a lot of the paper issues within the clinic and save time for all health-care professionals, including Dr. Ford.

If you were Candace, how would you approach Dr. Ford to propose this major change? What justifications would you list?

CALCANEO, Henry. R. 08/18/19--

Date of Onset	Date Recorded	PROBLEM LIST	Date Resolved	INACTIVE PROBLEMS
?	10/08/2---	1. Increased appetite, increased thirst	10/20/2---	
05/28/2---	06/30/2---	2. Dyspnea	07/10/2---	
05/11/2---	08/21/2---	3. Loss of job		

10/08/---

1. Increased appetite, increased thirst

S: "I eat all the time and never gain weight." "I didn't think about it, but yes, I drink water all the time, too."

0:   BP 120/88. T-R-P: 98 degrees F--80--18. Color good. Skin turgor adequate. Wt. 5# less than 3 weeks ago. Urine, 4+ sugar. FBS positive.

A: Uncontrolled diabetes; in family history.

P: Dx: Lab workup for diabetes. Tx: Begin on insulin; diabetic diet.

E: Instructed to enroll, attend next diabetic class; Taught importance of diet, exercise, insulin injections. Gave our 3 clinic-prepared brochures on diabetes (intro material). Gave 24 hr phone line to call if questions.

R: Seems to understand importance of learning about diabetes, injections, diet, exercise as 2 in family have disease. Asked good questions. MHL

7/10/---

2. Dyspnea

S: "I can't seem to get my breath. I'm weak all the time. It's worse when I lay down."

0:   BP 180/98. T-R-P: 99 degrees F--88--26. Chest x-ray negative. States he "awakens from sleep with respiratory distress." Cough; slight edema.

A: Congestive heart failure, left sided. History of hypertension and diabetes.

P: Hospitalize for cardiac workup.

E: Explain necessity of hospitalization.

R: States "I really don't want to go but if it'll help me breathe better, I'll do anything! I can't take this much more. It scares me." MHL

7/10/---

3. Loss of Job

S: "What can I do now? I'm not trained for anything but construction, and with this heart problem and diabetes, I'll never get back my old job."

0:   Heart condition improved; wt. gain 30#; brittle diabetic.

A: Is most upset that current job is not available as it's THE only job he wants. Money apparently not the issue. Off diabetic diet.

P: Return to diabetic classes w/spouse and son. Refer to Social Worker to discuss job situation.

E: Reviewed possible complications if unsuccessful in managing his diabetes. Talked about wt gain and what it means for diabetes.

R: Good interaction w/pt; willing to attend classes w/family; concerned about complications and said he wanted to prevent any, especially since one diabetic in family is nearly blind. MHL

Figure 9-2. Example of problem-oriented medical record (POMR)charting in the SOAPER format.

ELECTRONIC MEDICAL RECORDS

Electronic medical records (EMRs) contain the same information as found in a paper medical record, except in a digitalized format, and are replacing paper records.

As all medical records become electronic, there are two important terms: electronic "medical" records and electronic "health" records. Although some confusion still exists, for the purposes of this text, they are identified as follows: electronic medical record (EMR) is the computerized version of a client's medical chart in a single clinic or facility; electronic health record (EHR) is the combination of a client's care from multiple sources, such as a primary care clinic, hospital, pharmacy, and rehabilitation facility. As a result, a primary care provider (PCP) starts an EMR, but as the client acquires services from other sources, such as radiology, laboratory, pharmacy, and specialists, the EMR becomes an EHR, and the results are compiled in the PCP's record.

The Institute of Medicine (IOM) Committee on Data Standards for Patient Safety, in 2003, identified eight areas that should be included in an EMR to provide for quality care and client safety. These guidelines developed a common industry standard for EMR functionality. The suggested functions are:

1. Health information and data—complete client demographics and past medical history, including medications and allergies. This information should be arranged in a user-friendly display.
2. Order management—capability of ordering tests and prescriptions. This will eliminate lost orders, handwriting discrepancies, and other ordering mistakes.
3. Result management—all testing is computerized and more readily available to the provider. This quick return of results allows the provider to quickly treat the client, if needed, for abnormal test results.
4. Decision support—information should be accessible to aid a provider in his or her decision making. Some examples of topics covered in this area are drug interactions, allergies, and management of diseases and symptoms.
5. Patient support—instruction sheets and treatment plans are readily available for clients. This area also includes telemonitoring that could include such information as monitoring a client's electrocardiogram while they are wearing a Holter monitor.
6. Administrative processes and reporting—scheduling, billing, referrals, authorizations, and other administrative tasks need to interact with the medical record so that payment can be realized.
7. Electronic communication and connectivity—information would be accessible between all providers of health care, including providers, specialists, hospitals, and pharmacies. This type of information is an area that has not been perfected. (Further initiatives have been put into place to address this functionality and are introduced later in this chapter.)
8. Reporting and population health—this function would automate mandatory reporting to governmental agencies.

In 2004, President George W. Bush outlined a plan "to ensure that most Americans have electronic health records within the next 10 years." Also in 2004, the Certification Commission for Health Information Technology (CCHIT) was established to set standards for EHR software programs. The CCHIT reviews software programs to verify that they indeed meet the standards and are then deemed "certified." This certification is for a 3-year period. The CCHIT announces new standards annually. Each time a software program is due for recertification, an EMR company must pay approximately $28,000 for inspection of their program in hope of gaining recertification. If a software is updated significantly during those 3 years of certification, it must go through the process again (including the cost) to gain certification for the subsequent product release.

In 2009, President Barack Obama signed the American Recovery and Reinvestment Act. As part of this legislation, more than $19 billion was released to facilitate the implementation of EMRs. This money is available through the Medicare and Medicaid reimbursement systems to encourage providers to adopt certified EMRs. The stimulus money is available through the year 2014, with payments being reduced each year until 2014. It is to the providers' advantage to adopt an EMR sooner so that they can avail themselves of the funds for several years.

IN THE NEWS

Certification of EMRs was initiated to help guide providers to well-constructed, functional, and secure EMR software programs. CCHIT has credentialed approximately 55 out of a possible 300 software programs available on the market. This is eliminating the majority of EMRs from consideration by providers who want to take part in the federal stimulus money. Because of the expense ($28,000) and time needed to obtain a credentialed status, small companies are unable to pursue credentialing. It is feared that the certification process is stifling competition and will lead to higher prices, thus affecting providers' bottom line. This process will bear watching, especially once the stimulus money is no longer available in 2015.

To help meet the function set forth by the IOM regarding electronic communication and connectivity, the Consolidated Health Informatics (CHI) initiative was established. This is an initiative of the Office of Management and Budget that operates under the auspices of the Department of Health and Human Services (HHS). CHI is a collaboration between many federal governmental departments to adopt health information interoperability standards. CHI standardizes health information, including health-care vocabulary and messaging standards so that health-care software and health-care devices can interface and exchange information. This action brings hospitals, providers, clients, and other health-care entities together for the sharing of information. Information can be shared regardless of its location and EMR system and can improve health care.

The following computer guidelines to ensure confidentiality are important when instituting electronic records and fall under HIPAA guidelines:

• Computer hardware, servers, and network hubs are to be kept secure from intrusion.
• A list of users approved to access medical information must be identified and regularly updated.
• Robust firewalls and antivirus measures must be in place. Blocking of unauthorized intrusion must be a high priority.
• Passwords are to be changed at least every 90 days and created so that they are not easily guessed.
• Passwords are hidden when entered and are securely stored. They are not to be shared with anyone.
• The computer station should limit the number of invalid attempts to access information.
• Computer screens are to be out of view of the public and unauthorized staff.
• Screen savers should be used to prevent unwanted viewers' access. ●

Ideally, any time a computer workstation is vacated, even for a short period, the user should close out of the document, allowing the screen saver to activate. Upon returning, the user will again need to enter the protected password for access to the medical information. There are many advantages of EMRs.

Updated information and accessibility: Because all test results are received electronically, they are imported directly into the client's record. Access to the EMR is available at the client point of care.

Safety for the client: Prescription errors are reduced significantly by e-prescribing, which alerts providers of any allergies or interactions. All medical information is easily located. Chart notes are easily read because they are now typed and not handwritten. Health maintenance screenings can be prompted for appropriate age and gender and are easily tracked.

Better client care: EMRs provide alerts and notices to better practice guidelines. Health-care professionals can therefore consistently provide the most current standard of care to their clients. Appropriate client instruction sheets can be generated either by print or e-mail. Drug recalls can be easily handled and clients quickly notified.

Efficiency and savings: Electronic messaging systems within the EMR make communication between provider and other health-care specialists (clinic staff, consultants, pharmacies, and insurance carriers) an easy and efficient task. Savings are realized by the use of templates for clinic visits and the reduced time needed for any transcriptionists. At the completion of the visit, the EMR will generate the appropriate suggestion of an Evaluation and Management (E&M) code based on the documentation. EMRs encourage more detailed documentation that in turn leads to more accurate and often higher coding and reimbursement levels.

A Day in the Life of the Electronic Health Record

You are a 65-year-old woman going to a large multicare health setting for an annual physical examination. When your appointment was made with the primary care physician's nurse practitioner (NP), she noted that your physician will want fasting laboratory work, mammogram, and a dermatology screening. You explain that you also need a follow-up visit at the sleep clinic. All appointments are scheduled for 1 day. When you arrive, you go first to the laboratory for the blood draw and urinalysis. Then you have time for breakfast in the clinic's café before you see your primary care physician.

When you are in the examination room with the NP, she is able to pull the morning's laboratory results on her computer. She turns the computer toward you and is able to show you today's results on a spreadsheet with the last 2 years' results for comparison. Discussion follows. Your next stop is for a mammogram. The results of that test will be mailed to you. You hasten on to the sleep center, where the provider discusses your continuous positive airway pressure (CPAP) registry that shows on his computer how many hours a night you have successfully used the breathing apparatus. He comments that your primary care physician indicates in today's chart notes that you are using a new mask and nasal pillow system that you purchased on the Internet. The final day's visit is to dermatology, where you receive a full body screening for any changes in your freckles, moles, and aging spots. A suspicious mole on your lower cheek causes the dermatologist concern. She removes the mole and takes a biopsy and will notify you of the results. The dermatologist says, "I've looked at your chart; you've had a long day! Are you ready to go home now?"

LEGAL ASPECTS OF THE MEDICAL RECORD

Medical records, whether paper or electronic, are legal documents and as such become a vital piece of evidence in any malpractice case. Medical records that are relevant, accurate, legible, timely, informative, and complete withstand questioning from all sides. These types of records protect both the provider and the health-care professionals that work in the clinic.

CONFIDENTIALITY

As seen in Chapter 4, HIPAA, as well as state regulations, requires all health-care professionals managing records to protect the privacy of clients unless otherwise mandated by law. This involves both paper records and EMRs.

HIPAA has specific regulations about protected health information (PHI) related to EMRs. Under HIPAA, clients must grant written consent or permission to provide or disclose their PHI (electronic or paper format) for any reason.

Another law that emerged from the American Recovery and Reinvestment Act is the Health Information Technology for Economic and Clinical Health (HITECH) Act. This law extends the HIPAA data privacy and security regulations to support business associates, such as billing companies, accounting firms, and others. HITECH allows states to prosecute any individuals who have access to health-care files whether or not they are in the health-care setting. HITECH established that these "business associates" would face the same penalties as health-care providers.

IN THE NEWS

Huping Zhou, a cardiothoracic surgeon from China, who was working at the University of California, Los Angeles (UCLA) School of Medicine as a researcher, was sentenced in April 2010 to 4 months in jail after pleading guilty to accessing patient medical records that he was not authorized to view. Zhou, by his own admission, looked at the medical records of celebrities, his supervisor, and fellow workers. Zhou's jail time was the first in the nation for unlawful "peeking" at client files without authorization. Experts say that this should send a strong message to providers, health-care employees, and their business associates that HIPAA and HITECH violations will not be tolerated when it comes to a client's privacy.

RELEASE OF INFORMATION

A *release of information* signed by the client gives a provider authority to release certain medical information. Most clinics have created their own release of information form that a client must sign.

A release form includes the client's name, date of birth, and other demographic information. It authorizes the provider or clinic (specifically named) to release the medical record to a specific entity, which may be a clinic, provider, lawyer, or other specified individual. The form must include a portion that asks specifically if the client wants information to be released concerning the following topics: substance abuse, psychiatric or mental health issues, or HIV/AIDS testing or counseling. The client signs and dates the form that is then signed by a witness and placed into the medical record. To be legal, a clinic should have a form with an original signature; no faxes or e-mailed copies should be accepted. The medical record is then reviewed by the provider, and upon his or her approval, the staff may release only the information specified in the request (see Fig. 9-3).

Laws regulate who may sign a release of information form for clients who are underage or unable to sign for themselves:

- If the client is a minor, the parent or legal guardian may sign.
- If the parents are legally separated or divorced, the parent who has legal custody of the minor must sign all release forms.
- If the client is incompetent, the court-appointed guardian signs the release form.
- If the client is deceased, the legal representative of the estate signs the release form.

A standard procedure is essential for maintaining confidentiality and good client relations.

Providers and employees should remember that the medical record might be as valuable for what it does not say as for what it does say. "An act not recorded is generally considered an act not performed" by most courts of law. The necessity of using a medical record in a court emphasizes the importance of accurate records that honestly reflect the client's course of treatment. Also, some clinics do periodic audits of their charts to ensure good charting practices.

ERRORS IN MEDICAL RECORDS

If an error is made in a medical record, it must be properly corrected. Handwritten errors discovered later should be corrected by the following method: draw a line through the error using a red pen, write "correction" or "error," sign your initials, indicate the date, and write in the correction. An

AUTHORIZATION TO RELEASE INFORMATION

Please Print Clearly

Name _____
 (Last) (First) (M.I.)

Address _____
 (Street) (City) (State)

Phone_____ Date of Birth _____ Medical Record#_____

I authorize _____ to release medical information from my medical record to

Name of Doctor, Hospital, etc._____

Address _____

City/State/Zip Code_____

for the purpose of review/examination. I further authorize you to provide such copies thereof as may be requested. The foregoing is subject to such limitation as indicated below:

☐ Entire record

☐ Specific information: _____

☐ Old records from previous physicians: _____

I give special permission to release any information regarding: (initial on applicable line(s) below)

_____ Substance Abuse_____ Psychiatric/Mental Health Information _____ HIV information

Reason for request _____

This authorization will automatically expire 90 days from the date signed. I understand that I may revoke this content at any time except to the extent that action has been taken in reliance thereon.

Signed _____ Date _____

Witness _____ Date _____

FOR OFFICE USE ONLY

Received _____ Completed By _____

Completed_____ Fee Paid _____

Amount Billed $ _____ Amount Due_____

Disclosure Consisted Of _____
_____
_____

Name

Date:_____

Re: _____

Record #/Date of Birth _____

This is a multiple action form letter with only those items indicated by an "X" being applicable.

IN ANSWER TO YOUR REQUEST FOR MEDICAL INFORMATION

Please see attached medical record copies. NOTE: Request for copies of the entire record will include only the last 2 years of lab work. The attached medical information is CONFIDENTIAL. Subsequent disclosure is not authorized without the specific consent of the patient.

REQUEST FOR ADDITIONAL INFORMATION

☐ Your request is being returned for the following reason(s):

   ☐ We are unable to locate a record of treatment for this individual. Please provide additional information, such as full name of patient at time of treatment, date of birth, record #, or verification of spelling of name.

   ☐ No record on file for specified dates.

   ☐ Medical information is confidential and can be released only on written consent of patient/patient's legally authorized representative. Have the patient complete and return this form.

   ☐ Authorization date is over 6 months. Return your request with a more recently dated authorization signed by the patient/patient's legally authorized representative.

   ☐ The authorization received contained insufficient information for release of the information requested.

☐ Our charge for releasing records directly to the patient/patient's representative is $ _____ . If you provide us with the name and address of your new physician, we will send the copies there instead, thereby eliminating the charge. Otherwise, make check payable to _____, put patient's name on the check, and return a copy of this letter with check.

☐ Please remit _____, which is our fee for processing your request and photocopying the requested record. Make check payable to_____ , reference the patient's name on the check, and return a copy of this letter with check.

☐ Other:_____
_____
_____

Figure 9-3. Example of an authorization to release information form.

electronic error is made much the same way. Using the tracking device in the word processing software, a line is drawn through the error. The correction is then placed right after the information lined out, and the word "correction" or "error," the initials of the person making the correction, and the date the correction is made are added to the document.

When erasures or obliterations occur, confusion and suspicion may result. Poor or altered records can be detrimental to the provider's defense in court.

SUBPOENAS

At times during the course of medical practice, a court order or a subpoena may be received requesting a client's medical chart and/or specific information from the chart. If a health-care professional and the record are subpoenaed, it is called a *subpoena duces tecum* (see Chapter 6, Law for Health Professionals). Always notify the client before releasing the record in accordance with the subpoena. In some states, the attorney who subpoenas the medical record must notify in writing both the provider and the client and allow 14 days for a response. A certified photocopy of the medical record should be made for the courts. The person or agency issuing the subpoena usually covers the cost of making copies.

The medical record often becomes the center of a malpractice action wherein both attorneys involved bring in forensic document examiners to investigate the reliability of the record. These experts use specialized equipment that can detect different inks in the same entry, a fact that a jury could easily interpret to be an indication of the record having been tampered with or altered. Scientific equipment also can detect when pages have been added after the fact. Health professionals should never change a medical record unless correcting it properly. Never "leave room" for someone else to chart later. Such a space may cause suspicion. Finally, never remove a report or note from a medical record because it, too, may indicate that a record has undergone tampering.

All these problems can be avoided by having a compliance plan for documentation within the medical record. (Refer to Chapter 5, Professional Liability.)

Case Study

The medical assistant is catching up on the completeness of the practice's medical records. She notices that the provider wants a transcript of two telephone calls that had not been previously recorded. She now records them, post dates when the calls were made, and signs the entry.

Discuss.

A well-informed client discusses her marital problems with the provider and says, "Please do not put this in my record."

Discuss.

TELECOMMUNICATIONS

ELECTRONIC MAIL

Electronic mail (e-mail) is a useful tool for the health-care setting. It provides communication among providers and their employees and between provider and client. It creates a written record that information was shared, allows embedding of educational links, and can be used in malpractice suits to exhibit communication. However, e-mail has its disadvantages. Namely, e-mail is not a private or confidential means of communication; it is discoverable even after deleting; it may be necessary to obtain consent before sending; it may be misread and misunderstood; it can be monitored, accessed, and read by supervisors without liability for privacy invasion; and it is the property of the agency/facility. See Figure 9-4 for sample e-mail and fax confidentiality statements.

> **Confidentiality Notice:** This message and any attachments may contain confidential and privileged communications or information. The information contained in this e-mail/fax is transmitted for the sole use of the intended recipient(s). The authorized recipient of this e-mail/fax is prohibited from disclosing this information to any other party. If you are not the intended recipient or designated agent of the recipient of such information, you are hereby notified that any use, dissemination, copying or retention of this e-mail/fax or the information contained herein is strictly prohibited. If you received this e-mail/fax in error, please notify the sender immediately and permanently delete this e-mail/fax.

Figure 9-4. Confidentiality notice.

HIPAA requires specific consent for any electronic mail transmission of PHI. If e-mail is used in the practice, the following guidelines should be followed:

1. Establish time lines for reading and responding to e-mail.
2. Generate automated replies to acknowledge you have received e-mail.
3. Inform clients of the privacy risks of using e-mail.
4. Do not use e-mail without the client's informed consent.
5. Avoid using e-mail that requires an urgent reply.
6. Place e-mail correspondence in client records and ensure that the e-mails are properly identified.
7. Do not forward e-mail without permission.
8. Ensure that no one else has access to the e-mail account and do not leave the monitor unattended while signed onto the e-mail account.
9. Establish specific procedures for personal digital assistant devices if they carry e-mail and client information.
10. Frequently change passwords.
11. Have staff sign confidentiality contracts.

Case Study

A client e-mails her internist requesting permission to begin a water therapy class at the local YMCA that requires a provider's release. The internist responds to the e-mail within 24 hours and says, "Sounds like a good plan. Fax me the release form." The client faxes the release form to the provider's clinic. He completes it and faxes it directly to the therapist at the YMCA.

Discuss the advantages of this activity to the client and to the internist. Does it raise any problems?

FAX MACHINES

The facsimile (fax) machine can be especially useful if health-care information is needed more quickly than can be accomplished by mail, phone, or computer. Also, more detail can be given by fax than by phone. There are problems, however. The fax may inadvertently be sent to the wrong destination or retrieved by an unauthorized recipient. Therefore, careful attention to confidentiality must be considered when using a fax transmission for client medical records (see Fig. 9-4). Office policies should be initiated detailing proper procedures.

Use the following fax guidelines:

1. Use the fax machine only when there is not enough time for more secured measures such as mailing.
2. Use the fax machine only when machines are located in restricted-access, secure areas.
3. Obtain appropriate client authorization where required before the release of information.
4. Verify the recipient of the fax, the fax number, and the location of the fax machine. Include a statement to those who might receive the fax in error. Call to see if the fax was received.
5. Document the reason for any fax transmission and any misdirected fax.

Figure 9-4 illustrates a sample confidentiality notice to accompany any e-mail or fax.

OWNERSHIP OF MEDICAL RECORDS

The accepted rule is that medical records are the property of the person creating them and entering the data in them. Health-care providers are considered the owners of the medical records they have written. However, clients have access to the information in their medical records. Clients may be expected to make an appointment to obtain that copy and pay reproduction fees. Access should be withheld only when the law prohibits such access or when, in the provider's opinion, great harm would be done to the client.

Clients who request that their medical records be transferred to another provider must do so in writing. The original record must be retained in the clinic and the request honored with a photocopy of the complete record or the provider's summary. The continuance of medical records is important in a society that is so mobile. This continuity can be accomplished only with cooperation from providers. The important factor is to release the record promptly so that the client can receive proper care from the new provider.

Case Study

The use of "smart cards" has been suggested as a remedy for protecting clients' medical information. The encoded smart card contains a person's medical record, and only that person releases the information contained therein by sharing a personally chosen password.

Discuss the advantages/disadvantages of such a system.

STORAGE OF MEDICAL RECORDS

In today's computerized society, medical records are most likely stored electronically and do not pose a serious storage problem. However, most practices have a vast collection of medical records in a variety of media. All stored records need to be protected as carefully as active files.

Not all paper medical records need to be kept in the same location. Active records should be in readiness for providers. Closed or inactive files usually include records of clients who are no longer being seen by the provider, who may have moved away, or who have died. These files may be kept in a storage area separate from the current and active files. The clinic may have storage space or may rent storage space in another location. Some old medical files may be stored on microfiche and, if so, require a microfiche reader to access the information.

EMRs need to be backed up daily. The EMR software being used determines the back-up process and storage requirements. Some software is accessed through the Internet, and thus a back-up record is constantly being generated at the point of origin. If the EMR is installed on the clinic's server, a back-up record needs to be generated nightly. This record should be removed from the clinic to protect it from fire or other destruction.

RETENTION OF MEDICAL RECORDS

The question of how long to retain medical records is not easily answered. One guideline indicates that records should be retained until the statute of limitations for acts of medical malpractice has expired so that records are available for any possible litigation. This guideline may require a pediatrician to keep the record for as long as 7 to 10 years beyond the age of maturity. Most states have statutes that set retention guidelines for medical records. When a state has no statute regarding retention of medical records, state medical associations and insurance carriers are the best resources for this information. Hospital medical records and provider medical records have different retention time limits. Health-care professionals should know the limits for the state in which they are employed.

 ## DESTRUCTION OF MEDICAL RECORDS

Once records have reached the limits of retention, follow procedures to purge aged data. Whether the medical records are paper based or electronic, their destruction should follow specific guidelines suggested by the American Health Information Management Association (AHIMA) and the Healthcare Information and Management Systems Society.

A destruction log is developed to keep track of all destroyed medical records. It includes the client's name, date of birth, and date of last encounter. The log should also include the date and method of destruction, a statement that the records were destroyed in the normal course of business, and the signatures of the individuals supervising and witnessing the destruction. These records are to be kept permanently.

One method of destruction for paper medical records is to have them picked up by a company specializing in record destruction. Upon completion of the task, a signed certificate is returned to the clinic indicating the contents and date of the destruction.

Depending on the amount of material to be destroyed, another method involves on-site destruction. A large truck that is fitted with an industrial shredder arrives at the clinic, and the records are placed into the shredder and destroyed. For some clinics this is a preferable method because a health-care employee can observe the actual destruction. Thus, the records are destroyed before they are removed from the property.

AHIMA suggests that the preferred method of destroying computerized data is to degauss the data. This is a technique that alters the way data align in the magnetic storage field and renders the previous data unrecoverable and impossible to reconstruct. To keep current on the latest medical record destruction methods, the AHIMA recommends reassessing the process annually based on current technology, accepted practices, and availability of timely and cost-effective destruction services.

SUMMARY

Medical records carry pertinent client information and data that, in part, determine the care given. Medical records have very sensitive information and must be kept private and confidential; any information released must be done so only with the consent of the client and/or on a "medical need to know" basis. Health-care professionals must always remember that medical records may become a critical document in litigation of what was or was not performed. Careful documentation in medical records that is complete, organized, sequential, and kept confidential and private tells a story of meticulous client care.

 Watch It Now! How do you protect the medical record and its contents? at http://davisplus.fadavis.com/lawandethics

Questions for Review

SELECT THE BEST ANSWER

1. Who owns the medical record?
   a. The client
   b. The hospital where the provider is associated
   c. The clinic
   d. The provider
   e. None of the above

2. A Privacy Notice should address the following topics:
   a. Restrictions of PHI
   b. Request of confidential information
   c. Request of any amendment to the PHI
   d. Opportunity to receive an accounting of PHI disclosures
   e. All of the above

3. Which of the following is not a purpose of the medical record?
   a. Serves as a legal basis for litigation
   b. Protects only the legal interest of the provider
   c. Documents total health care from birth
   d. None of the above
   e. Only a and c above

4. Weeding out inactive charts that are older than their retention time frame is called
   a. Relinquishing.
   b. Purging.
   c. Instituting.
   d. Microfiching.
   e. None of the above.

5. POMR is an acronym that stands for
   a. Policies on Medical Records.
   b. Protected Office Medical Records.
   c. Problem-Oriented Medical Records.
   d. Problem Office Management Reports.
   e. None of the above.

TRUE OR FALSE

T   F   1. Regardless of the storage medium in which a medical record is saved, inactive charts should be protected with the same safety measures as active charts.
T   F   2. In all cases, medical records should be kept for a minimum of 5 years since first seen.
T   F   3. Proper and complete documentation is a provider's best defense against litigation.
T   F   4. As long as a client has signed a medical records release form, the health-care professional can make copies of the appropriate parts of a record without the provider's approval.
T   F   5. Faxing of medical records is preferable over mailing a copy of the records.

CLASSROOM EXERCISES

1. A fax was received in a private home where no fax was expected. The fax has come from a nearby long-term care facility, is addressed to a provider, has personal information about a resident of the facility, and requests a medication change. What should the home owner do? What responsibility and action does the long-term facility have?

2. The following report was phoned in and charted: "05/14/2- Urinalysis reveals RBC too numerous to count." When the written report is received, you note it as WBC, not RBC. How would you make this correction in a paper record? How would it be made in an EMR?

3. You are preparing a medical record after it has been subpoenaed. Describe the procedures you would follow. What do you do with medical information from a referring provider?

4. A client becomes angry when refused permission to hand-carry medical records when moving out of state. What alternatives can an employee suggest?

5. Describe what might be done when there is simply no room for any more medical records in the clinic.

6. Refer to the vignette "A Day in the Life of the Medical Record." As a client, how did the availability of the medical record facilitate the care received? As a health-care provider, what are the advantages of having up-to-the-minute information on the client? Discuss the legal implications of a medical record used in this manner.

INTERNET ACTIVITIES

1. The provider that you work for has announced his retirement. Go to the American Medical Association's website and find out what steps need to be taken with regard to medical records.

2. Go to your state's Department of Health Web site. What is the law regarding retention of medical records?

WEB RESOURCES

American Health Information Management Association (AHIMA)
   www.ahima.org

Consolidated Health Informatics
   www.hhs.gov/healthit/chi.html

User Satisfaction with EHRs: Report of a Survey of 422 Family Physicians
   www.medscape.com/viewarticle/570380

 DavisPlus | For additional resources please visit
http://davisplus.fadavis.com

CHAPTER 10

Reimbursement and Collection Practices

"Even if you're on the right track, you'll get run over if you just sit there."—Will Rogers (1879–1935); American cowboy, humorist, social commentator, actor

KEY TERMS

capitation Providers are paid a fixed monthly amount for each health maintenance organization (HMO) member in their care.

co-payment An amount that a member of an insurance plan must pay for certain medical procedures and provider visits.

COBRA Consolidated Omnibus Budget Reconciliation Act of 1985; mandates that continuation of group insurance coverage be offered to covered persons who lose health or dental coverage due to a qualifying event.

coordination of benefits An agreement between insurance carriers that if a client has two insurance plans, neither the provider nor the subscriber will receive more than 100% of the covered charges.

Current Procedural Terminology (CPT) codes A list in which each procedure performed by a provider is given a specific number to universally identify it for billing purposes.

deductible A cost-sharing arrangement in which the member pays a set amount toward covered services before the insurer begins to make any payments.

diagnosis-related group (DRG) A classification system that groups together clients with similar diagnosis, treatment, and consumption of hospital resources, thus allowing comparisons of resource use across hospitals with varying mixes of clients. Used primarily in the United States as a method of funding hospitals.

Evaluation and Management (E&M) codes A section of the *Current Procedural Terminology, 4th Edition* (CPT-4) manual that lists codes for office visits. Each level of visit dictates how much is charged by the provider and paid by the insurance carrier.

***International Classification of Diseases,* 9th Revision, *Clinical Modifications,* Volumes 1, 2, and 3 (ICD-9-CM)** Listing that identifies the diagnostic categories, specific DRG numbers, and relative values for those categories. The relative value is how U.S. hospitals and providers are reimbursed unless there are extenuating circumstances. (ICD-10 is anticipated to be effective in 2013. These new codes will be more specific.)

medical savings (or spending) account (MSA) A method for companies with 50 or fewer employees, self-employed persons, and uninsured individuals to purchase medical insurance by making tax-free deposits to an MSA.

TRICARE Federal insurance plan that covers military personnel and retirees and their families.

usual, customary, and reasonable fee (UCR) Describes how providers are reimbursed for their services; is widely accepted by insurance carriers.

LEARNING OUTCOMES

Upon successful completion of this chapter, you will be able to:

10.1 Define key terms.

10.2 Explain, in a short paragraph, the importance of appropriate reimbursement and collections.

10.3 List at least five guidelines related to reimbursement.

10.4 Recall the laws that have an impact on reimbursement.

10.5 Describe five government insurance programs.

10.6 Discuss the suggestions that help clients be financially responsible for their health care.

10.7 List at least five items to be covered in a collection policy.

10.8 Identify the appropriate procedures to follow when collecting a bill by telephone or by mail.

10.9 Identify the seven "collection don'ts" established by the Federal Trade Commission.

10.10 Discuss solutions to collection problems.

10.11 Explain the one important procedure to follow if a client is denied credit because of a poor credit rating.

10.12 List steps to follow in selecting a collection agency.

10.13 Discuss ethical implications regarding reimbursement and collections.

COMPETENCIES

CAAHEP

• Discuss procedures for collecting outstanding accounts. (CAAHEP VI.C.11)

• Describe the impact of both the Fair Debt Collection Act and the Federal Truth in Lending Act of 1968 as they apply to collections. (CAAHEP VI.C.12)

• Perform collection procedures. (CAAHEP VI.P.2.c)

ABHES

• Perform risk management procedures. (ABHES 4.e)

• Collections. (ABHES 8.q)

VIGNETTE

Can You Afford This?

A general surgeon practicing in a metropolitan area loves his work. He spends only 1 day of the week in the clinic and performs about six operations a week. He no longer covers night emergencies. Early in his career, he determined that insurance carriers were totally dictating his compensation, so he stopped accepting any insurance. To see this general surgeon, clients must pay cash. If clients want to file for reimbursement from their insurer, it is up to them. His fees are based on what the market will bear. His net income for at least a decade has been nearly $1.2 million per year.

What does this practice say about the state of health care in the United States?

Billing, reimbursement, and collections are sensitive areas for many clients and health-care professionals. The best way to manage finances within a clinic is to have set policies and procedures in place within a compliance plan and to be sure that both clients and employees understand those policies. Policies and procedures related to finances that are both legal and client-oriented will lead to client and employee satisfaction. A major task within a clinic is the appropriate billing and collecting for services performed. It is also a major concern for clients who may not seek medical attention if they feel they cannot afford to pay.

 ## COMPLIANCE PLAN

Compliance plans (see Chapter 5, Professional Liability) are an excellent way to avoid litigation and to help prevent problems from arising in the delivery of health care. When a compliance plan for billing and reimbursement is in place and used appropriately, areas of concern will be noted that the accounts manager (the compliance officer for a billing and reimbursement plan) can correct before they become a major problem. When an insurance carrier audits a clinic's activities in the billing area, it looks for intentional fraud. With a written compliance plan and proof that the compliance plan has been adhered to, a clinic can show that it is making a good faith effort to avoid fraud. This action will work in the clinic's favor.

 ## HOW PROVIDERS ARE PAID

The medical reimbursement system in the United States will change with the passage of the Health-care Reform Bill of 2010. This bill, passed in 2010, is still meeting opposition and likely will face a number of changes throughout its progression toward its goal to reform the health-care system. Some responsibility for that reform may shift to the states, with Utah and Massachusetts leading the way, in the ongoing efforts to insure all residents. The ultimate goal of this health-care reform is for all Americans to have health insurance. For the purposes of this book, we will explore the current reimbursement system.

Health-care providers will receive reimbursement for their services from many different sources. Successful practice management, billing, and collections require knowledgeable personnel who understand the complex characteristics of how reimbursement is made.

Recall from Chapter 2, Medical Practice Management, that 70 years ago, clients expected to pay physicians the full fee for services at the time they were rendered. Out of courtesy, some physicians would send a statement at the end of the month. Insurance of any kind was rare. Today, providers receive reimbursement in any number of ways. Payment may be made by (1) funds received through a client's insurance plan, probably receiving only a percentage of allowable charges; (2) a set fee for a client's services in a capitation arrangement regardless of the costs; (3) funds from a client in the form of cash, check, or credit or debit card; (4) a bonus if providers perform well in giving service across a spectrum of quality measures in a pay-for-performance (P4P) method; or (5) funds from an automatic-payment program in which clients permit an insurance carrier to make payroll deductions for their medical expenses.

PRIVATE PAY

Private pay may come from clients who have no work-related medical insurance, have insufficient medical insurance, or do not qualify for government health-care coverage. These clients may be working only part-time, never having enough working hours to qualify for insurance benefits, or they may choose a medical service that is not covered by insurance. Payment is usually made at the time of service unless other arrangements are made.

THIRD PARTY PAYERS

Usual, customary, and reasonable fee (UCR) describes how providers are reimbursed for their services from third party payers.

- The usual fee is a provider's average fee for a service or what is usually charged for a procedure.

- The customary fee is the average of fees within a particular geographic area for a described service or procedure and performed by the same kind of provider.
- The reasonable fee is what is normally acceptable for services that are unusually difficult or complicated.

The UCR is widely accepted across the country by insurance carriers and provides a basis for reimbursement to providers. Diagnostic (ICD-9), procedural (CPT), and DRG code sets also help determine the amount of reimbursement by a third party payer.

Insurance funds for medical expenses may come from more than one source:

- *Individual policies* are a kind of personal insurance in which clients often must submit to a physical examination and give a detailed medical history to qualify. Premiums are generally expensive, and benefits may be less than with other plans.
- *Group policies* are designed for a group of individuals covered under a master contract issued to their employer. Both employers and employees pay a percentage of the premiums. Deductions may be made from salaries to help pay the costs of group plans. Premiums are less costly than individual policies, and benefits are greater. A physical examination is not normally required.

Government plans include the following:

- TRICARE (Formerly known as Civilian Health, and Medical Program of the Uniformed Services [CHAMPUS]). This program was formed in 1956 to provide medical treatment to authorized dependents of military personnel and has been known as TRICARE since 1994. TRICARE covers active-duty personnel and their families and military retirees and their families; former spouses are covered if they have not remarried; and children, if unmarried, continue to be covered. The program is managed by the military in concert with civilian hospitals and clinics. The Civilian Health and Medical Program of the Department of Veterans Affairs (CHAMPVA) was formed in 1973 to provide benefits to veterans and their dependents.
- *Medicaid,* in 1965, made agreements with states to provide health care to the medically indigent. The federal government provides funds to the states that, in turn, decide how to use those funds in providing medical care. Thus, Medicaid is funded by both the federal and state governments. Medicaid also covers certain individuals receiving federal and state aid, persons who receive supplemental Social Security payments, recipients of Aid to Families with Dependent Children. Medicaid pays Medicare premiums for some low-income elderly persons and provides COBRA coverage for low-income persons who lose employer health insurance benefits. In most states, a provider must accept the Medicaid payment as payment in full. The client cannot be billed for any remaining balance.
- *Medicare* is a federal insurance program established in 1966 for people ages 65 years and older, for individuals who are blind or disabled, and for people on kidney dialysis or who have had a kidney transplant. There are several parts to this plan: Part A is hospital insurance and is mandatory for all individuals who receive Social Security. Premiums are paid from the client's monthly social security check. Part B is medical insurance that will help to cover ambulatory care and requires a larger monthly premium. Part C, now known as Medicare Advantage, offers HMO plans to augment Medicare payments. This part also requires additional premiums. Part D provides everyone with Medicare access to prescription drug coverage with a range of different plans, all requiring a premium to be paid by recipients. Only part A is mandatory; the others are optional additions to the Medicare coverage. Medicare is what is known as an 80/20 plan. Medicare will pay 80% of the allowed amount for a service, and the client is responsible for the other 20% unless the client has Medicare Advantage or another supplemental plan, in which case the HMO will cover most of the remaining charges.
- *Workers' compensation* programs were established in all states to cover the cost of medical care resulting from accident or illness related to a person's employment. Loss of income benefits is also included. The provider of services must accept the workers' compensation as payment in full and cannot bill the client.

- *The Health Maintenance Organization Act of 1973* defined the characteristics of managed care. Managed care insurance plans attempt to reduce costs by limiting where and from whom clients can receive medical services. Some plans limit any type of specialty care. Managed care plans provide health care within a network of providers for a predetermined and set fee.

In some instances, a client may have more than one health insurance plan. Through coordination of benefits, an agreement is made between insurance carriers that if a client has two insurance plans, neither the provider nor the subscriber will receive more than 100% of the covered charges.

OTHER PAYERS

Providers may receive reimbursement by other methods as well. Clients who have long-term care insurance may be able to use a portion of those benefits to pay medical bills, especially if they have a life-threatening illness. Some life insurance policies allow clients to draw from the policy benefit to pay medical indebtedness. Disability insurance, whether or not work related, can be used to pay for related medical expenses. Medical savings (or spending) accounts (MSAs) provide a method for companies with 50 or fewer employees, self-employed persons, and the uninsured to purchase medical insurance by making tax-free deposits to an MSA. Clients can use the funds in their MSA to pay for routine medical expenses. Any money in the account at the end of the year earns tax-free interest. Some states will have similar accounts for state employees. In Massachusetts a client contributes only the dollar amount that will be used in 1 year. Unlike the MSA, at the end of the year, all money that has not been used by the client in this state plan is removed from the account by the state and not returned to the employee.

The complexity of medical reimbursement has created a bookkeeping and accounting nightmare for health-care providers. The most successful facilities in the arena of reimbursement likely have at least one individual, or several individuals in a large clinic, whose sole responsibility is payment and collections. They have computerized their billing and spend several hours weekly in appealing denied insurance claims.

 ## CLIENTS' RESPONSIBILITY FOR REIMBURSEMENT

With or without the involvement of an insurance plan for health-care costs, clients are still responsible for the payment of their medical bills. There are a number of guidelines to keep in mind related to client reimbursement, some of which may be a part of the compliance plan. They include, but are not limited to, the following:

- If there is no insurance, expect payment at the time of service, and offer installment payments if necessary.
- Request payment for any coinsurance, deductibles, or exclusions at the time of service. Offer debit or credit card payment for services provided. Remember that you cannot charge clients the fees the facility pays for the use of debit or credit cards.
- Help clients understand their medical services and how much they cost.
- Clearly identify what clients are expected to pay and when. You cannot expect payment up front if clients have not been provided this information.
- Expect to explain to clients at least the basic principles of insurance reimbursement according to their individual plan.
- Never bill for a service that is not clearly identified and appropriately charted.
- Carefully adhere to all laws pertaining to reimbursement and collections.
- Establish a reimbursement and collection policy and then follow a compliance plan with regard to billing, reimbursement, and collections.
- Treat all clients equitably and fairly.
- If clients are to be denied services because of inability to pay, offer and discuss alternatives.

However billing and collection is accomplished, there are numerous legal aspects to consider. A brief presentation of applicable laws for reimbursement and collections is given. Ethical concerns are addressed later in this chapter.

LAWS FOR REIMBURSEMENT AND COLLECTIONS

TRUTH IN LENDING ACT

Regulation Z of the Consumer Protection Act of 1968 is also known as the Truth in Lending Act. This act is enforced by the Federal Trade Commission and, when applied to the health-care setting, deals with collection of clients' payments.

Briefly, the regulation requires that an agreement by providers and their clients for payment of medical bills in more than four installments must be in writing and must provide information regarding finance charges. Even if no finance charge is involved, the agreement must be in writing and stipulate no finance charge.

If consumers decide to pay their bills by installments unilaterally with no established agreement with providers, Regulation Z is not applicable as long as the provider continues to bill for the full amount.

Situations in which the Truth in Lending Act is often used include arrangements for surgery, prenatal or delivery care for fee-for-service plans, or other medical services not covered by insurance. The amount owed by the client is often more than a client can pay in one installment or is more than is covered by medical insurance. Health-care employees then can discuss with the client appropriate installment payments, put the agreement in writing, and provide a copy for the client. Few providers will charge a finance fee in this situation, although to do so is both legal and ethical. If bilateral installment agreements are common or if computer billing automatically includes a finance charge after a certain period, the wording should be approved by a legal representative.

Truth in Lending Consumer Credit Loss Disclosure is similar to the Truth in Lending Act but goes a step further. It requires providers to disclose all additional costs, such as interest and late charges, and to include them on the billing statement.

EQUAL CREDIT OPPORTUNITY ACT

The Equal Credit Opportunity Act ensures that all consumers are given an equal chance to obtain credit so that when providers extend credit for one client, all clients must be offered the same opportunity. Providers may deny credit to clients based on their inability to pay and inform their clients that credit has been denied. Clients then have 60 days to request the rationale for the denial in writing.

FAIR CREDIT BILLING ACT

The Fair Credit Billing Act states that clients have 60 days to complain about any error in their billing. The health-care employee must document, acknowledge the complaint, and respond within 90 days to the complaint. The response may be to correct any error or to explain to the client why the bill was accurate.

FAIR DEBT COLLECTIONS PRACTICES ACT

The Fair Debt Collections Practices Act, a federal law governed by the Federal Trade Commission, addresses the communication that occurs when collecting debts in the manner a collections agency might. According to the law, its purpose is to eliminate abusive debt collection practices by debt collectors, to ensure that those debt collectors who refrain from using abusive debt collection practices are not competitively disadvantaged, and to promote consistent state action to protect consumers against debt collection abuses. This act is discussed in detail later in the chapter.

FEDERAL WAGE GARNISHING LAW

Garnishment of salary is one method that can be used to collect a fairly large delinquent account. The Federal Wage Garnishing Law addresses payment of debts using employee salaries. Garnishment means to attach a person's property or wages by court order to pay debts. The law limits the amount of money that can be garnished and protects an employee from being dismissed because of garnishment.

Federal employees, however, are exempt from this law. Some state laws may differ from the federal law, so it is best for the health-care professional to contact either the Department of Labor or legal counsel for clarification.

TAX EQUITY FISCAL RESPONSIBILITY ACT

The Tax Equity Fiscal Responsibility Act is a federal law that addresses hospitalization payments for Medicare. It specifies provisions relating to savings in health and income security programs. This includes changes in payment for services, benefits, and premiums of Medicare as well as changes in provisions under Medicaid and other specific programs covered by Social Security.

The prospective payment system using diagnosis-related groups (DRGs) reimburses hospitals on a lump sum rather than a fee-for-service basis. DRGs classify clients who are medically related according to diagnosis, treatment, and length of hospital stay. The *International Classification of Diseases, 9th revision, Clinical Modification* (ICD-9-CM) identifies the diagnostic categories, specific DRG numbers, and relative values. The relative value is how U.S. hospitals and providers are reimbursed unless there are extenuating circumstances. The role of the health professional is important in this type of reimbursement because the initial hospitalization diagnosis generally comes from the admitting provider who is in ambulatory care. In 2013, the 10th revision of the ICD will be released. It will be more specific than the 9th version. Reimbursement will be affected, but to what degree has yet to be determined.

STARK I, II, AND III REGULATIONS

Stark I and II Regulations prohibit a physician or provider from referring a Medicare client for services to an entity with which the provider or an immediate family member has a financial relationship through ownership or compensation, unless the referral is protected by one or more exceptions provided in the law. The third phase of the Stark Law went into effect in 2007. It further specified and clarified the rules for referrals. More information on all three phases of the Stark Law can be found at the Web site of the American Academy of Family Practice: **http://aafp.org.**

DEFICIT REDUCTION ACT

The Deficit Reduction Act was enacted in 1984 and revised in 2005. It addresses Medicare reimbursement by increasing provider service payment rates. In 2005 it brought an increase to the reimbursement rates. In ensuing years, the health professional has seen continuing adjustments in Medicare rates. Unfortunately for the providers, the Medicare rate has dropped, with the biggest change occurring in January 2010 whereby Medicare no longer pays for consultations. This area will bear watching because constant changes are taking place.

CIVIL MONETARY PENALTIES ACT

The Civil Monetary Penalties Act addresses Medicare and Medicaid fraud and provides for prosecution in such cases. Physicians or providers who falsely bill clients' services or incorrectly code services can be liable for their acts under this regulation. Hence, health-care employees must be current in Medicare and Medicaid policies and be honest in their coding and billing procedures.

ENFORCEMENT OF THE LAWS

The Department of Justice and the Department of Health and Human Services (DOJ-HHS) have joined together to form the DOJ-HHS Medicare Fraud Strike Force. It is a multiagency team of federal, state, and local investigators designed to combat Medicare fraud through the use of Medicare data analysis techniques and an increased focus on community policing. The Medicare Fraud Strike Force has now moved to television with a commercial blitz urging senior citizens to protect their cards and numbers and report any suspicious charges to their Medicare accounts. They continue to police Medicare billling and its abuses.

> **IN THE NEWS**
> In July 2010, according to the Department of Justice's New Releases, the Medicare Fraud Strike Force brought charges against 94 doctors, health-care company owners, executives, and others for billing Medicare for more than $251 million in alleged false billing.
>
> According to the court documents, the defendants charged participated in schemes to submit claims to Medicare for treatments that were medically unnecessary and, often, never provided. In many cases, indictments and complaints alleged that beneficiaries accepted cash kickbacks in return for allowing providers to submit forms saying they had received the treatments that were unnecessary or never provided. These sting strikes took place in Miami, New York, Baton Rouge, and Detroit.

COLLECTION GUIDELINES

Collection procedures may be necessary to obtain full payment of services provided to clients. Collection procedures must be firm but temperate enough not to irritate otherwise satisfied consumers who intend to pay. If they feel comfortable doing so, providers should not hesitate to discuss directly with consumers the fees for their services. Many times, a client more readily accepts a statement of fees from a doctor than from an employee.

Medical managers must establish an appropriate collection policy for employees to follow (Fig. 10-1). Clients need to be informed in writing of the policy. That policy should state how insurance claims are managed. Will the clinic file claims for all insurance carriers, or only a certain few? Does the client in a managed care plan ever receive a bill; if so, under what circumstances? The policy should state how and when co-payments and deductibles are collected. The policy will detail whether and at what point collection letters will be sent. Will there be a minimum payment schedule? Will the collection letter be different for every account? Are collection telephone calls to be made; if so, by whom? How many? When? What procedures will be followed? Will delinquent accounts ever be turned over to a collection agency or pursued through the local courts? A clearly defined or stated policy gives employees the support necessary for successful collections.

It is important to build a professional and cooperative relationship with insurers to prevent billing problems and delayed or inaccurate reimbursements. Medical personnel should meet periodically with insurance representatives to learn their rules and billing processes. When specific problems arise, discuss with the representatives and pose possible solutions. Gather and analyze these computerized payment records and identify those insurers who are chronically late with payments. Use these data with the insurer to negotiate a better reimbursement time line. Clinics have a right to reimbursement within 90 days on accurately submitted bills.

Establishing a good procedure for collecting fees can eliminate headaches later.

- Establish fees
- Discuss fees
- Have a written fee policy
- Expect payment at time of service
- Provide a brochure describing fee policy
- Ask for payment before client leaves the office
- Provide a stamped, addressed envelope for payment
- Provide accurate, itemized statements
- Have a follow-up policy
- Have a collection policy

Figure 10-1. Collecting fees.

COLLECTION DO'S

The following guidelines are provided to suggest possible procedures for collections in the health-care setting, quite possibly identified in the compliance plan:

- Discuss fees with clients the first time they present themselves or call for treatment. A written payment policy is essential. Explain to consumers their responsibilities in a managed care plan.
- Provide clients with a clinic brochure that gives them information about hours, emergency contacts, the providers' services, how billing is managed, and whom to call if there is a question about a bill. Identify the insurances accepted by the providers.
- Provide an opportunity for the client to pay before leaving the clinic. The charge slip or encounter form is an ideal way for the provider to indicate charges and services as well as the diagnoses. The bill is then presented to the client, who is asked to stop at the bookkeeper's desk on the way out. The bookkeeper can say, "Mrs. Lotta M. Bucks, your charge today is $165. Would you like to pay by cash, check, debit card, or credit card?" Some clinics have been successful in providing clients with a stamped, addressed envelope in which to mail the fee when they return home or are billed at the end of the month.
- Have an established practice for mailing statements, and follow that practice. Statements should be itemized, accurate, and easy to understand. Make sure all credits have been posted up to the closing date. Statements should be mailed to arrive the first of the month. Statements that include envelopes, especially colored ones, are paid faster.
- When your collection policy dictates that an unpaid bill should be followed with a letter or a telephone call, do it. Be consistent, pleasant, and firm. The sooner you follow through on a delinquent account, the more likely it will be collected.
- Employees responsible for collections should have certain phrases and the wording of possible letters at their fingertips for quick and easy referral. They also need the authority to carry the collection process to its completion.
- Suggested procedures for mail or telephone collections include the following: (1) Introduce yourself. (2) Establish that you are speaking to the proper person, if it is a telephone call, or address the letter to the proper person. (3) State the reason for the call or the letter. ("Your account is past due.") (4) Be pleasant, but be firm. ("You are generally prompt with your payments; we wondered if this has been overlooked.") (5) Get a commitment. Make it specific. ("May we expect $150 from you by next Monday?") Then mark that commitment in your tickler file and follow up next Monday if there has been no response. (6) End the contact graciously. Do not get pulled into all the financial problems of the client. (7) Be prepared to offer a payment plan that is suitable to both the client and the clinic.
- Have a clearly established practice of when, if ever, to turn the account over to a collection agency or to collect the balance due in small claims court.

 COLLECTION DON'TS

The Fair Debt Collection Practices Act is a federal law that governs the actions of parties acting as debt collectors for personal debts. The Federal Trade Commission has specific regulations for debt collection. They include the following:

- Do not misrepresent who you are or why you are contacting a person.
- Do not send postcards; rather, mail a collection letter.
- Do not use deception in any form in your contact.
- Do not telephone at odd hours or make repeated calls or calls to the debtor's friends, relatives, neighbors, employers, or children. Acceptable hours to call are 8 a.m. to 9 p.m.
- Do not use obscene, profane, or abusive language.

- Do not make calls or send letters demanding payment for amounts not owed.
- If a contact must be made to the debtor's place of business, do not reveal to a third party the reason for the contact. All calls to a workplace must be stopped if so requested (written or verbal) by the client. The client's privacy and reputation must be protected.

If your clinic denies credit to a client on the basis of an adverse credit report from a credit bureau or similar agency, you must tell the client the name and address of the agency providing the information, even if you are not asked. Failure to do so could result in legal action. Let clients know that it is their right to obtain a copy of their credit report to see if all the information is correct. A form letter should be available in your clinic that courteously informs the client that credit has been denied, leaving blanks for the name and address of the agency that supplied the credit information. Mail a copy to the client and keep a copy for your records.

 ## COLLECTION PROBLEMS

An up-front, matter-of-fact approach to collections will increase the cash flow in the health-care setting and make collections easier for everyone. However, every clinic has slow payers, hardship cases, skips, and a few who never intend to pay. Move slow payers to a cash basis as soon and as often as possible and yet maintain good public relations.

Hardship cases pose another problem. Anyone might have a time when the payment of a medical bill is nearly impossible. Care must be taken to be understanding at all times. Try to work out payment plans with the clients so that they, too, are able to take pride in themselves and their ability to pay. Social agencies may be suggested if necessary.

There will always be a small percentage of clients who never intend to pay their bills. Some of these individuals leave the area, "skipping" out on their financial responsibilities. All possible resources should be exhausted to find the skips and to seek reimbursement. If the client has not skipped but still does not intend to pay, consider taking action in small claims court. Providers often withdraw themselves formally from these cases and encourage the clients to seek treatment elsewhere.

Chapter 6, Law for Health Professionals, gives information about the procedures to follow for collecting a bill from the estate of a client who has died. Chapter 6 also provides an explanation of the steps to follow for taking a client to small claims court. Both of these situations are fairly uncomplicated and will produce results worth the effort if employees are consistent and conscientious in these dealings.

Another problem can occur in reimbursement when insurance claims are denied for one reason or another. Successful medical practice management suggests that spending a couple of hours a week appealing denied claims is well worth the effort.

Case Study

Jenna works as an insurance biller for a large clinic. She delays calling the responsible party of a large family whose members are clients of the clinic because she knows she will become involved in a complex "hard luck" story that probably is true.

What are Jenna's options in this case? Will the delay cause more problems? Discuss.

 ## COLLECTION AGENCIES

If you have diligently followed billing and collection procedures and come to the conclusion that the client is not going to pay, you can refer the account to a collection agency. Obviously, this decision must be consistent with clinic policy. Collection agencies generally are employed as a last resort. Most people, including clients and those who work in clinics, tend to have a negative attitude toward collection agencies. However, the agency can be valuable to those who choose to use such professional services.

Selection of an appropriate agency should be made as carefully as one would choose a bank. Considerations should include the following:

1. Does it handle medical and dental accounts exclusively?
2. What methods does it use to collect?
3. What is the agency's financial responsibility?
4. What percentage will the medical clinic receive?
5. How promptly does it settle accounts?
6. Does the agency have a good bank reference?
7. How much cost versus goodwill will the clinic incur by using this agency?
8. Will it provide you with a list of satisfied customers or references?
9. Will you have the ability to end the agency's collection efforts?

Check with the Better Business Bureau or the local medical association for possible recommendations. An agency that is a member of the American Association of Credit and Collections Professionals will generally adhere to high ethical standards.

Once the agency is selected, all delinquent accounts are turned over to it, including any useful nonclinical data. A record should be kept of accounts given to the agency, as well as a running account of the agency's progress. Any contact with the client regarding these bills, whether in person, by phone, or by letter, must cease once the account has been turned over to the collection agency. If the client sends payment to the clinic, report it immediately to the agency. If the client calls regarding the account, courteously refer the client to the agency.

The collection agency represents the clinic. Employees should work with the agency to collect the accounts.

REIMBURSEMENT ATTITUDES

Reimbursement for providers in the health-care setting is in constant transition. Although a large portion of today's society is covered by some form of health plan, many in managed care, a number of clients are covered by no plan at all. Often these clients will not seek health care or will request detailed information about your clinic's billing practices. Payment plans may need to be established. Also, providers serving in any number of managed care plans will find some plans struggling to find a better method of curbing health-care costs. Medicare is constantly being explored to lower reimbursement rates to providers. As of January 2010, Medicare no longer covers consultations, causing many specialists to opt out of caring for Medicare clients.

Regardless of the reimbursement plan, financial status has no bearing on the kind of treatment clients should receive. The Medicare or Medicaid client should receive the same care as the client who pays cash. Providers and employees need to be careful of their attitudes toward those clients who have difficulty paying their bills, for whatever reason. Actions often speak louder than words, and clients easily perceive their true meanings.

ETHICAL IMPLICATIONS

ETHICS CHECK

Reimbursement and collection issues bring to the forefront ethical implications for discussion. Consider the following questions. None has a simple or easy answer.

• Is health care a right or privilege?
• Should providers be able to deny care to anyone?

- What is the driving force behind increasing costs of medical care?
- Who pays for medical insurance and why is it so costly?
- What is the role of government in providing health care, if any?
- Who controls client health care—the client, the insurance carrier, the primary care provider, or the government? ●

Ethics in medicine has received attention with regard to the recent Medicare changes. As mentioned previously, Medicare no longer pays for consultations, forcing the specialists to charge Evaluation and Management (E&M) codes (from the CPT-4 manual) for visits. These codes receive much lower reimbursement than the consultation codes. This has been done by Medicare as a cost-saving measure. As a result, some specialists refuse to see Medicare clients. Where will this leave our elderly population? Can this be perceived as discrimination? Will specialists be sacrificing their financial security and their reputation in the long run? This is an area that should be watched carefully. Many insurance carriers usually follow behind Medicare in making policy changes. If all insurance carriers refuse to pay for consultations, how will a specialist be paid? Will specialists now refuse to see anyone with Medicare insurance? As health-care professionals, watch these areas closely because they will affect your clinic and how your clients are referred.

Case Study

Often, employees in health care believe they have more client contact when performing clinical procedures. After reading and understanding the complexity of this chapter, discuss the importance of client contact when helping clients understand reimbursement.

SUMMARY

Providers and health-care professionals receive payment for their services through numerous means. There are more than 100 different insurance plans to cover clients' costs. The complexity of reimbursement challenges both the health professional and the client. Education is paramount for the client; however, there also are numerous laws related to reimbursement and collections that health-care professionals must understand.

 Watch It Now! Can you be successful in collections? at http://davisplus.fadavis.com/lawandethics

Questions for Review

SELECT THE BEST ANSWER

1. The _____ prohibits a provider from referring Medicare clients for services to a laboratory in which the provider has a financial interest.
   a. Truth in Lending Act
   b. Equal Credit Opportunity Act
   c. Deficit Reduction Act
   d. Stark Laws
   e. None of the above

2. This regulation requires that any payment plan that is for more than four installments must be in writing.
   a. Truth in Lending Act
   b. Equal Credit Opportunity Act
   c. Deficit Reduction Act
   d. Stark Laws
   e. None of the above

3. A CPT manual contains which of the following information?
   a. Diagnostic codes
   b. Procedure codes
   c. HCPCS codes
   d. Only a and b above
   e. None of the above

4. Co-payments should be paid
   a. Within 30 days of the visit.
   b. At the time of service.
   c. After the insurance carrier has paid its portion.
   d. Never, because the provider gets enough money from the insurance carrier.
   e. None of the above.

5. A provider may receive reimbursement in which of the following ways?
   a. By a client
   b. By an insurance carrier
   c. As a bonus
   d. All of the above
   e. None of the above

TRUE OR FALSE

T   F   1. Clients are responsible only for the copayment portion of their bill.

T   F   2. A compliance plan can help prevent charges of fraud.

T   F   3. Once a visit has been denied by an insurance carrier, the provider has no other options for payment.

T   F   4. A health-care professional may need to help a client understand his or her insurance policy.

T   F   5. A procedure that is not clearly identified and appropriately documented cannot be billed.

CLASSROOM EXERCISES

1. As a newly employed medical clinic manager, you discover that one of the providers in the clinic does not follow the written collections policies and is more lenient about clients paying their bills. What problem does this create for you and the other providers?

2. A provider overhears the receptionist say to a client, "Well, you know, we can take only so many welfare clients." How can the client now be put at ease?

3. Correct the following telephone conversation:

BOOKKEEPER (BK):	"Hi, this is Dr. Erythro's office. Who's this?"
CLIENT (CL):	"This is Laura Phagocyte."
BK:	"You owe us $46.25. Can you pay us $10 today?"

CL:	"Yeah, I'll put it in the mail."
BK:	"Will it be check or money order?"
CL:	"Check."
BK:	"Fine, I'll expect it in a few days. Thank you. Good-bye."

4. You are a bookkeeper for a very busy two-provider clinic. Managing client accounts that are covered under a myriad of insurance plans providing differing reimbursement rates is taking an increasing amount of time and energy. The providers have already determined not to take any more Medicare or Medicaid clients and are discussing dropping other insurance plans. What are the legal and ethical implications?

5. You have been asked to do the collection calls in your large medical clinic. Although you work in insurance coding and billing, you are not sure you have the skills to do so. This assignment will also include appealing denied insurance claims. What must you do to be prepared and to be successful?

INTERNET ACTIVITIES

1. Go to the CMS Web site and check the "Compliance Timelines" for implementation and testing dates for both ICD-10 and Version 5010.

WEB RESOURCES

Centers for Medicare and Medicaid Services: Deficit Reduction Act of 2005.
www.cms.gov/deficitreductionact/

Debt Collection Laws and Publications by State.
www.privacyrights.org/fs/fs27plus.htm#Georgia

Medicare.
www.medicare.gov

Medical Group Management Association.
www.mgma.com

Medical News Today, Medical Malpractice/Litigation News.
www.medicalnewstoday.com

Stark Law Overviews
Phase I: www.aafp.org/fpm/2003/1100/p27.html
Phase II: www.aafp.org/fpm/2004/0200/p41.html
Phase III: www.aafp.org/fpm/2008/0300/p25.html

 DavisPlus | For additional resources please visit
http://davisplus.fadavis.com

CHAPTER 11

Employment Practices

"To be successful, the first thing to do is fall in love with your work."—Sister Mary Lauretta; American nun and science teacher

KEY TERMS

Americans With Disabilities Act (ADA) Prohibits discrimination of individuals with physical or mental disabilities from accessing public services and employment.

Family Medical Leave Act (FMLA) Requires public employers and private employers of 50 or more employees to provide up to 12 weeks of job-protected unpaid leave for such family-related issues as birth or adoption, care of a seriously ill family member, or serious illness of employee.

Occupational Safety and Health Act (OSH Act) A 1970 act with the goal to ensure a safe and healthy workplace environment; a division of the U.S. Department of Labor. Important components identified below:

    Bloodborne Pathogen Standard Requires the use of engineering and work practice controls to eliminate or minimize employee exposure to bloodborne pathogens from needlestick injuries and other sharps-related injuries.

    Chemical hygiene plan (CHP) Regulation that addresses training, information requirements, and provisions to be implemented for chemical exposure in the ambulatory health-care setting.

    Protecting America's Worker Act Updates OSH Act to protect all state and local public employees, federal workers, and millions of other workers inadequately covered by other laws; increased civil and criminal penalties for job safety violations.

Quid pro quo The plan to get something of value in return for giving something of value.

LEARNING OUTCOMES

Upon successful completion of this chapter, you will be able to:

11.1 Define key terms.

11.2 Discuss the importance of policy manuals.

11.3 Describe the information in personnel policies.

11.4 Explain, in your own words, the importance of correct hiring practices.

11.5 List at least four necessary components of personnel policies.

11.6 Identify the three necessary elements of job descriptions.

11.7 Discuss clinic hours, workweek schedule, benefits, and salaries.

11.8 Explain where and how to locate prospective employees.

11.9 List eight techniques for effective interviews.
11.10 Identify five potential discrimination problems to consider when hiring.
11.11 Describe sexual harassment.
11.12 Explain the four parts of the Occupational Safety and Health Act.
11.13 Discuss the importance of the Americans With Disabilities Act for employer and employee.
11.14 Outline the Family Medical Leave Act and its use in the medical practice.
11.15 Recall procedures for selecting the right employee.
11.16 Recognize steps that encourage employee longevity.

COMPETENCIES

CAAHEP

- Identify personal safety precautions as established by the Occupational Safety and Health Administration (OSHA). (CAAHEP III.C.4)
- Identify how the American With Disabilities Act (ADA) applies to the medical assisting profession. (CAAHEP IX.C.11)
- List and discuss legal and illegal interview questions. (CAAHEP IX.C.12)
- Complete an incident report. (CAAHEP IX.P.6)

ABHES

- Define scope of practice for the medical assistant and comprehend the conditions for practice within the state that the medical assistant is employed. (ABHES 1.e)
- Perform the essential requirements for employment such as resume writing, effective interviewing, dressing professionally, and following up appropriately. (ABHES 11.a)

VIGNETTE

Must Amy Go?

Amy Porter, RMA, steps into the office of her manager at the Sheraton Medical Center to submit her resignation as the administrative MA. Amy has thoroughly enjoyed all their clients, being responsible for busy telephones, scheduling appointments, and helping clients with their insurance, but she has taken another position in a day-surgery center near the hospital. Jeff Lyon, CMAS, her clinic manager, is shocked about her decision. Amy has been with them only for 2 years, and he never dreamed she was looking for another position. Jeff asks, "Why would you leave after such a short time?" Amy hesitates a moment, but decides to tell Jeff. "I have been here this long without any kind of evaluation, no increase in salary even though my responsibilities have increased, and no opportunity for advancement or additional training. I can do nothing more for this position. I need a challenge, and the surgery center provides that for me. I will miss everyone, especially the clients, but it is time for me to go."

HIRING EMPLOYEES

Providers do not function alone in the health-care setting. Even providers who are just starting their practice hire an assistant as soon as possible. Selecting appropriate personnel is an important business task. As a practice grows, a clinic manager, in cooperation with the clinic providers, is usually the one responsible for hiring personnel. Current employees commonly are influential in the process of obtaining additional employees. Hiring and preparing employees to function in specific roles are both expensive and time-consuming tasks. Therefore, it is important to perform the tasks effectively the first time. For example, a new doctor arrives in a small town and hires a certified medical assistant (CMA) as a first-hire because the CMA can perform both administrative and clinical responsibilities in the clinic. In just a short time, the practice has grown and more staff is needed. The likely candidate to become the clinic manager to oversee the staff is the CMA who has been there from the beginning. It is important to understand, in some situations, that you might become a manager within a short time after being hired.

There are a number of important areas of consideration and tasks to perform before successful and effective hiring takes place. They include the following:

1. Creating a policy manual
2. Establishing personnel policies
3. Determining job descriptions for each position
4. Locating the best employee for the position
5. Conducting effective interviews
6. Selecting candidates to fulfill the practice's needs
7. Evaluating employees on a predetermined and regular basis
8. Keeping employees for the long term

POLICY AND PROCEDURE MANUAL

Policy manuals identify the policies of the practice. This manual sets the tone for the practice and expresses the philosophy of the providers regarding client care. Policy manuals will identify the scope of client services, providers' specialty areas, clinic hours and workweek schedule, insurances accepted and processed, and biographical and educational information about each provider and staff member. The biographical and educational information often becomes part of a clinic brochure that is made available for clients. Many brochures of this nature only identify the specifics of each provider. However, including background information about each staff member not only heightens the level of importance of each staff member, but it helps clients to identify those individuals with whom they have a great deal of contact during their care.

The policies should be updated from time to time to reflect any changes in the clinic, but they should always be in writing and available to employees. Computerizing the policy manual makes changes and updates quite easy to accomplish.

A *procedure manual* details (usually in steps) how to perform certain procedures, both in the administrative and clinical areas. It is much different from a policy manual but is equally important to a safe and efficient medical clinic.

PERSONNEL POLICIES

Personnel policies are established to identify and address concerns of employees and state the desires of management. Without established personnel policies, providers soon lose control of the management of their own practices when or if they begin to make decisions in an arbitrary and inconsistent manner. Larger clinics will have personnel policy manuals, often called employee handbooks. Smaller practices most likely include personnel policies in a separate location of the policy manual.

Personnel policies will identify workweek schedule and hours, salary and benefits, overtime reimbursement, sick leave and vacation policies, employee and client safety, employee conduct and discipline, and employee evaluation and salary review. A most critical personnel piece relates to total confidentiality of all client information. Figure 11-1 gives an example of a policy statement regarding a confidentiality and nondisclosure agreement that employees may be asked to sign. Such a document should be reviewed with employees yearly.

Before a person is hired, staff needs are to be determined and job descriptions written. Determine in advance if employees are to be generalists or specialists in their skills, or if employees with a combination of these skills will be more effective. It is important, too, to decide if employees will be cross-trained and, if so, for what specific positions.

CLINIC HOURS AND WORKWEEK SCHEDULE

Clinic hours and the workweek schedule are fairly easy to establish. Hours may be determined by the medical specialty and the dictates of the community. The long and often inconsistent hours of

CONFIDENTIALITY AND NONDISCLOSURE AGREEMENT

I, _____, do affirm that I will not divulge
_____[PRACTICE NAME]_____ DATA TO ANY UNAUTHORIZED PERSON FOR ANY REASON.
Neither will I directly use, or allow the use of, _____[PRACTICE NAME]_____ DATA for any
purpose other than that directly associated with my official assigned duties.
I understand ALL CLIENT INFORMATION, including financial data, is strictly confidential.

Furthermore, I will not, either by direct action or by counsel, discuss, recommend, or suggest to
any unauthorized person the nature or content of any _____[PRACTICE NAME]_____ information.

Violation of confidentiality is cause for disciplinary action, including immediate dismissal.

I understand that signing this document does not preclude me from reporting instances
of breach of confidentiality.

Signed _____ Date _____

Figure 11-1. Example of a confidentiality and nondisclosure agreement.

a medical practice should be addressed; for example, will every employee stay late, will hours be staggered, and will overtime be compensated? Will the workweek schedule be the same as or longer than clinic hours? How will a policy be established that provides for the needs of clients, is fair to employees, and allows all tasks to be performed?

Employees become unhappy if they are told upon hiring that the workweek schedule will be 40 hours and it turns out to be closer to 50 to 60 hours. Planning for overtime is essential. Being honest with employees is a must. Employees are expected to plan for their out-of-clinic responsibilities so that they do not interfere with their employment. Therefore, firm policies on overtime make accommodating for day care, family needs, and out-of-clinic responsibilities easier.

JOB DESCRIPTIONS

Job descriptions indicate minimum qualifications required, a description of the job to be performed, and to whom the employee is responsible. Job descriptions must be developed for each position in the clinic. These job descriptions are often shared with candidates at the time of interviews.

The established health-care clinic will find its employees to be the best resources when writing job descriptions by having the employees put in writing descriptions of the tasks they perform in a normal workday. This exercise becomes the basis for the job descriptions.

When developing a specific job description, education and training requirements must be included. Equally important, job descriptions should also contain any specific physical requirements necessary for the job. The frequency with which each physical requirement is used should be established. *Rarely, frequently,* and *regularly* are terms that may be used. For example, an application for a position in a sports medicine clinic might indicate: "Assistance with ambulation is regularly required." This practice helps ensure that the Americans With Disabilities Act (ADA) is followed and that the right employee is hired to do a specific job.

BENEFITS AND COMPENSATION

Benefits and compensation are of concern to both employees and employers. Providers will want to pay a salary that is commensurate with the responsibilities of the task to be performed and that reflects the education, training, credentialing, and experience of the employees. Another consideration can be the prevailing wage of the community. It is important to have a method of evaluating salaries yearly. Some tie salary to performance reviews; others review salaries at the end of each calendar year.

Often, benefits are as important to employees as salary. Benefits to consider include medical insurance, sick leave, vacations, holidays, retirement, and profit-sharing plans. Other incentives may include payment of approved educational courses, seminars, professional memberships, a uniform allowance, and possibly a gas allowance. An important benefit, especially in the city, may be free parking or bus passes.

An important consideration for vacation time often occurs when the provider is a sole proprietor. It may be preferable to have an assistant working to direct clients to another source for their care and to provide some catch-up time for administrative tasks such as billing and collecting while the provider vacations. Other clinics, however, will give staff members leave whenever the provider takes leave. The difficulty with this plan is that the provider's vacation leave may not be the best time for the assistant's vacation to occur. If the assistant's vacation period is different from that of the provider, a temporary MA can be hired. However the issue is resolved, it is important for an honest discussion that includes problem solving from both provider and staff to occur.

THE EMPLOYMENT PROCESS

LOCATING EMPLOYEES

A valuable resource for clinics seeking employees may be the county medical society. Some sponsor a medical employment agency. Schools in the community that have accredited education programs for MAs, medical secretaries, or other professionals often have names of graduates seeking employment. Social media is often used for job contacts.

Professional national organizations for MAs, such as the American Association of Medical Assistants and the American Medical Technologists Association, may have local chapters in geographic areas that are able to provide possible candidates for employment.

Other providers and their employees often know of potential candidates. Employment agencies specializing in medical and dental employment can be a resource. Newspaper advertising may also be successful but should specifically identify that a résumé be sent as the first step.

In an established medical practice, the initial screening of candidates is likely performed by a clinic manager or a specific person other than the provider.

INTERVIEWING CANDIDATES

With a printed job description and a list of possible candidates, the interview process can begin. The interview is a time to meet with each candidate personally. A job application is often completed at this point.

 Commonsense techniques to make the interview more effective and satisfy any legal concerns include the following steps for the interviewer to keep in mind:

1. Identify the purpose of the interview and describe the position being filled.
2. Avoid interruptions during the interview. Do not rush; however, it is prudent to inform the interviewee that you have a set amount of time for the interview.
3. Use effective communication skills and listen carefully to the candidate.
4. Match the candidate to the job. Look at the total qualifications of the candidate. Do not pick a clone similar to yourself. Look for diversity.
5. Observe nonverbal behavior.
6. Ask each candidate the same questions. This is important and makes the comparison of more than one candidate as fair and unbiased as possible (Fig. 11-2).
7. Remain objective.
8. Maintain control of the interview.
9. Present possible scenarios requiring a solution to help determine skill level and communication style.
10. End on a positive note; summarize, allow for questions from the candidate, and provide the candidate with a possible date for a decision.

Questions may include:
A. What are your qualifications?
B. Why are you leaving your present position?
C. When can you begin work?
D. What salary do you expect?
E. What do you expect to be doing in 1 year? In 5 years?
F. Why do you want to work here?
G. Do you foresee any difficulties that may prevent you from doing a good job?
H. What prompted you to become an employee in the medical field?
I. What is your major strength?
J. What is your major weakness?

Figure 11-2. Possible questions to ask potential employees.

Once the interview has ended, time should be taken to make notes that will serve as a reminder later when considering all the candidates. Inform applicants that you will be taking notes during the interview; otherwise, they may be concerned.

IN THE NEWS

The American Association of Medical Assistants (AAMA) predicts that medical assistant employment will grow 35% by the year 2016. This is a much faster rate than the average for all occupations. Much of the reason for this rapid growth is the increase demand for health-care services and the flexibility of the multiskilled medical assistant whose education and training are most appropriate for ambulatory health care.

SELECTING EMPLOYEES

After completion of the interview process, make a careful study of all candidates and their responses to your questions. If you have not already done so, read the employment applications and contact references. Contacting references is one task that 75% of employers do not do. Yet talking with former employers and individuals named as references is an important part of the decision-making process. Ask permission from any prospective employee before checking references or include a permission request on the job application form. Possible reference check questions follow:

1. Can you share information about this applicant?
2. Our applicant has listed a position with you as _____. Is this correct?
3. Does the applicant work best as a member of a team or alone?
4. Can you give an example of this applicant's exemplary performance?
5. How does the applicant perform under stress?
6. Would you rehire this person? Why or why not?
7. Would you recommend the applicant for this specific position?
8. Is there anything else we should know about this applicant?

How each candidate will function with other staff members is to be considered. If candidates have been asked to perform any skill functions, check the tests for accuracy. Candidates may be asked to do some keyboarding, take a spelling test (medical and nonmedical words), or perform a clinical function. Telephone candidates or ask them to call the clinic at a later time to screen their telephone personalities. The manner in which candidates handle the telephone is important because the client's first contact with the provider's clinic is often made via the telephone.

Once a decision is made, contact the chosen candidate to offer the position. Once the position has been filled, *all* candidates should be informed. This courtesy is often overlooked. Set a start date for employment and establish a probationary period for the new employee; 3 months is usually adequate time to determine whether the working relationship is a good one. At the end of this period, either employee or employer should be free to end the employment agreement. Salary paid during the probationary period may be less than that offered for permanent employment.

Case Study

An MA who is morbidly obese is interviewed for a position as a clinic assistant. The receptionist sarcastically comments to the clinic manager, "That's a good role model to have in a cardiologist's office."

What effect, if any, does the obesity of this candidate have on likelihood of being hired? What legal ramifications must be kept in mind?

EVALUATING EMPLOYEES

Evaluation of employees is an ongoing task throughout the individual's employment. Probably the biggest mistake in health-care employment is not making evaluation a formal process. A clearly established and written evaluation policy and form should be developed and carefully explained to employees, with a copy given to each. At regular intervals during the course of employment, evaluations should be conducted. New employees should be evaluated at 3 months, thus ending the probationary period. Another evaluation is conducted 6 months later. Thereafter, yearly evaluations on the date of original hire are conducted. If problems surface or an employee is assigned a new major responsibility, evaluations may change and increase in frequency. Strengths and weaknesses should be documented. The evaluation then becomes part of the employee's personnel file after it has been reviewed and discussed with the employee. Also, the employee and supervisor should both sign and date the document.

An adequate evaluation enables employees to improve job performance and serves as a tool for employers to discuss salary increases, provides background for any necessary dismissal, and establishes a record for future referral. Samples of employee evaluation forms may be available through the American Medical Association and resources provided by Medical Group Management Association. One is provided for you on Davis*Plus.*

Although the evaluation records may assist a manager in determining salary increases, a change in salary is best made at the end of each year and discussed with each employee. Salary changes and evaluations should be kept separate. Salary raises attached to evaluations tend to make the whole process a punitive one. When evaluations are separate from salary increases, the whole intent of the evaluation is to make the employee a better one, to praise what has been done well, and to challenge the employee to learn more. When salary raises are given at the end of the year, they encourage management to consider how well the business has done and what profits have been made. Also, less friction occurs among employees when personnel receive a percentage raise related to their base salary. Also, when the economy is in a slump and salary increases may not be possible, that statement to everyone at the end of the year is better than giving no raises at the time of performance evaluations. However, a wise manager recognizes the value of an excellent employee and will make the salary reimbursement or other benefits an encouragement for the employee to remain with the practice.

Case Study

In the vignette at the beginning of the chapter, identify steps that might have been taken by the clinic manager to prevent the resignation.

EMPLOYEE DISMISSAL

When evaluating employees, the decision may be made to dismiss an employee. Dismissal is a difficult, unpleasant situation, but steps must be taken to protect the clinic while minimizing the stress for the employee who is dismissed.

If the evaluation process has been effective, documentation exists in the employee's personnel file detailing the problem behaviors. The file should include dates the problems were discussed with the employee and specific actions discussed for correction of the problems. It is best to have the employee sign the documents to ensure that the employee has been informed and understands the problem areas and what specific actions are required for correction. Such written documentation will be essential should the terminated employee later seek litigation.

The employee's progress or lack of progress should be evident in the personnel file. Dismissal should take place during the probationary period if possible. Warnings (both verbal and written) to the employee help ward off surprise when dismissal is made. During the dismissal conference, it is best to be brief, to the point, and honest without degrading the employee.

There are likely three reasons requiring immediate dismissal of employment: (1) breach of client confidentiality, (2) disregard for client safety, and (3) fraudulent or criminal actions. The clinic's policy and/or personnel manual must clearly identify and define these reasons for immediate dismissal. Also, it may be best to take any dismissal action late on a Friday afternoon so that disruption is minimized and there is no opportunity for the employee to compromise the medical clinic. Larger clinics with a personnel department will also have the dismissed employee escorted from the building and will make sure to receive any keys, codes, or clinic property that the dismissed employee may have. Computer passcodes are immediately changed.

Managers can learn from the dismissal experience. Was the job description clear and accurate? Was the probationary period long enough? Was the evaluation process fair, clear, and well documented? How and when were the problem areas communicated to the employee? However unfortunate dismissal is to both the employee and employer, it is best to use good human relation skills, express empathy, and communicate clearly all expectations to employees. All matters regarding the dismissal are confidential.

WHEN EMPLOYEES CHOOSE TO LEAVE

There is any number of reasons for employees to leave a practice. They may find a better job, move, have a change in family responsibilities, or retire. An exit interview should be conducted. This is a time to gather specific information about closing the employment relationship. It is also a time for both employer and employee to evaluate the position and identify any potential changes. Some of the questions to ask of the employee who is leaving include the following:

1. What did you like best about your job?
2. What did you like least?
3. What would you change about your position?
4. Did you receive the support that you needed to do your job?
5. What would improve the workplace for someone in your position?
6. Did you receive the feedback you needed?
7. Was your supervisor's management style a key to your leaving?
8. Is there anything else you would like to comment on?

These questions can help to formulate any changes in the job description when seeking a replacement for the position.

RETAINING EMPLOYEES

Retaining employees is as important as selecting them. Salaries that are commensurate with work performance and the qualifications of employees are a must. Salary is not a place to try to cut clinic expense. The old adage "You get what you pay for" is especially true in employment. Replacing an employee can cost as much as three to four times a monthly salary.

As important to employees as an adequate salary is the assurance that their work is appreciated and is necessary for efficient functioning in the health-care setting. The simple "thank you" and "well done" are compliments that foster goodwill and motivate employees to greater effectiveness. Finding out what each staff member likes to do best and allowing him or her to perform that task will enhance employee satisfaction. Good employees merit trust and increased responsibilities. Encourage employees to improve their education and knowledge and provide incentives for them to do so.

If employees are to be corrected or disciplined, never do so in front of other employees or clients. Most will accept tactful criticism well. Few will forget if they are embarrassed before their peers or the clients. Remembering birthdays and employment anniversaries with simple gifts or cards takes little effort but does much for employee morale.

Employees in the health-care setting can make or break a medical clinic. It is a good idea to take the time and effort to ensure that the staff functions as a team to create an atmosphere conducive to good provider-client relationships.

Individuals involved in the hiring process must be knowledgeable of state and federal work and employment regulations. The U.S. Department of Labor, Wage, and Hour Division will answer questions regarding minimum wages, use of child labor, and length of workday. A state's human rights commission can answer questions on possible discrimination in the interview or hiring process. ●

Case Law

Naiel Nassar, MD, plaintiff, double-board-certified in internal medicine and infectious disease medicine, brought suit against University of Texas Southwestern Medical Center alleging that Dr. Beth Levine, Chief of Infectious Diseases Medicine, made numerous discriminatory comments about him and other physicians of various racial and religious backgrounds. Dr. Nassar is a Muslim and Egyptian native. Trial testimony showed that Dr. Levine delayed promoting Dr. Nassar based on his race and religious beliefs and then blocked his move to another position at Parkland Hospital by refusing to give a favorable recommendation and warning Parkland not to hire him.

Jurors found in favor of the plaintiff, Dr. Nassar, and awarded $3.6 million in damages.

Naiel Nassar, MD v University of Texas Southwestern Medical Center at Dallas. Civil Action No. 3:08-CV-1337-B, U. S. District Court, May 24, 2010.

Federal law states that an employer of 15 or more people must not discriminate on any form of application for employment. The discrimination includes age, sex, race, creed, marital status, national origin, color, or disabilities (sensory, mental, or physical). Many states have adopted laws that are more strict than federal law. For example, in the State of Washington, an employer of eight or more cannot discriminate. Massachusetts, however, goes several steps beyond the federal guidelines, stating that employers with six or more employees are prohibited from discriminating against employees based on race, color, religious creed, national origin, ancestry, sex, age, criminal record (applications only), handicap (disability), mental illness, retaliation, sexual harassment, sexual orientation, and genetics. In addition, employers in some states have an affirmative responsibility to provide maternity leave to biological and adoptive parents even though it is not mandated by federal law.

Nothing in either the federal or state discrimination laws is intended to prevent the employer from hiring only the most qualified person. Obviously, to protect this right, a well-written job description is essential, followed by impeccable attention to personnel issues. ●

Potential discrimination problem areas include the following:

- *Age*—Any inquiry implies a preference and is prohibited.
- *Marital status*—No inquiries are permitted.
- *Race or color*—No inquiry concerning race or color of skin, hair, eyes, and so forth is permitted.
- *Sex*—No inquiry is permitted.
- *Disabilities*—No inquiry is permitted if disabilities or health problems are not related to job performance. If the employer needs to take a special need or handicap into account in determining job placement or fitness to perform, an inquiry can be made.

Most laws permit employers to talk about the job, its duties, and its responsibilities but prohibit any questions unrelated to the job. For example, it is not job related to note that the applicant has children, but it is job related to note whether the applicant indicated problems getting to work or working overtime. Managers preparing for an interview who bring a structured outline of subjects to cover with all applicants and who treat the candidates alike in all respects will have greater success in the hiring process and will prevent legal repercussions.

Even though some health-care settings may not have 15, or even 6, employees, it is best to follow the state and federal requirements, not only for protection but also for ethical reasons and for good public relations. See Figure 11-3 for valid reasons for declining applicants.

FAMILY AND MEDICAL LEAVE ACT

Another law that may affect medical clinics is the Family and Medical Leave Act (FMLA) of 1993. The law applies to organizations with 50 or more employees and will most likely be seen in large medical centers, hospitals, and hospital-affiliated clinics. The act provides employees up to 12 weeks of job-protected and unpaid leave for family and medical reasons. The reasons include (1) birth and care of a child as well as adoption or care of a foster child; (2) care of an immediate family member who is seriously ill; and (3) care of an employee's own serious health condition. Employees must have been employed at least 12 months and worked at least 1250 hours during the 12 months before the FMLA leave begins.

SEXUAL HARASSMENT

Title VII of the Civil Rights Act of 1964 protects employees from sexual harassment that may occur on the job. The guidelines from the Office of Equal Employment Opportunities make the employer strictly liable for the acts of supervisory employees as well as for some acts of harassment by coworkers and clients of the company. A written policy on sexual harassment, detailing inappropriate behavior and stating specific steps to be taken to correct an inappropriate situation, should be established. Such a statement can be placed in the policy manual and referred to in personnel policies.

The traditional form of harassment is the scenario in which sexual favors are implicit and demanded of an employee by a supervisor in exchange for job advancement. This is known in legal terms as *quid pro quo,* which means "this for that." For example, the provider says to an employee, "You know, there's a hefty raise for you if you spend the weekend with me on my boat." A second, probably more common form of harassment, a hostile work environment, occurs when the work environment interferes with the employee's work performance. The conduct must be severe or pervasive and may take the form of a series of sexual questions, comments, jokes, inappropriate touching by coworkers, or verbal belittling

Valid reasons for declining employment applicants:

- There is a health problem that would preclude the applicant from safe and efficient job performance.
- Applicant is not available for the required work schedule for the particular job (observance of religious holidays not included).
- Applicant lacks sufficient skills, training, or experience to perform the required duties of the job.
- Another applicant is better qualified.

Figure 11-3. Valid reasons for declining employment applicants.

and teasing (refer to Case Law in Chapter 1). For example, a male MA is always making comments in the front office about "my girls," teasing them about premenstrual syndrome (PMS), and letting them know that they are inferior to men. When the harassment is commonplace and the supervisor or employer does not correct the situation, the employer and the clinic manager are liable under Title VII.

Generally, the easiest way to end harassment is to tell the harasser to stop the behavior. This works in some cases. Telling another colleague or threatening the harasser that you will tell another person is the second best tactic. Ignoring the offensive behavior does not work, and it is illegal not to take corrective action. If the harassment continues, employers must make it easy and safe for those being harassed to seek help, and the harassment must stop.

The policy on harassment should include at least the following:

1. A statement that sexual harassment of employees and a hostile work environment will not be tolerated.
2. A statement that an employee who feels harassed needs to bring the matter to the immediate attention of a person designated in the policy.
3. A statement about the confidentiality of any incidents and specific disciplinary action against the harasser.
4. The procedure to follow when harassment occurs. ●

OCCUPATIONAL SAFETY AND HEALTH ACT

Congress passed the Occupational Safety and Health Act (OSH Act) to prevent workplace disease and injuries. This statute applies to virtually every U.S. employer. The general purpose of the act is to require all employers to ensure employee safety and health.

Occupational Safety and Health Administration (OSHA) mandates that employers:

- Encourage employers and employees to reduce workplace hazards and to implement new and improved health programs.
- Establish "separate but dependent responsibilities and rights" for employers and employees for the achievement of better safety and health conditions.
- Maintain a record-keeping system to monitor job-related injuries and illnesses.
- Develop mandatory job safety and health standards and enforce them effectively.
- OSHA representatives may make unannounced visits to the workplace and may issue citations or penalties per violation to an employer who does not provide a safe environment.

Penalty rates changed in 2010. The maximum penalty for a serious violation had been only $7000 and for a willful violation was $70,000. The Protecting America's Worker Act raised these penalties to $12,000 and $250,000, respectively. The average penalty for a serious violation increased from an average amount of $1000 to an average of $3000 to $4000. Contained in the OSH Act are two regulations especially important in the health-care setting: the Bloodborne Pathogen Standard and the Occupational Exposure to Hazardous Chemicals Standard or the chemical hygiene plan (CHP).

The Bloodborne Pathogen Standard became effective in 1992. Its primary goal is to reduce occupational-related cases of HIV/AIDS and hepatitis B and C infections among health-care workers. The procedure or policy manual should carefully detail the following steps addressed in the Bloodborne Pathogen Standard and identify early updates and employee education:

1. Control and determination of exposure
2. Universal precautions
3. Hepatitis B virus vaccine
4. Postexposure follow-up
5. Labeling and disposal of biological wastes
6. Housekeeping and laundry functions
7. Employee training for safety and documentation

In 2001, in response to the Needlestick Safety and Prevention Act, OSHA revised the Bloodborne Pathogens Standard. The revised standard clarifies the need for employers to select safer needle devices and to involve employees in identifying and choosing these devices. The updated standard also requires employers to maintain a log of injuries from contaminated sharps.

The chemical hygiene plan addresses training, information requirements, and provisions that must be implemented for chemical exposure in the ambulatory health-care setting. Chemical inventories must be taken, a material safety data sheet (MSDS) manual has to be assembled, and employers are required to provide a hazard communication education program to employees within 30 days of hire.

The Occupational Exposure to Hazardous Chemicals Standard requires the following tasks to be performed by employers:

1. Inventory any and all hazardous chemicals regarding quantity, manufacturer's name, address, and chemical hazard classification.
2. Assemble MSDSs from manufacturers. The sheets should be kept in a manual and reviewed regularly. Label the chemicals using the National Fire Protection Association's color and number method.
3. Provide educational training to all employees who handle any hazardous chemicals within 30 days of employment and before an employee is allowed to handle the chemicals.
4. Develop and evaluate a chemical hygiene plan to address how to handle any spills or exposures.

For the safety of employees and all clients, carefully following and monitoring these regulations is essential. Job descriptions should identify any position that may cause exposure to hazardous chemicals, bloodborne pathogens, and needlesticks.

AMERICANS WITH DISABILITIES ACT

The Americans With Disabilities Act (ADA) was passed in Congress in 1990 to eliminate discrimination in employment against a qualified individual with a disability. The statute applies to all persons with substantial impairment that significantly limits a major function. This includes hearing, seeing, speaking, walking, breathing, performing manual tasks, caring for oneself, learning, and working. It also protects persons with a history of cancer in remission, persons with a history of mental illness, and persons with AIDS or who are HIV positive.

Also, ADA covers individuals with a drug addiction who are currently in a drug rehabilitation program or have successfully completed rehabilitation and have not used drugs illegally for some time. However, an employer may be able to dismiss or refuse to hire a person with a recent history of illegal drug use, even if the person no longer uses drugs, in such specific occupations as law enforcement or public transportation when an employer can show that this policy is job related and consistent with business necessity. This exemption may apply to a health-care setting if controlled substances are regularly kept in the facility. For the most part, however, except in the case of such health-care settings as surgery centers, pain clinics, and oncology centers, very few clinics keep controlled substances on site.

If an employee who has a disability meets all of the qualifications of the job, the employer must make "reasonable" accommodation for the disability. The employer is not required to make an accommodation that imposes "undue hardship" or requires an action with significant difficulty or expense. Reasonable accommodations might include the following:

• Handicap parking
• Ramps or elevators
• Electronic or easily opened doors
• Hallways with at least 36 inches of clearance
• Accessible bathroom and lunchroom facilities
• Reception counters low enough for a wheelchair (34 inches maximum)

For example, if the best qualified applicant for receptionist has permanent and serious facial scarring, the applicant cannot be denied the position simply because of the fear of negative reactions from others. A medical transcriptionist in a wheelchair should be hired if she or he is the best candidate for the job. In all probability, reasonable accommodation can be made for this individual.

Case Study

An MA comments to another employee confined to a wheelchair in the medical practice, "You know, when we first hired you, I was concerned. But you complement our practice more than any other employee we have ever had."

What does this case study say about bias and opinions?
Are there other professions that may hold the same issue?

The employment provisions of the ADA are enforced under the same policies of discrimination under Title VII. Remedies may include hiring, reinstatement, back pay, and the order to stop discrimination. Most employers with the foresight to hire persons with disabilities and to make the necessary accommodations have found that those employees are among the best.

SUMMARY

Outside of concern for appropriate client care, treatment, and comfort, one of the most important functions of the manager and provider will be hiring employees and keeping them. Legal implications of not having good hiring and employment practices and keeping good employees are far reaching and essential to the process.

State laws and regulations concerning employees must be considered. Some states regulate MAs or require certain certification to practice. Some states require a license, a registration, or a certification for certain special or invasive procedures that MAs perform. In employment practices, the smartest step that can be taken is to hire the best educated and credentialed individuals for the positions. Refer to Chapter 3, The Health-Care Team in the Ambulatory Setting, for further information on credentialing and education.

Watch It Now! Can you treat everyone fairly and without discrimination?
http://davisplus.fadavis.com/lawandethics

Questions for Review

SELECT THE BEST ANSWER

1. Employee evaluations
   a. Are the only way to determine salary increases.
   b. Are best performed by the providers.
   c. Establish a background for any necessary dismissal.
   d. Follow no established form or plan.
   e. Are completed biannually.

2. The OSH Act
   a. Is known as the Occupational Safety and Health Act.
   b. Includes the Bloodborne Pathogen Standard.
   c. Requires training to all employees handling any hazardous chemicals.
   d. All of the above.
   e. Only a and b above.

3. Job descriptions should indicate
   a. Minimum qualifications required for the job.
   b. A description of the job to be performed.
   c. To whom the employee is responsible.
   d. The salary scale.
   e. Only a, b, and c above.

4. In an employment interview
   a. Each candidate is asked the same questions.
   b. Salary is never discussed.
   c. Nonverbal behavior is less important than the application.
   d. The employment candidate is in charge.
   e. The telephone personality is checked.

5. The ADA covers individuals who
   a. Have substantial impairment that limits major function.
   b. Have AIDS or are HIV-positive.
   c. Are in recovery from drug addiction.
   d. May be discriminated against in employment.
   e. All of the above.

TRUE OR FALSE

T F   6. The policy manual describes how to perform each procedure.

T F   7. The best place to find potential employees is in newspaper ads.

T F   8. It is important to check references of potential employees.

T F   9. Breach of client confidentiality is a likely cause for immediate dismissal.

T F   10. No inquiry regarding age is permitted in the employment process.

CLASSROOM EXERCISES

1. In the case study about the morbidly obese candidate, identify the conversation that might be held between the clinic manager and the receptionist. Describe what might happen if the applicant overhears the conversation.

2. The provider says to the assistant in the hall, "I'm tired of telling you how to do things and having you mess it up during an exam. Pick up your check at the end of the week and don't come back." How could this situation be prevented by using wise employment practices? What are the implications of how this was handled?

3. Under what conditions might clinic hours and an employee's actual workweek be different? Why?

4. Your supervisor makes lewd remarks and obvious sexual advances. What will you do?

5. Dream a little. You have the "perfect" employee and want to show your appreciation. What might you do?

6. As a potential employee, answer the candidate questions listed in number 6 under the section "Interviewing Candidates" found earlier in the chapter.

7. You find the right candidate for the job who is wheelchair dependent. What will you do?

8. For the position of clinical medical assistant, identify standards related to hazardous chemicals, bloodborne pathogens, and needlesticks that must be in place.

INTERNET ACTIVITIES

1. Search the Internet for your state's law regarding discrimination related to employment. Is your state more or less restrictive than the federal law? If you live in a city or large metropolitan area, you might also research antidiscrimination laws in that area.
2. This chapter identifies ADA regulations in employment. Search the Internet to determine what kind of accommodations a medical clinic must have to be in compliance with ADA.

REFERENCE

Harris, D.M.: *Contemporary Issues in Healthcare Law and Ethics, 3rd Edition.* Chicago: Health Administration Press, 2008.

WEB RESOURCES

Human Resources: Business and Legal Reports
  http://hr.blr.com

Occupational Safety and Health Administration
  www.osha.gov/dep/administrative-penalty.html

U.S. Department of Labor
  www.dol.gov/whd/

 Davis*Plus* | For additional resources please visit
http://davisplus.fadavis.com

CHAPTER 12

A Cultural Perspective for Health Professionals

"As different as we are from one another, as unique as each one of us is, we are much more the same than we are different. That may be the most essential message of all, as we help our children grow toward being caring, compassionate, and charitable adults."

—Fred Rogers, American educator, Presbyterian minister, songwriter, and

television host

KEY TERMS

ageism Discrimination based on age.
bias A point of view that prevents impartial judgment on issues relating to the subject.
ethnic Pertaining to groupings based on the same race or nationality, sharing a distinctive culture.
gender Society's meaning of the roles of male and female.
internal milieu Environmental condition.
prejudice Opinions determined with no knowledge or examination.
sexual orientation The attention of a person's sexual interest toward members of the same, opposite, or both sexes.

LEARNING OUTCOMES

Upon successful completion of this chapter, you will be able to:
12.1 Define key terms.
12.2 Discuss the impact of cultural influence on health care.
12.3 Identify the levels of sensitivity to cultural diversity.
12.4 Recall the components of cultural diversity.
12.5 Give an example of each component of cultural diversity.
12.6 Examine the concept of a new culture in health care.
12.7 Evaluate self as related to cultural sensitivity.

12.8   Identify any personal prejudice or bias and determine a strategy to address it.

12.9   Facilitate cross-cultural communication.

COMPETENCIES

CAAHEP

- Identify resources and adaptations that are required based on individual needs, i.e., culture and environment, developmental life stage, language, and physical threats to communication. (CAAHEP IV.C.7)
- Discuss the role of cultural, social, and ethnic diversity in ethical performance of medical assisting practice. (CAAHEP X.C.3)
- Demonstrate awareness of diversity in providing patient care. (CAAHEP X.A.3)

ABHES

- Analyze the effect of hereditary, cultural, and environmental influences. (ABHES 5.g)

VIGNETTE

Who Is the Healer?

In a southwestern region of the United States, a Native American healer was called at the same time as an ambulance. Before the ambulance crew could begin their work, the healer performed a "purification" or "healing ritual" on the afflicted person.

"Smudging" or making a "sacred smoke bowl blessing" is the common method for healing and cleansing likely used in this example. Smudging is a powerful cleansing technique from the Native American tradition when herbs, such as lavender, mugwort, and white sage, are tied into a bundle and allowed to dry, making a "smudge stick." Native Americans consider the herbs used for smudging to be sacred, and the smudge stick is treated with great respect. A candle flame is used to light the smudge stick. Once a flame is created, it is blown out so that the smudge stick smolders, freeing the smoke to circle in the air. During healing work, the smoke is fanned over the person by hand or with feathers to clear out unhealthy energies and to bring in the special attributes of the herbs.

In today's increasingly mobile society, clients come from all cultural backgrounds seeking health care. Every health-care professional is a member of a particular cultural heritage that is always with them, defines who they are, and includes bias, prejudice, and preconceived notions about others whose culture is different. Sometimes cultural variances are obvious by color, dress, stature, or action. However, cultural differences may also be obscure. Health professionals who understand and appreciate their own culture are better able to embrace individuals from very differing cultures.

 ## UNDERSTANDING CULTURAL DIVERSITY

To understand more about culture and its effect, ask yourself these three questions: (1) Do you understand clients' traditions and customs that differ from your own? (2) Are you accepting of both differences and similarities? (3) Are you open-minded? The many facets that create cultural differences are relative to age, gender, sexual orientation, ethnic background, educational preparation, life experiences, spiritual influences, role models and mentors, economic influences, values, internal milieu, and health and illness.

Being aware of cultural differences must be a goal for all health professionals who desire to perform legally, ethically, and therapeutically in their employment environment. Refer to the sphere diagram in Figure 12-1 to note that every aspect of a person's culture is related. Each cultural aspect points to every other aspect on the sphere; they are impossible to separate.

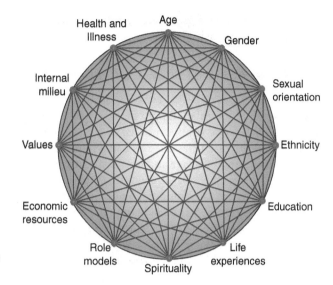

Figure 12-1. Cultural differences that make us unique.

Figure 12-2 is based on information from Larry D. Purnell and Betty J. Paulanka in their book, *Transcultural Health Care*. In the first level, individuals are unaware that they lack knowledge of cultural diversity. In the second level, individuals learn that they lack knowledge of diversity. In the third level, individuals begin to learn more about cultural diversity, verify known generalizations of the culture, and begin to provide culturally sensitive care. In the fourth and last level, individuals automatically provide culturally sensitive care without thinking about it.

These levels are continuous and never ending. To be culturally sensitive implies that there is always learning and growing. Stop a moment to reflect on your own culture and your level of

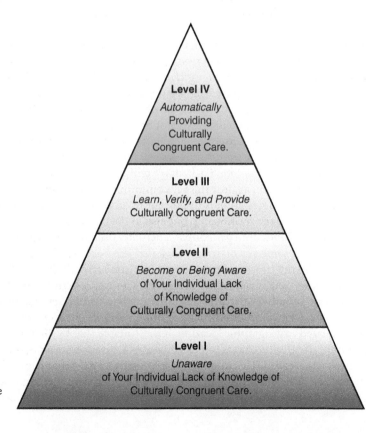

Figure 12-2. Cultural congruent care levels.

development as you progress through this chapter. The goal is to function in the third and fourth levels of cultural sensitivity.

 ## COMPONENTS OF CULTURAL DIVERSITY

Ageism is any form of prejudice, bias, or discrimination that negatively targets the person on the basis of age. For example, children may be viewed as property to possess; adolescents may be seen as individuals who have strange moods, who seldom listen to others, and who are difficult to understand. Elders are often classified as being hard of hearing, forgetful, opinionated, and set in their ways. The importance of age and how differently it is viewed varies among cultures.

The Wang family is elderly. They are Chinese. Mrs. Wang has difficulty walking and has severe kyphosis. Mr. Wang loves his garden but has circulatory problems. He finds it increasingly difficult to cultivate his vegetables and help his wife. The Wang children are moving their mother and father into the home of the eldest son, who has already prepared his house for the two of them.

Next door to the Wang family is another elderly couple. Mr. and Mrs. Johnson are struggling to stay in their home. The house is too large, the yard work is getting away from them, and they have stairs to climb. Their children are pressing them to enter an assisted living facility where their meals will be prepared for them, there is no yard work, and someone will make sure they take their medications. Mr. Johnson worries that he will have to give up his car.

How do these examples show a variation on the ideas of care for elderly people? Explain.

Gender issues arise from prejudices, biases, and discrimination based on sexual identity, whether you are a woman or man. Gender is sometimes used to refer to sex-based categories. For example, in some cultures men may be seen as dominant, athletic, mathematically inclined, and physically superior, whereas women may be seen as intuitive, caregiving, nurturing, and physically weak. Cultures often differ in their views of gender. Medical research in the United States has predominantly centered on men. More recently, studies now include women. In some cultures, women take the lead in raising children, whereas in other cultures, the men may. In the United States, some professions are predominantly male, but women are not barred from entering those fields. In some countries, women do not work out of the home. In other countries, there is no distinction between men and women in the work they perform or the pay they receive for that work.

Your son plays soccer with a teenager from Iran. In the locker room, Mahyar tells your son about his latest escapade with a teenage girl in his class. He brags that it is cool American girls are so "willing" but that his own sister must still be a virgin when she marries.

What does this tell about the role of young women in different cultures?

Sexual orientation addresses issues of heterosexuals, gays, lesbians, bisexuals, and transvestites. Of recent use is the word *transgendered* to refer to individuals as gay, lesbian, bisexual, or transsexual. In the United States, some states address sexual orientation in law. Until overturned in May of 2010, the rule in the military was "don't ask, don't tell" if you were gay and serving in the armed forces. Widespread discrimination against the gay community is common and is often bitterly debated. However, a person's sexual orientation is important to an individual's health care not only in what pathology may be unique to the relationship but also in the effects of illness on significant others.

Gerry and Chuck are a gay couple. They have been together for many years. When the opportunity came for legal same-sex marriage, they tied the knot. Their parents don't think much of this relationship and tell everyone that they are just good friends, but as the legality of same-sex marriages comes under increased scrutiny, Gerry and Chuck are actively involved in the legislation.

How do members within your culture view sexual orientation? Discuss.

Ethnic background or ethnicity is one's national heritage, race, tribe, clan, and language; it is often related to geographic location. It is estimated that by 2050 Hispanics will be the largest ethnic group in the United States, yet not many U.S. citizens speak Spanish, and many Hispanics speak only a little English. The language barrier often implies that people have not yet learned to "think" in English; rather, they think in their native language and then translate into English. Physical space, form of greeting, and eye-to-eye contact vary greatly with cultures. Some professionals are respected more than others in differing cultures. In the United States, as in many other countries, if the native language is not spoken easily and correctly, there is often bias that the individual lacks intelligence.

A 15-month-old Puerto Rican child enters the urgent care center with a history of persistent, productive cough, fever, sleeplessness, and congestion. The child is diagnosed with pneumonia and is to be hospitalized. The child is wearing a pretty bracelet with black and red stone beads. The mother explains that this bracelet is what protects the infant from the evil eye. Two hours later, a hospital nurse removes the bracelet.

Discuss the implication.

Case Law

The Patient Self-Determination Act (PSDA) was passed as part of the Omnibus Budget Reconciliation Act of 1990 (further discussed in Chapter 16, End of Life Issues). The law requires all health-care facilities receiving reimbursement from Medicare and Medicaid to ask individuals, on admission, if they have an advance directive. The law requires that individuals be given written information explaining advance directive documents if they so choose and the opportunity to create an advanced directive.

Since 1990, research regarding the role ethnicity plays in end-of-life decisions has been conducted. This research shows that regardless of the specific ethnicity, members of minority groups are generally less desirous of completing advance directives than are whites. The research suggests that end-of-life choices are more related to race, ethnicity, and culture than to age, education, or socioeconomic status.

Barriers made by the law that surfaced during the research are that (1) the PSDA is based on written communication and assumes all clients can read and write; (2) there is the assumption that clients will trust the medical community to make every possible attempt to save a life before "pulling the plug," but not all clients hold that belief; and (3) the law assumes that personal choice is of higher importance than family or communal choice.

Describe the conflicts surfaced by this law related to cultural differences.

What might you do as a health-care professional to "bridge the gap" in cultural communications related to end-of-life issues?

Educational preparation is one's formal education, such as kindergarten through high school; some cultures provide children with only 4 or 5 years of formal education and educate only the males. In other cultures, privately funded education is the norm. Such differences may include private, public, or parochial education or home schooling. People moving to the United States may come with a high level of skill and education that is recognized in their country but are forced to take low-paying, menial jobs because of language barriers or lack of recognition for their level of accomplishment. An example of this is seen when doctors coming from another country must reeducate themselves in the United States before taking the licensing examination. Others may come with limited education and are able to reap benefits from the U.S. education system.

In today's dollars, a bachelor's degree is worth more than $2.1 million over 40 years. "Having that post-secondary diploma can make such a difference in lifetime earnings," said Washington, D.C.–based Employment Policy Foundation President Ed Potter. It seems that during a recession, obtaining a college degree becomes even more important. According to the U.S. Department of Labor, all seven of the job categories that are predicted to grow faster than average during the next decade require a college diploma. One of those seven is a career in health care.

Two expectant mothers come to the women's clinic for their prenatal care. One woman of Appalachian heritage has limited educational preparation. The other woman holds a Ph.D. from the nursing department in the local university. Each is having her first child.

What are the implications for each of these women and/or for the health-care professional?

Life experiences include such events as death, divorce, disability, chronic illness, family crises, adoption, and surrogacy. Some people have siblings; others may be an only child; some may have been raised with extended family members. These experiences shape how individuals adjust to life's challenges. Survivors of the Holocaust and survivors of "ethnic cleansing" in other countries have seen and experienced persecution that few can comprehend. Veterans of wars experience events that shape their lives forever. They experience death and destruction few know. Divorce may be impossible in some cultures yet simple to obtain in others. Some cultures view disabilities as shameful, and people with disabilities may be hidden away or killed. Other cultures give a person with disabilities great respect.

Jared was 18 when he went into the military. He wanted nothing more than to serve his country. He had his wish. He spent time in Croatia, Bosnia, and Afghanistan. Few can imagine the violence and devastation that Jared saw and experienced while helping to retrieve bodies from the war zone. He returned home after two tours of service, disillusioned with the entire military experience. He felt his future was in question and found it difficult to integrate back into society. His former friends were strangers to him. He was diagnosed with post-traumatic stress disorder.

How does the health-care professional relate to this client?

Spiritual influences may include any of the major religions or no specific religion. A person's belief system may be a separate and unique spiritual support system. Individuals with a belief in a supreme deity seem to be better prepared for surgery. They tend to "let another take charge." Some individuals are more ready for death and accept it more easily because of their religious beliefs. Sometimes, too, people may view illness or disease as a "punishment" because of their religious views. Consider two varying views below of the impact religion has on one's life.

Reverend Jesse Morris is a retired clergyman. His faith has been strong for more than 70 years. He has a serious illness that will take his life in a short period of time. His nurse has tears in her eyes as she gives him a shot for pain. Reverend Morris says, "It is okay. I am fine. I am ready. God has a better place for me where there is no pain."

Aarif Faraj is a member of a certain cult and sect of Islam who believe suicide is not self-sacrifice but is legitimate and highly commendable when undertaken for reasons of jihad (holy war). Aarif understands that going into war knowing with certainty that he will die is martyrdom, a much praised form of self-sacrifice in the path of God, a way to win the eternal affection of one of the beautiful virgins of the Koranic paradise.

Is there a place for spirituality in health care? Justify your response.

Role models and mentors may be family members, teachers, famous persons, pacifists, or warriors, and they may have a positive or a negative effect on individuals. Role models and mentors differ within cultures; however, the way in which health care is viewed by a person's role model is often the way one will view their own health care. For example, if health care is seen as a right by parents, children often will expect the same or more. If health care is a luxury, however, then it is not expected or sought.

Cherylinn's stepbrother was addicted to drugs. He had a couple of pit bull dogs who guarded his house while he made meth. His life was a mess, but after his suicide, Cherylinn's Dad took her to see his place. It was both shocking and sad. Cherylinn's response to the experience was, "I will never use drugs as long as I live. It is hard for me to understand how someone could get to such a place."

What kind of statement did Cherylinn's stepbrother make for her as a role model? What did Cherylinn learn from this visit? Can health care offer any answer to Cherylinn's question?

Economic influences stem from resources available, wealth and its distribution, the developing world versus industrial or informational affluence, and dictatorship versus democracy. Individuals who do not have the economic resources to pay for their health care may do without. It may be difficult for people who come from a socialist health-care system to adjust to a democracy. The third party payer idea is an economic consideration. Some people may be able to pay cash and receive the care needed, whereas in other countries, it would be impossible to receive such services. In preventive medicine, inoculations are required, whereas in underdeveloped countries, people die from diseases these inoculations can prevent.

A young mother works for a community service agency. She receives little or no child support from her former husband. She has no health insurance other than Medicaid. She has an abscessed tooth. The dentist says she needs a root canal. She has no funds for the antibiotics to treat the abscess or to have the root canal. The dentist can only pull the tooth.

Why is adequate dental care not accessible to this mother?

Rene Helbling is a wealthy philanthropist. She has been on the kidney transplant list for some time. In her desperation, she turns to India in search of a kidney match and the surgery. Money is not an issue, and she has decided not to tell her nephrologist of her plans until after she returns from India.

What difference does economic influence make in this situation? Explain your answer.

Values are morals or standards that are acceptable and practical in a culture. The value of life versus the value of death is a standard set by a culture. Values are determined by culture, family, religious beliefs, school, friends, and mentors. They are shaped by life experiences. Values are difficult to modify. They are one way in which to identify culture.

In some societies, people will advertise to sell a kidney for money. In other societies, people will offer to donate a kidney or bone marrow to someone unknown to them.

What value do you place on your body? From where or what influence does that value come?

Internal milieu cannot be seen by people, but it affects one's daily life. Many of the influences addressed previously affect one's internal milieu and how one reacts to life. A person may be diabetic, have a chronic heart condition, or suffer from very low self-esteem, but this is not always obvious. A person's internal milieu affects how health care is approached.

Cultural differences exist. Every standard and influence is culture bound. What is "right" in one culture may be considered "wrong" in another. We feel most comfortable in our own culture working within our own values.

Ron Harrison is a 68-year-old man. He is active and slender; he plays golf and eats very healthy food. No one knows that he is a walking time bomb with a cholesterol level of 385.

Bess Thor is 53. She parks in a handicap parking place and has a handicap license, but she walks into the grocery store with ease and without aid. The shopper who sneers at her and points to the disabled parking sign cannot know that Bess has chronic obstructive pulmonary disease (COPD) that will limit her shopping time to only 10 minutes before she will have to return to her car to rest.

What do these examples tell us about assumptions we sometimes make?

The way a person reacts to **health and illness** is an attitude and a perception that encompasses all of the other cultural components identified here. Although some diseases are endemic and specific to ethnic groups, all cultures share the threat of death from illness or disease.

Some individuals are intensively private about their health issues; others may broadcast them to anyone who will listen. Some ignore their health challenges.

What implications do these examples have for each of us? For health professionals?

Rather than accentuate cultural differences, the question is, "How can we learn to complement them?" Our culture is one among many. It has no special status. It is important to develop a knowledge base and acceptance for differences in cultural traditions and standards.

ESTABLISHING A NEW CULTURE IN HEALTH CARE

Every exchange with a client is a cross-cultural one. Each person brings to that exchange a diverse background, experience, education, age, gender, race, ethnic origin, physical ability, religious belief, and sexual orientation. Developing a new culture, if that is what it might be called, where there is mutual respect, acceptance, and an environment conducive to teamwork among clients, physicians, other health-care providers, and health-care personnel must be the goal. Health-care professionals must recognize that the failure to accept such diversity among clients and each other or the inability to embrace one's own differences becomes a barrier to health-care communication and quality health care.

Entering into a new culture of mutual respect, acceptance, and teamwork does not require total agreement with another person's differences; it merely requires acceptance of those persons for who they are and what they believe. It also gives them the right to their beliefs and values. One must be nonjudgmental, which means seeing each person with a "clean and open slate," not one that has been tainted by one's own prejudice and bias. For example, we do not have to alter or change our sexual orientation in order to respect and accept someone of a differing sexual orientation. We must be able to see each person as a unique and special human being who has a right to culturally sensitive treatment.

Such a culture demands that each of us become more accepting and inclusive in our interactions with others. It requires that we become informed and knowledgeable of others' cultures. If several clients are Spanish speaking, we can learn Spanish so that at times we may converse in their language or more clearly understand what is being said. Not only is respect gained, but we learn how hard it is to "think" in a second language.

Case Studies

A male caregiver who is about 6 feet, 3 inches and 250 pounds brings a 5-year-old boy into the clinic. The child is injured, and it appears that he has been struck pretty hard. While the pediatrician is attending to the child's injuries, the very nervous caregiver paces to the receptionist's desk, leans over, and says, "My God, what have I done? I did not mean to hit him; I got so mad when he wouldn't mind me!" Your response might be, "Get out of my face; the police will take care of you!" Or it might be, "How could a brute like you hit a child so small?" Or struggling to be therapeutic, remembering that the abuser is also a victim, and trying to accept this person, obviously distraught and upset, as another human being of equal value, you might reply, "As hard as this is for me, you've taken the first step in realizing your mistake. We're treating the boy now. Please just have a seat, try to remain calm, and I'll have the doctor speak with you as soon as she's finished."

Identify the conflicting values expressed. What would you say if you were the receptionist?

A young Navajo woman employed in the medical clinic where you work is expecting her first child in a month. The staff is anxious to have a baby shower for her during lunchtime. When you tell the woman of the plans for her, she is embarrassed but tells you she does not want a shower. She explains that in Navajo culture, preparing for the birth is taboo and forbidden. Together you decide it would be fun to have a shower after the baby is born when she can return to the clinic during lunch and everyone can see the baby.

Identify the positive outcomes of this scenario. How might it have been different?

A middle-aged man comes out of the examination room and stops to make a follow-up appointment. You notice the tears in his eyes and ask how you can help. He sobs, "Not only must I go home and tell my wife I've been leading a life as a bisexual, I must also tell her I'm positive for HIV." You can respond by saying, "You play with fire, you're going to get burned. I pity your wife." Or, "Personally, I'd never go home. I'd drive my car off a cliff." Or again you can strive to put your prejudices and biases aside and respond, "This must be very difficult for you. I am sorry. Would it help if you asked your wife to talk with us or to make an appointment with the doctor? What can I do for you?"

Can you see yourself making any of these responses? Justify your response. Might you just ignore the client's obvious distress? Why or why not?

Your clinic's provider is treating a woman of Chinese ancestry. She is elderly and has been in this country only a few years. She is often temperamental and angers easily. She tells you as she waves the prescription paper in your face, "No make me take this! Dr. Chin's herbs much better—much cheaper, too!" You can say, "You crazy old lady, just go see your Dr. Chin. Don't bother us anymore. Insurance won't pay for him anyway!" Recalling your knowledge of the Chinese culture, and the importance of herbal medication, you can say, "You feel like Dr. Chin's herbs really help more? Did you share that with the doctor? It may be OK to take both the herbal medicine and the prescription. Let's ask the doctor just to be safe. We want you to get well."

Identify both the negative and the positive outcome of this situation.

EVALUATING SELF

Cultural competence begins with the honest desire to treat everyone with respect regardless of their cultural heritage. This requires an honest assessment of positive and negative assumptions about others. This is not easy because no one wants to admit that he or she is culturally ignorant or harbors negative stereotypes and prejudices. Examine each prejudice or bias you hold. On what assumptions is it based? Do those assumptions have any merit? Ask someone whose judgment you value to assist you in this examination. Recall someone with whom you have great differences. Can you foster the kind of respect and acceptance of that person to enable you to see him or her as a human being with equal merit rather than as a person with whom you disagree?

 ## CROSS-CULTURAL COMMUNICATION

Facilitating cross-cultural communication requires sensitivity to differences, attentive listening, and a respectful, nonjudgmental attitude. However, conflicts will arise. To deal with cultural conflicts, pay close attention to body language, language barriers, and tone of voice. The use of a translator who is not a family member may prove to be beneficial. A nonfamily member is less likely to do more than interpret and give advice.

 It is the responsibility of health-care providers to make certain that an interpreter is available when necessary to ensure the client's full understanding of procedures and treatment. ●

When negative emotions expressed during a cultural conflict are yours, it is a good idea to step back, breathe deeply, and control your own emotions first. Then ask clients to express their experiences and feelings, if possible, and acknowledge them. Help clients find options suitable to them, and compromise over treatment goals and modalities whenever possible.

SUMMARY

Cultural diversity has been examined in this chapter, and personal feelings were explored in order to recognize the importance of cultural diversity in every client interaction. Continually evaluate your behavior so that your actions reflect an automatic sensitivity to cultural differences. In the next section on bioethical issues, your culture and your belief system will be challenged. In each situation, strive to remain as free from prejudice as possible, thus allowing open examination of all sides of an issue.

Consider the following quotes:

"The real act of discovery consists not in finding new lands, but in seeing with new eyes." Marcel Proust, French novelist and critic.

"A new idea is first condemned as ridiculous and then dismissed as trivial, until finally, it becomes what everybody knows." William James, American psychologist and philosopher.

 Watch It Now! Are you sensitive to other cultures? at
http://davisplus.fadavis.com/lawandethics

Questions for Review

SELECT THE BEST ANSWER

1. Ethnicity refers to
   a. Those who are gays and lesbians.
   b. National heritage, race, tribe.
   c. Language, geography.
   d. None of the above.
   e. Only b and c above.

2. Role models and mentors
   a. Can be positive or negative.
   b. Have little or no influence on a person's culture.
   c. Refer to religious leaders.
   d. Are dependent on educational preparation.
   e. None of the above.

3. The cultural congruent care levels
   a. Identify five levels or stages.
   b. Are achieved over a period of many years of trial and error.
   c. Is one diagram that illustrates how individuals may become culturally sensitive.
   d. Were designed by the authors of this text.
   e. Simply do not work in real life.

4. Gender cultural issues may
   a. See men as dominant and athletic.
   b. View women as intuitive and nurturing.
   c. Refer only to gays and lesbians.
   d. All of the above.
   e. Only a and b above.

5. Being nonjudgmental means
   a. Seeing every person with a "clean and open slate."
   b. Total agreement with the other person's differences.
   c. Being exclusive in our belief system and interactions with others.
   d. Creating an environment for disagreement.
   e. Accentuating cultural differences.

FILL IN THE BLANK

1. _____ is the part of culture that cannot be seen by people but affects daily living.

2. Death, divorce, disability, chronic illness, and family crises are all part of

   _____.

3. In Purnell/Paulanka's cultural congruent care levels, an individual in Level 1 is
   _____ of culturally congruent care.

4. _____ implies discrimination because of age.

5. Entering into a new culture in health care will require _____,
   acceptance, and teamwork.

CLASSROOM EXERCISES

1. In each of the case studies given in the chapter, what would be your response? Is your response accepting and nonjudgmental?

2. Interview two persons who are of a different culture than your own. Ask them how they access health care. What is the influence of the family unit? Who makes health-care decisions?

3. Recall a time when you personally have been discriminated against in the health-care setting or some other setting because of your culture.

4. What role models and mentors have influenced your choice of health care?

5. Identify the largest ethnic minority in your geographic location. How are the health needs of this group addressed?

INTERNET ACTIVITIES

1. What are the laws in your state addressing discriminatory actions related to sexual orientation?

2. Related to Classroom Exercise number 5 above, search the Internet to determine as much about that culture as you can. Identify its customs and traditions. How do people of that culture celebrate births, birthdays, and weddings? What kind of custom is followed on the death of a loved one?

REFERENCES

Baker, M. E.: Cultural differences in the use of advance directives: A review of the literature. Department of Social Work, Wright State University, 2005. Available at: www.rcgd.isr.umich.edu/prba/perspectives/fall2000/mbaker.pdf.

Purnell, L. D., Paulanka B. J.: *Transcultural Health Care: A Culturally Competent Approach, 3rd Edition*. Philadelphia: F. A Davis, 2008.

WEB RESOURCE

Gift of a College Degree. www.salary.com

Davis*Plus* | For additional resources please visit http://davisplus.fadavis.com

Bioethical Issues

CHAPTER 13

Allocation of Scarce Medical Resources

"Due to budget cuts, light at the end of tunnel will be out."—Bumper sticker on car

KEY TERMS

Apgar score System of scoring newborn's physical condition 1 minute and 5 minutes after birth. Heart rate, respiration, muscle tone, response to stimuli, and skin color are measured. Maximum score is 10; those with low scores require immediate attention if they are to survive.

concierge medical service Medical care that provides "over and above" medical services to clients for fee.

diagnosis-related groups (DRGs) Categorization of hospital medical services to standardize prospective medical care.

macroallocation System in which distribution decisions are made by large bodies of individuals, usually Congress, health systems agencies, state legislatures, and health insurance carriers.

microallocation System in which distribution decisions are made by small groups or individuals, such as hospital staff and physicians.

LEARNING OUTCOMES

Upon successful completion of this chapter, you will be able to:

13.1 Define key terms.
13.2 Compare/contrast allocation and access of health care.
13.3 Describe how "defensive medicine" occurs.
13.4 Explain concierge medical coverage.
13.5 Provide examples of how politics, economics, and ethics influence allocation of scarce medical recourses.
13.6 Explain the phrase *microallocation and macroallocation of scarce resources.*
13.7 Describe how decisions are made at the microallocation and macroallocation level.
13.8 Outline both systems of selection.
13.9 Formulate a personal understanding of the impact scarce medical resources has on clients.

COMPETENCIES

CAAHEP

• Differentiate between legal, ethical, and moral issues affecting health care. (CAAHEP X.C.1)
• Identify the effect personal ethics may have on professional performance. (CAAHEP X.C.5)
• Develop a plan for separation of personal and professional ethics. (CAAHEP X.P.2)

- Examine the impact personal ethics and morals may have on the individual's practice. (CAAHEP X.A.3)

ABHES

- Advocate on behalf of family/patients, having ability to deal and communicate with family. (ABHES 5.e)

VIGNETTE

Who Decides?

You are employed by a team of transplant surgeons in a major city when a call comes from a hospital that donor organs are available. The wheels move quickly to determine proper matches among the clinic's clients. Your surgeons discover that two equally needy clients are waiting for the donor liver. One is an 18-month-old infant whose first liver transplant is being rejected. The other possible recipient is a 7-year-old recently diagnosed with liver failure.

Allocation of scarce medical resources and access to medical care are major bioethical concerns in today's society. *Allocation* refers to the distribution of available health-care resources. *Access* refers to whether people who should have health care are able to receive that care. Winners in the arena of access to health care are most likely healthy and well-insured individuals with good corporate coverage. Losers in this dilemma are often children, persons of color, and those who are poor and powerless. It is reported that 46 million Americans are living without health insurance. Many more are underinsured.

ALLOCATION AND ACCESS IN TODAY'S HEALTH-CARE ENVIRONMENT

Many examples of allocation and access concerns can be found in today's health-care environment. Six million children younger than 18 years are without adequate health care. Prenatal care is an unaffordable luxury for most of the uninsured. Often, adequate care is unavailable even after infants are born. There are a number of individuals working full-time and part-time jobs who "fall through the cracks" for coverage with medical insurance. Elderly people are increasingly having difficulties obtaining adequate health care and paying for their prescription medications. Medicare, with its increasing costs and decreasing coverage, is inadequate. Without a quality Medicare supplement program, elderly persons, like many of the nation's children, will go without. The number of Medicare recipients without supplemental insurance is about 34.2 million.

The Healthcare Reform Bill of 2010 made some changes in insurance coverage. By 2014, 32 million more Americans should have heath insurance coverage, but approximately 14 million Americans will still be left with no health benefits.

ETHICS CHECK

Access and allocation of heath care often relate to geography. There are vast rural areas in many parts of the United States with few providers of heatlh care and/or hospitals in which to provide necessary services. Clients may drive more than 100 miles to reach medical care that is clustered in cities and suburban areas. The ethical question has to be, What value is placed on human life in America when basic health care is not available to those in need? ●

Case Study

A young boy in a rural Maine dies in a small hospital after an automobile accident. The family practice physician, on emergency call at the hospital when the ambulance brings in the boy, works feverishly for more than an hour to save him, but the boy dies. The next morning the doctor shares with you the feeling of hopelessness knowing the boy's life might have been saved if a neurosurgeon and more sophisticated equipment had been accessible to the hospital.

Why does geographic location often dictate who lives and who dies?
Is there anything that might have made a difference in this young boy's treatment?

With the ever-changing health-care climate, health professionals in all facets of the industry, ambulatory as well as inpatient care, are required to do more with less, forcing hospitals and acute care centers to radically alter their health-care delivery system. For example, a surgical nurse with 10 years of experience may be moved to the role of circulating nurse while a surgical technician with only 9 months of recent training steps in to assist the surgeon. The circulating nurse is removed from the actual operation yet is ultimately responsible for the supplies and equipment in the room and must document any incidents that might occur. Responsibility and accountability issues in all areas of health care are shifting toward cost containment.

The hospital has become a massive business entity whose financing comes from government programs, private insurers, bond issues, loans, donations, and the personal pockets of clients. Medical supply houses and pharmaceutical manufacturers develop new devices and drugs, market agressively to the public, and gain a stronger foothold in the total health-care climate. Legal regulations abound, and malpractice is a continued concern. This threat leads providers into practicing "defensive medicine" by ordering tests and procedures that normally might be considered unnecessary—just to make certain that all bases are adequately covered.

All clients are directly affected by increased health-care costs, and some must make difficult choices about what to eliminate from their health–care–pay $1200 a month for medication that is really needed, or pay the rent? Those who are older often lose the option to move closer to family when the only available providers do not take new Medicare clients and turn away all Medicaid recipients because of inadequate reimbursment. At the same time, well-insured and financially successful clients are able to purchase nearly any kind of health care they desire. This has been proved by the numbers of individuals who readily purchased "concierge" or "premier" medical service as soon as it was made available by their medical providers. Such services provide guaranteed access to their provider, telephone and e-mail contact, hospital-stay coordination, and prompt follow-through on any ordered tests. Some concierge services even provide house calls to their clients. It is interesting to note that in the 1940s and 1950s, with the exception of e-mail access, this type of service was provided to all clients.

Continual innovation in medical technology has made it possible to replace body parts; create new drugs for mental distress; refine diagnostic procedures to quickly determine fractures, tumors, or infections; and supply complex pharmaceutical regimens for many chronic illnesses. Nonessential reconstructive surgery, assisted reproduction, and experimental therapies are available, whereas the less fortunate are either denied access or are given no choice in their health-care treatment. The result is there are medical luxuries for a few, but others do without.

INFLUENCE OF POLITICS, ECONOMICS, AND ETHICS ON HEALTH CARE

Inadequate access to health care is a complex problem. It is a political issue; it is an economic problem; it is an ethical dilemma. This influence leads to a number of questions.

The political questions are, Who will pay for basic health care? Who decides what kind of benefit package everyone should receive? and How can I maintain status quo in an election year?

The economic questions are, How can scarce medical resources be allocated in light of the necessary costs and human needs or desires? How can costs be curtailed? and Is the Healthcare Reform Bill of 2010 a step toward a solution or an economic disaster?

The ethical questions are, Is medical care a right or a privilege? and How will these scarce resources be justly and fairly distributed?

HEALTH-CARE LEGISLATION

In an attempt to make health care more accessible and more affordable, states entered into the political arena hoping to answer these questions.

In 1999, Oregon passed the first program for rationing health care in the United States. The Oregon legislature created the Health Services Commission, which presented a prioritized list of health services they believed warranted diagnosis and treatment. Illnesses below a certain number were not covered because it was believed that either the persons would get well on their own or treatment would be futile. Today, the Oregon Health Plan extends Medicaid eligibility to all state residents with incomes below the federal poverty level; establishes a high-risk insurance pool for people refused health coverage because of preexisting health conditions; and addresses small businesses by offering them options to provide their employees with the ability to change jobs without losing their health insurance coverage. The controversial plan was successful in spreading insurance coverage and decreasing the numbers of the uninsured in the state.

Maine passed a a similar law in 2003 to expand health care to its underserved population. In 2006, Massachusetts lawmakers required all its 500,000 uninsured citizens to have some form of health insurance. Every citizen earning $9500 or less yearly is covered at no cost. Businesses that do not offer health insurance pay a $295 annual fee per employee. Other states with similar actions include Tennessee and Minnesota. ●

The Healthcare Reform Bill of 2010, finally enacted after decades of debate and a great deal of opposition, further identifies and mandates health-care services for many of the underserved and may alter some of the states' plans. To say that the health-care reform legislation was political is an understatement. The vote taken followed strict Republican and Democratic party lines with just a few exceptions and passed only because the Democrats controlled Congress.

Some say such legislation is long overdue; others see these plans as examples of government controlling health care. In any instance, the plans provide for treatable health-care coverage, however limited, to increased numbers of residents. Only time will address their effectiveness, efficiency, quality, and cost.

Whenever health-care access and allocation decisions are made, improving health care should be the primary goal. Health professionals, researchers, and members of nearly all academic disciplines have been formally debating such issues for many years. For discussion, it is easier to define the problem in terms of macroallocation and microallocation of scarce resources.

MACROALLOCATION AND MICROALLOCATION

Allocation decisions deal with how much shall be expended for medical resources and how these resources are to be distributed (Fig. 13-1).

Macroallocation decisions are made by larger bodies, such as Congress, health systems agencies, state legislatures, health organizations, private foundations, and health insurance carriers. For example, Congress determined that Medicare should provide medical care for the client with chronic renal disease, yet no other chronic disease is specifically named in the Medicare program. Macroallocation decisions also are evident when determinations are made regarding funding of medical

Figure 13-1. A brief description of how resources are allocated.

research. How much should be allotted for cancer research, for preventive medicine, or for techno-logical advances in medical equipment? The health insurance industry largely determines the "rea-sonable and customary" charges in medical care and therefore what will and will not be covered by health insurance premiums.

In addition, Congress instituted a Medicare prospective payment system in 1983 that reflects macroallocation called diagnosis-related groups (DRGs), used in hospitals to categorize clients' conditions by number. Payment is made on the basis of a predetermined rate or average cost. The intended effect of the DRGs was to encourage facilities to be better stewards of their time and re-sources in treating individuals in the hospital and to equalize Medicare payments made to facilities and providers. The prospective payment system has inadvertently encouraged providers to be more specific in documenting their services so that their coders find no gaps in documentation for the correct and most appropriate diagnoses and procedures.

Case Study

The family at 913 Twelfth Street will be saved from financial ruin because Medicare will help defray the costs of their young son's kidney dialysis. The family at 909 Twelfth Street may suffer great financial stress because of increasing medical bills for the treatment of their daughter's juvenile-onset diabetes mellitus, which has left her blind and nephrotic.

How does the government determine that one medical problem warrants financial assistance and another does not?

Microallocation decisions concerning who shall obtain the resources available are made on an in-dividual basis, usually by local hospital policy and doctors. Decisions at the microallocation level cut deeper into the conscience, because of their personal closeness to everyday living. Examples of ques-tions requiring these decisions include, Who is allowed to occupy that one available bed in intensive care? Does the Medicaid client receive the same care as the local VIP? Does a 60-year-old Medicaid client have an equal chance at the kidney transplant as the foreign visitor who has cash to pay for the procedure? Who gets the flu shots when there is not enough vaccine for all those at risk?

Case Study

Review the vignette at the beginning of the chapter.

How will the decision be made regarding the available liver?
Who makes the decision?
How much time might be available before a choice is made?

SYSTEMS FOR DECISION MAKING

How are the criteria established that attempt to answer such questions of allocation? Two prominent systems have arisen. The first system identifies three possible selection processes. The second system identifies five principles for a fair selection process.

An outline of the two systems follows:

SYSTEM I

1. *Combination criteria system.* Those who satisfy the most criteria ought to receive treatment. Such criteria might include the following:
   a. Capacity to benefit from treatment without complications
   b. Ability to contribute financially or experimentally as a research subject
   c. Age and life expectancy
   d. Past and potential future contributions of the client to society
2. *Random selection system.* This system is more like "first come, first served," or a simple chance selection or drawing of lots.
3. *No-treatment system.* This system is based on the premise that if all cannot be treated, treatment should be given to none.

SYSTEM II

Decisions should be made on the following basis:

1. To everyone an equal share
2. To everyone according to their individual needs
3. To everyone according to their individual efforts
4. To everyone according to their contributions to society
5. To everyone according to their abilities and merits

A summary of the American Medical Association's Council on Ethical and Judicial Affairs suggests that, when making allocation decisions of scarce resources, the only ethically appropriate criteria to consider are quality of life, benefit and duration of benefit, and urgency of need. Such factors as age, ability to pay, client contribution to illness, or social worth should not be considered. If the allocation decision poses little disparity among clients who will receive treatment, then practitioners should use the "first come, first served" approach.

There has been much debate about whether individuals with unhealthy lifestyles should pay more for their health insurance premiums than healthy individuals. (Unhealthy lifestyles are defined as smoking, obesity, and not exercising.) There is a strong belief that it is fair to require higher premiums in much the same manner as car insurance increases or is cancelled after a certain number of accidents. In addition, it seems fair to seek higher co-payments and deductibles from unhealthy individuals. Insurance carriers are making offers to subscribers to influence good health—partial payment of exercise club memberships and financial bonuses for not smoking or for losing excess pounds.

Case Study

When a 58-year-old employee, Sam, loses his job because his company is downsizing, he is unable to maintain his health insurance premiums for more than 6 months. He also finds it impossible to find employment with similar pay and benefits. His wife, receiving care for cancer, is now left without insurance. Sam pays more than $160,000 for his wife's care before her death, which occurred just 3 months after the health-care coverage was lost. Sam is nearly bankrupt.

Case Law

Cheryl Matthews, plaintiff, brought suit against Blue Cross/Blue Shield of Michigan for wrongfully refusing to pay $38,000 in insurance claims stemming from Applied Behavior Analysis (ABA) treatment for her autistic son. Blue Cross defendants argued that ABA therapy was not covered under the policy held by Matthews and filed to dismiss the case.

Judge Prentis Edwards denied the motion, forcing Blue Cross to either settle the claim or go to court. Blue Cross was ordered to pay $125,000 to Matthews based on the fact that Mathews' inability to access ABA therapy for her son will increase his life care costs.

Matthews v Blue Cross, Case No. 09-018750-CK.

 HOW WOULD YOU DECIDE?

To appreciate more fully the difficulties in making choices related to the allocation of scarce medical resources and to assist in establishing a criterion for selection, the following examples are given for you to ponder.

ALLOCATION OF RESOURCES

Example 1

On the advice of the staff nurse in an assisted living facility, an 82-year-old woman is transported by Medic 1 to the nearest hospital with suspected fractures after a fall in her bathroom at 9:30 p.m. Two miles from the hospital, Medic 1 is advised that the hospital emergency room is overflowing and is on divert. Medic 1 continues to the second hospital, 10 additional minutes away. The second hospital emergency area is so busy that two individuals on hospital beds are placed in the hallway. After x-rays and a long wait for an examination, it is discovered that there are no fractures, only bruises. The doctor sighs, "I'm so glad to send you back to your home. If you needed hospitalization, I'd have to send you to another hospital an hour's drive away. We do not have one empty bed."

Example 2

You have just given birth to a 20-oz infant of 6 months' gestation. The Apgar score is -2. The infant cannot suck and has no muscle tone, no gag, and no reflux. There is a need to protect the brain and the nervous center. The attending physician approaches you and the infant's father with the news that the only chance of survival is to transport the infant to a neonatal center in the nearest city, 200 miles away from home.

What is your response? How might the infant's father respond? What problems do you foresee? What are the legal implications of your decision?

Consider this case a second time, only 6 months later and with more facts. The decision was made to send the infant to the neonatal center. After 2 weeks, your medical bill is well over $300,000, and you know you have only enough money to add to your medical insurance to cover a normal labor and delivery. It appears that the infant will be unable to come home for several weeks, if ever. The infant has now been diagnosed with the following problems: cerebral palsy; blindness; hydrocephalus, which has been alleviated with a shunt in the brain; and seizures.

What choices are available to you and the infant's father now? Who is responsible for the increasing hospital bill? Is medical care a right or a privilege under these circumstances? Who makes the decisions involved in this case?

It quickly becomes obvious that no established criteria provide clear-cut solutions to the afore-mentioned examples. None would be easy to follow. Factors other than those mentioned in the two systems will also influence decisions. They include personal ethics, personal preferences, religious beliefs, geographic location, legal requirements, and the political climate. Many problems and few solutions are evident when considering how and to whom scarce medical resources are to be allocated.

SUMMARY

Many times allocation and access to scarce medical resources pose more questions than answers. Influences, such as economics, geographic location, availability of health-care professionals, politics, and insurance coverage, determine both allocation and access to health care. How decisions are made and who decides are critical questions to be asked. As a health-care professional, it is important to help clients recognize what services are available to them and to help them determine where or how to access other services if needed. If time has not been spent thinking through some of these difficult choices, responding ethically becomes a challenge.

 Watch It Now! How do you choose when there really is no choice? at http://davisplus.fadavis.com/lawandethics

Questions for Review

SELECT THE BEST ANSWER

1. Microallocation
   a. Decisions are made on an individual basis.
   b. Uses the DRGs for decision making.
   c. Is used by insurance carriers to determine coverage.
   d. All of the above.
   e. Only b and c above.

2. The "first come, first served" system for decision making
   a. Is a combination criteria system.
   b. Identifies the random selection system.
   c. Is not approved by the American Medical Association's (AMA's) Council on Ethical and Judicial Affairs.
   d. Considers capacity to benefit.
   e. Only a and b above.

3. Macroallocation
   a. Decisions are usually made by hospitals.
   b. Determines who gets the flu shots where there is not enough vaccine for all who are at risk.
   c. Helps to determine how much money is spent on medical research.
   d. Gives to everyone an equal share.
   e. Considers age and life expectancy in decision making.

4. Allocation of scarce medical resources is a bioethical issue because
   a. Everyone does not have access to health care.
   b. It is important to determine how health care is distributed.
   c. Questions of economics, ethics, and politics must be addressed.
   d. All of the above.
   e. Only c above.

5. Action by state legislatures making decisions about allocation of medical care is an example
   of _____ at work.
   a. Microallocation
   b. Bioethics
   c. Economics
   d. Politics
   e. System II

TRUE OR FALSE

T   F   1. "Access" refers to the distribution of health-care services.

T   F   2. "Concierge" or "premier" health care is enhanced medical services provided to those
              who can afford it.

T   F   3. A random selection system of health-care resources means that those who satisfy the
              most criteria ought to receive treatment.

T   F   4. In 1999, Virginia passed the first program for rationing health care in the
              United States.

T   F   5. Who will pay for basic health care is a political rather than an economic question.

CLASSROOM EXERCISES

1. Consider each of the case studies in the chapter and answer the following questions:
   a. At what level (macroallocation or microallocation) is a decision made?
   b. Can one of the selection systems be applied?

2. On what basis do you decide who gets the last open slot of the provider's appointment
   schedule? What system of selection is followed?

3. Two clients desperately need the use of one remaining hemodialysis machine. One is an
   elderly Medicaid client. The other is a young college student who has full health insurance
   benefits. Which client would you choose to treat? Support your answer.

4. What suggestions do you have to make health care available to all? How would your plan be
   funded?

5. Bioethicist, Dan Callahan, states that the root of the allocation problem in modern medicine is "our cultural inability to acknowledge limits to life and to face the reality of death."
   Comment on this statement, describing your personal feelings and giving an example of
   this philosophy.

INTERNET ACTIVITIES

1. Research the Internet for examples of allocation of scarce medical resources. Pay close attention to litigation involving insurance carriers' denial of medical coverage.

2. Go to http://latimesblogs.latimes.com/booster_shots/2010/07/aclu-letter-to-cms-regarding-abortion-rights.html. You will find comments in an article related to the influence of religion on medical decisions and ethics committees. With a classmate, discuss the ramifications of such actions as identified in the article.

REFERENCES

Beauchamp, T. L, & Walters, L.: *Contemporary Issues in Bioethics, 4th Edition.* Belmont, CA: Wadsworth, 1994.

Furrow, B. R., Greaney, T. L., Johnson, S. H., Jost, T. S., & Schwartz, R. L.: *Bioethics: Health Care Law and Ethics, 6th Edition.* St. Paul, MN: Thomson West, 2008.

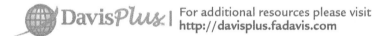

DavisPlus | For additional resources please visit
http://davisplus.fadavis.com

CHAPTER 14

Genetic Engineering

"It is not easy to be a pioneer—but oh, it is fascinating! I would not trade one moment, even the worst moment, for all the riches in the world."—Elizabeth Blackwell (1821-1910); the first female doctor in the United States

KEY TERMS

amniocentesis Method of prenatal diagnosis in which a needle is used to withdraw fluid from the amniotic sac within the uterus of a pregnant woman; the fluid withdrawn is tested for genetic anomalies.

autosomes Non–sex-determining chromosomes; humans have 22 pairs.

blastocyst An outer and inner cell layer from which an embryo develops; the stage at which implantation in the uterus lining occurs.

chorionic villus sampling (CVS) A method of genetic testing whereby a flexible catheter inserted through the vagina and cervix sucks out a tiny piece of chorionic villi tissue on the outermost layer of the amniotic sac.

chromosome A threadlike strand of DNA that carries genetic information.

chronic myeloid leukemia (CML) A cancer of the blood characterized by increased numbers of certain cells; results from the translocation or swapping of genetic material between chromosomes 9 and 22.

deoxyribonucleic acid (DNA) A type of molecule that encodes genetic information.

Down syndrome Genetic disorder causing a moderate to severe mental disability. It is marked by a sloping forehead, short broad hands with a single palmar crease, a flat nose or absent bridge, low-set ears, and generally dwarfed physique. Also called trisomy 21 because individuals have an extra chromosome number 21.

eugenics Improving a species through genetic engineering.

genetic engineering The alteration, replacement, or repair of genetic material by artificial means.

genome All the hereditary material possessed by an organism.

genomics The study of genes and their function.

homologous Having similar structure and anatomical position in different organisms suggesting a common ancestry or origin.

Huntington chorea or disease A rare inherited disorder that causes part of the brain to degenerate; symptoms usually are not obvious until adulthood. Dementia and death usually occur between ages 25 and 55 years.

liposome A synthetic, microscopic globule consisting of layers of lipids to encapsulate certain substances.

pharmacogenomics The study of how variations in the human genome affect the response to medications.

phenylketonuria (PKU) Hereditary disease caused by an enzyme deficiency; requires immediately starting a special diet to prevent complications such as mental retardation.

sickle cell anemia Hereditary, chronic form of anemia, affecting principally people of Mediterranean and African ethnic origins.

spina bifida Neural tube defect involving incomplete development of the brain, spinal cord, and/or their protective coverings caused by failure of the spine to close properly during development.

ultrasound Sound waves of extremely high frequency used to examine structures inside the body for diagnostic purposes; produces an image or photograph of an organ or tissue.

vector In medicine, a carrier; usually an insect; can be a virus.

LEARNING OUTCOMES

Upon successful completion of this chapter, you will be able to:

14.1   Define key terms.
14.2   Describe the work of the International Human Genome Sequencing Consortium.
14.3   Discuss the implications of genetically informed medicine.
14.4   Name at least six diseases that can be detected by genetic testing.
14.5   Compare voluntary and mandatory genetic screening.
14.6   Explain six reasons for genetic screening/testing.
14.7   Discuss the possible components of genetic counseling.
14.8   Identify uses for gene therapy.
14.9   Compare/contrast the following stem cells: embryonic, adult, umbilical cord, and amniotic fluid.
14.10   Identify the use of stem cell research in treating disease.
14.11   Trace the political conflict of stem cell research.
14.12   Discuss the use of stem cells in creating "new" organs and tissues.
14.13   Discuss the legal and ethical implications of genetic engineering.
14.14   State special considerations for health-care employees concerning any area in genetic engineering.

COMPETENCIES

CAAHEP

• Differentiate among legal, ethical, and moral issues affecting health care. (CAAHEP X.C.1)
• Identify the effect personal ethics may have on professional performance. (CAAHEP X.C.5)
• Develop a plan for separation of personal and professional ethics. (CAAHEP X.P.2)
• Examine the impact personal ethics and morals may have on the individual's practice. (CAAHEP X.A.3)

ABHES

• Comply with federal, state, and local health laws and regulations. (ABHES 4.f)

Do You Really Want to Know?

Maryann just turned 70. Every year on her birthday, she identifies goals for the coming year. This birthday is a major milestone. She realizes more than ever, even though her health is quite good, she has lived the better part of her life. Will she have 10 more years, perhaps 15, or only 5? She recalls her genetic heritage. She is an only child, and both parents are deceased—her father at age 88 and her mother at 85. Maryann worries about Alzheimer disease. Her mother began showing symptoms in her 70s. By the time of her death, she could not speak and did not recognize anyone. Maryann's aunt on her mother's side died of Alzheimer disease, and a cousin now is afflicted, also. Two of her dad's brother's had Alzheimer disease before their deaths. Maryann keeps her mind active, but she wonders about being tested to see if she has the genetic trait.

GENETIC ADVANCES

Recent advances in genetic engineering raise legal and ethical concerns never before considered. Giant strides have been made in the field of genetics since DNA (deoxyribonucleic acid) was first isolated, analyzed, and recognized in the nucleus of the cells in 1869 by Friedrich Miescher. In 1928, experiments showed that DNA carried genetic information, and its role in heredity was confirmed in 1952 by Alfred Hershey and Martha Chase (see Fig. 14-1.)

Genes are the pattern for heredity. Each gene directs cells to produce proteins and enzymes. The human genome is the complete set of genes present in virtually every body cell that is inherited from parents. Genes are organized in stringlike structures called chromosomes. Every individual inherits

Figure 14-1. DNA strand.

two sets of 23 chromosomes, one from each parent. There are two sets of 22 autosomes and one set of sex chromosomes.

In October 2004, the International Human Genome Sequencing Consortium, led by the United States with the Human Genome Research Institute and the Department of Energy, began working on encoding genes. Interestingly enough, it was originally estimated that there were more than 100,000 genes to encode; however, the Consortium later reduced that number to about 20,000 protein-coding genes in the human genome and identified another 2000 DNA segments that were predicted to be protein-coding genes. Scientists then discovered that the DNA segments were important; they learned how genes were switched on and off and that each human genome was different.

Scientists soon confirmed that to use genetics in the treatment of disease is quite complicated. However, even with this complexity, gene sequencing has allowed the investigation of genes to prevent or cure some diseases and to trace heritage. Many diseases are the result of a complex set of genetic and/or environmental causes. Inheriting certain harmful gene mutations increases the chance that a person will develop a specific disease. Much more research remains to be done, especially in the use of gene therapy to predict, prevent, and treat diseases.

GENETICALLY INFORMED MEDICINE

Genomics enables the analysis of every cell to better understand its growth, how its environment is invaded, and how, in the case of a cancer cell, it metastasizes. This research is then applied to targeting the damage in cells with treatment or medications that may result in correction. In some cancers, remission or sustained absence of tumors may result. In other words, it is now possible in some circumstances to learn enough about individual characteristics in a cell's DNA to specifically tailor a client's treatment. Such genetically informed therapy and medicine also look at the genome inherited from parents for markers that might be useful in determining risks for certain diseases.

Genetic research has made it possible for scientists to identify genes that play a major role in some cancers when the genes are damaged by mutations, rejoined, amplified, or inappropriately expressed in some way. For example, genetically influenced cancer medicine became quite successful in treating chronic myeloid leukemia (CML) once it was learned that the disease is dependent on a single mutation found in more than 95% of clients with that cancer. As a result, the drug Gleevec is now used for treating CML in clients with the mutation.

This type of research has shown effectiveness in the field of pharmacology, opening a new field in science called pharmacogenomics, the science of determining how genetics influences a medication's response. Pharmacogenomics is often able to determine whether a client will benefit from a particular drug, suggest the medication dosage, and identify possible effectiveness of the drug.

GENETIC SCREENING AND TESTING

Genetic research accompanies or is quickly followed by decisions related to genetic screening and testing. Approximately 4000 genetically related disorders have been identified. In some cases, genetic testing is helpful in determining treatment of a client's disorder. In others, no treatment or cure is possible even if genetic testing can detect both the carriers and the sufferers of many disorders.

A genetic disease or disorder is a disease caused by an abnormality in an individual's genome. The abnormality can range from minuscule to major—from a discrete mutation in a single base in the DNA of a single gene to a gross chromosome abnormality involving the addition or subtraction of an entire chromosome or set of chromosomes. Some genetic disorders are inherited from the parents. Other genetic diseases result from acquired changes or mutations in a preexisting gene or group of genes. Mutations can occur randomly or from some environmental exposure.

A DNA sample for genetic testing can be obtained from any tissue, but blood or a swab from inside the cheek is most often used. Cost of testing can range from about $100 to more than $2000 depending on the nature and complexity of the test. Health insurance plans may pay for the testing when recommended by a primary care provider. Genetic tests are used for several reasons and are identified here.

CARRIER SCREENING

Carrier screening is used to identify unaffected individuals (adults) who carry one copy of a gene for a disease requiring two copies for disease expression. Carriers are individuals who have an abnormal gene for a disorder but do not have any symptoms or visible evidence of the disorder. Risk is higher when one or both partners have a family history of certain disorders or have characteristics that increase the risk for having certain diseases. In this case, the screening is often performed to allow couples to make a choice about passing on a genetic abnormality to any offspring.

PREIMPLANTATION GENETIC DIAGNOSIS

Preimplantation genetic diagnosis (PGD) is used to detect genetic abnormalities before in vitro fertilization (see Chapter 15, Reproductive Issues). Developed in the 1980s, PGD is an alternative to prenatal diagnosis. PGD tests a single cell from the **blastocyst** for genetic disorders before implantation in the uterus. Not all genetic disorders can be diagnosed, however. PGD is likely used for couples with repeated pregnancy loss as a result of genetic disorders, couples with one child with a genetic disease who are at high risk for having another, and couples who wish to identify a tissue match for a sick sibling who can be cured with transplanted cells.

PRENATAL DIAGNOSTIC TESTING

Pregnant women often choose some form of prenatal diagnostic testing. **Ultrasound** can identify the size and gestational age as well as examine structures inside the fetus. It can detect some visible fetal anomalies, such as spina bifida and heart defects. A sampling of the mother's blood for serum alpha-fetoprotein testing can detect protein that may indicate neural tube defects, or Down syndrome. Chorionic villus sampling (CVS) is a test used to detect genetic defects as early as the 10th week of gestation. This test can detect chromosomal defects. It cannot test for certain brain and spine birth defects, however. In amniocentesis, a sample of amniotic fluid surrounding the fetus is taken. The fetal cells are then studied for genetic defects. The procedure is performed no earlier than at 14 weeks' gestation and is generally done between 16 and 18 weeks' gestation.

NEWBORN GENETIC SCREENING

Genetic testing of newborns is increasingly common, even required in most states. Phenylketonuria (PKU), a congenital disease resulting in serious neurological deficits in infancy, can be detected when infants are screened within 24 hours of delivery. PKU can be effectively treated with a diet that does not contain phenylalanine (an amino acid) or is low in phenylalanine.

Mandatory screening of all newborns for PKU began in 1960 and is now a law in most states. Also, 49 states and the District of Columbia mandate the testing of sickle cell disease in all newborns.

IN THE NEWS

In 2010, the National Collegiate Athletic Association (NCAA) Division 1 announced the requirement that all athletes be screened for sickle cell trait. This action was intended to help prevent sudden deaths of athletes who carry the trait. Persons with the trait are believed to be at higher risk for death from intensive exercise when their kidneys fail. This is especially critical when the athlete is not hydrated enough and is exercising in hot and humid weather. At least eight football players who carried the trait have died during intensive training since 2000.

PRESYMPTOM GENETIC TESTING

Presymptom genetic testing is performed to predict such adult-onset disorders as Huntington disease, cystic fibrosis, breast cancer, and Alzheimer disease. Diseases linked to a gene mutation are predictable if the mutated gene is inherited from a parent, causing offspring to have a 50% chance of getting the disease. Women who have the breast cancer susceptibility genes *(BRCA1* or *BRCA2)* are about five times more likely to develop breast and/or ovarian cancer than women without the mutation.

FORENSIC IDENTITY GENETIC TESTING

Forensic identity genetic testing is not done to detect disease; it is performed for legal purposes using DNA sequences to identify an individual for legal purposes, parentage, or in criminal investigations.

 ## GENETIC COUNSELING

Counseling most likely is a major component in any form of genetic testing and screening to determine the following:

- If there are family members with the disorder identified by the testing
- The cause of death in family members
- The health of all living first-degree relatives (parents, siblings, and children). In some cases the health of second-degree relatives (aunts, uncles, and grandparents) is also important.
- Ethnic background in which certain ethnic groups are at higher risk for certain disorders

Counselors who specialize in genetic counseling are often members of the National Society of Genetic Counselors (NSGC). These are individuals with knowledge and skills in both counseling and genetics. The NSGC and its members can help counsel individuals to:

1. Review family and medical histories.
2. Explain how genetic conditions are passed down through families.
3. Determine who is at risk for a disease.
4. Provide information about genetic conditions.
5. Offer guidance to help in making informed choices or life plans.
6. Provide information about testing options.
7. Assist in finding medical specialists and advocacy and support networks.

Genetic counseling can be especially pertinent if a particular disease detected is very debilitating or lethal. Surveillance can be increased when it becomes known that an individual is likely to develop a particular genetic disorder, hopefully catching a disease early while it may be most treatable. In some cases, such as breast or ovarian cancers, women have chosen prophylactic surgery to remove healthy breasts or ovaries and fallopian tubes to avoid the disease. Certain drugs have been created to reduce the risk for developing some cancers; such is the case with raloxifene, approved by the U.S. Food and Drug Administration (FDA) for postmenopausal women at higher risk for breast cancer.

 ## ETHICS CHECK

The results of genetic testing often pose difficult decisions. Individuals may choose not to have children when they learn their offspring will suffer a debilitating genetic disease. Pregnancies may be terminated if it is known that the fetus is unhealthy, malformed, or seriously compromised. Many prospective parents have neither the funds nor the stamina to face such an issue. If the results of the testing are positive but there is no prevention or cure, as in Huntington disease or Alzheimer disease, is there an advantage to be gained by knowing? Some will suggest that there is. Others will argue that not knowing is far less stressful. ●

Case Study

Bert Schurr is in the clinic of his primary care provider with a health insurance application. Bert has decided it is time to purchase a long-term health insurance policy to help defray expenses of any long-term illness in his later years. As the doctor looks over the application, he makes the comment, "Bert, you know, this might not work for you. Remember when we did the DNA testing for Huntington disease a few years back? You were concerned that if your older brother had it you could have it, too." "Yeah, but the test showed I was OK." "True, but the insurance carrier may still look at you as high risk." "Well, then just take that information out of my medical record."

What, if anything, can the doctor do at this point? Can Bert be discriminated against in this manner?

GENETIC DISCRIMINATION

Individuals seeking genetic screening or testing may be discriminated against when the results of their testing appears in medical records. There is a law to prevent discrimination based on genetic information in relation to health insurance and employment, but the law *does not* cover life, disability, or long-term care insurance. It also does not cover members of the military. The Genetic Information Nondiscrimination Act (GINA) of 2008 became fully effective in May 2010. However, life, disability, and long-term care insurance providers are skilled at "seeing through the haze" of blood testing reported in a client's health record to be able to determine whether the tests were likely ordered for genetic reasons. Because of this risk, some individuals will choose to pay for genetic testing out of pocket rather than to risk the results affecting their life, disability, or long-term care insurance coverage. Also, clients have the right to ask that providers not include any discussion related to genetic screening or testing in their medical record (see Chapter 9, Medical Records.)

GENE THERAPY

Identifying genetic causes of disease points in one direction—altering the human genome. A number of possibilities exist to change, prevent, and treat potentially harmful genes that put offspring at risk or put people at risk for disease in adult years. When gene mapping leads to any change or manipulation of the gene identified that causes illness or disease, this is known as gene therapy. There are a number of different approaches in gene therapy. It is possible to:

1. Place a normal gene within the genome to replace an abnormal one. (This is the most common technique.)
2. Swap an abnormal gene for a normal gene through homologous recombination; this is known as DNA crossover between two homologous DNA molecules.
3. Repair an abnormal gene through reverse mutation to return it to normal function.
4. Regulate the degree to which a gene is turned on or off or altered.

When a normal gene replaces an abnormal one (number 1 above), a vector is used to deliver the therapeutic gene to a client's target cells. Viruses are the most common vectors to date. Viruses have an effective way of encapsulating and delivering their genes to human cells to cause disease. Scientists have been able to manipulate the virus genome to replace the disease-causing genes with therapeutic genes. There are a number of nonviral options for gene delivery, but they either require large amounts of DNA, require the creation of an artificial liposome to transport the therapeutic DNA, or require chemically linking the DNA to a molecule that will bind to special cell receptors. Researchers are also experimenting with the creation and introduction of a 47th artificial chromosome into target cells.

Gene therapy is not without concern, however. If genes are to be replaced in the ovum or sperm, the replacement gene is passed on to the next generation. This can be beneficial or harmful. For example, two copies of the gene for sickle cell trait cause sickle cell disease. If you replace the two sickle cell genes with two normal genes, you also eliminate protection from malaria, which is provided by a single copy of the sickle cell.

ETHICS CHECK

With all the potential genetic research promises, ethical and legal dilemmas are raised. Some genetic tests do no more than tell persons that some day they will suffer from a dreadful and progressive disease. Genetic tests may force wrenching decisions to be made by parents who may choose to abort rather than give birth to a child carrying a gene for a lethal disease or a severe genetic defect. The questions in this arena that have not been addressed are "What is normal?" "What is a disability?" and "Who decides?" If genetic testing is done later in life and there is nothing to do to prevent or treat the disease, what has been accomplished? Is gene therapy performed in the adult cells of persons known to have a disease more or less ethical than gene therapy that selectively chooses the "healthiest" blastocyst and eliminates the unhealthy ones? Also, preliminary attempts at gene therapy are very expensive. Who is able to afford the expense? Who pays? ●

As research progresses in gene therapy, there is the potential to alter specific characteristics and appearance. At this point, technology conceivably moves from the genetic therapy for the correction of disease into social engineering for the creation of a "superior" human being. This is known as eugenics. Some are so fearful of this possibility that they believe all genetic research should be ended now. Others believe that the genetic age will create a society that is healthier and free from a number of debilitating illnesses.

Another question being debated is the use of patent rights to DNA. In fact, about 20% of the human genome is patented by the U.S. Patent and Trademark Office. The U.S. Department of Health and Human Services currently holds a gene patent that makes the protein the hepatitis A virus uses to attach to cells. About one-half of the genes that affect cancer are patented. A private corporation has patented a gene that plays a key role in early spinal cord development. Governments, private individuals, corporations, and research institutes have rushed to patent particular genes in order to claim ownership for future use and research. ●

The ethical debate is intense. Ethical questions arise. How can someone "own" my genes? More private corporations have gene patents in the United States than public entities. Whose right is it to own a gene? Who decides? Can laws keep up with gene technology?

STEM CELL RESEARCH

A major piece of genetic engineering relates to stem cell research. Stem cell research strives to cultivate and nurture stem cells, the basic cells of the body, so that they might be reproduced to other specific parts of the body. With the raw material for virtually every kind of human tissue, new treatments for a wide range of human diseases (diabetes, heart disease, some forms of cancer, and Parkinson disease) are now possible (Fig. 14-2). The controversy in stem cell research is not so much related to the method of research as it is to the source of the stem cells.

TYPES OF CELL TISSUES

Terms are defined below to explain some technical concepts presented throughout the following discussion on stem cell research.

- **Stem cells** are single cells that can regenerate and turn themselves into any one of the body's more than 200 cell types. They come from adult tissues (mostly blood and bone marrow), embryonic cells, and umbilical cord blood.

Figure 14-2. Stem cell manipulation.

- **Embryonic stem cells** are stem cells derived from embryos that develop from eggs that have been fertilized in vitro and then donated for research purposes with the consent of the donors.
- **Adult stem cells** are those that are found in many kinds of tissue, such as bone marrow, skin, and liver. Scientists more likely use the term *somatic* stem cell instead of *adult* stem cell because somatic refers to body cells rather than to germ cells, sperm, or eggs.
- **Umbilical cord stem cells** are collected from the umbilical cord at birth; they can produce all the blood cells in the body. Studies indicate that cord blood is useful in restoring blood cells to individuals who have undergone chemotherapy to destroy their bone marrow.
- **Amniotic fluid stem cells** are collected from amniotic fluid when an amniocentesis is performed. Scientists believe that cells at the very early stage of prebirth development can be directed to become virtually any cell in the human body.

Many expectant mothers plan to store their umbilical cord blood and/or fluid obtained through amniocentesis for future use in the life of their child should stem cell transplantation be warranted. Stem cells from a single placenta are enough to restore the blood and immune system of a child with leukemia. The stem cells in cord blood can help restore red blood cells in people with sickle cell anemia. Human cord blood contains as many stem cells as bone marrow and is much easier and safer to use as a transplant.

Of all these cells, the embryonic cells are the most versatile and the most controversial.

IN THE NEWS

The FDA gave a green light for a treatment derived from embryonic stem cells in July 2010. The University of California at Irvine and the Geron Corporation will test cells on clients with recent spinal cord injuries. Thomas B. Okarma, Ph.D., M.D., Geron's president and CEO, said, "Our goal is unchanged—to achieve restoration of spinal cord function by the injection of cells directly into the lesion site of the patient's injured spinal cord." The study will also explore other degenerative central nervous system (CNS) disorders, such as Alzheimer disease and multiple sclerosis.

Adult stem cells have shown promise in many arenas. In June 2010, vision was restored to individuals whose eyes had been damaged by caustic chemicals. Stem cells were taken from the person's healthy eye to be grown and multipled in the laboratory before being transplanted into the damaged eye. The cells were able to grow into healthy corneal tissue. In another example, out of desperation, an orthopedic surgeon at Boston University Medical Center drew bone marrow from his client's pelvic bone, condensed it to about 4 teaspoons of red liquid, and injected it back into the same client's ankle. The ankle had been broken but still refused to heal even after several surgeries. In four months, the ankle was healed.

Early in 2010 the Vatican announced it was funding research at the University of Maryland, where research was ongoing related to adult stem cells from the intestines. Maryland researchers said the Vatican is interested in supporting stem cell research that does not destroy embryonic stem cells, which the Catholic Church and religious conservatives have long opposed. Also, doctors in Italy have successfully transplanted two windpipes injected with the recipients' own stem cells. German doctors reported in 2010 that 191 persons with heart disease treated with their own bone marrow adult stem cells showed significant improvement in heart function, with decreased death and no side effects.

FETAL TISSUE RESEARCH

As early as the 1950s, scientists knew that fetal tissue cells held promise for medical research and advances in the treatment of numerous diseases and medical conditions including, but not limited to, Parkinson disease, Alzheimer disease, Huntington disease, spinal cord injury, diabetes, and multiple sclerosis.

Fetal tissue research, however, has had a rocky road. Federal funding for such research was severely restricted from the late-1980s to 1993. In 1993, President William Clinton issued an executive order lifting the ban on federal funding for research involving fetal tissue cells, especially those coming from induced abortions. The action was reversed, however, in 2001 when President George W. Bush said there would be no federal funding for stem cell research except for present existing cell lines. There would be no destruction of embryos (even spare frozen embryos, some abandoned and destined for disposal) used for stem cell research or human cloning.

President Bush took additional action in December 2005, in creating a new federal program to collect and store cord blood and expand the current bone marrow registry program to also include cord blood. The Act was known as the Stem Cell Therapeutic and Research Act of 2005. President Obama cleared the way in 2009 for new government spending on scientific research using embryonic stem cells. In doing so, he overturned the 8-year-old ban on government financing for the research first imposed by President Bush.

Major conflict still exists, however. ●

Case Law

In August 2010, Royce Lamberth, a federal district judge in Washington, D.C., overturned President Obama's decision to relax funding rules for research using embryonic stem cells and to allow the National Institutes of Health (NIH) to set the boundaries for that research. The judge wrote in his decision that the NIH guidelines, as well as the more restrictive Bush administration policy, violate the 1996 Dickey-Wicker amendment banning federal funds for research that destroys human embryos. Appeal from the White House was denied, and Lamberth said that to temporarily stay the injunction would violate Congress's will as expressed in the amendment. Lamberth wrote, "Congress remains perfectly free to amend or revise the statute. The court is not free to do so."

Such a decision should be no surprise because of the conflict in the United States between a medical community anxious to move forward on the frontiers of stem cell research and conservative activists who have moral and religious objections to any research that tampers with "human life."

A number of states have enacted legislation related to fetal tissue research. State laws may restrict the use of embryonic stem cells from some or all sources or specifically permit certain activities. The laws vary widely. California, Connecticut, Illinois, Iowa, Maryland, Massachusetts, New Jersey, and

New York encourage embryonic stem cell research. South Dakota and Nebraska strictly forbid research on embryos regardless of the source.

China, Japan, South Korea, Singapore, Israel, and the United Kingdom receive generous government support for fetal tissue research and have less political controversy than the United States. The conflict in the United States has created a strong trend toward private funding rather than government funding for research. The University of California at San Francisco and Stanford University have received substantial private grants. In addition, millions of dollars have come from the Howard Hughes Medical Institute, the Juvenile Diabetes Foundation, and the Michael J. Fox Foundation.

TISSUE AND ORGAN ENGINEERING

It is quite possible that cells can be cultivated from human embryonic stem cells that have the potential one day for allowing researchers to build custom-made organs. Somatic cell nuclear transfer (SCNT), or therapeutically cloned tissues, is very effective and more viable in terms of being accepted by a recipient because the tissues themselves can contain the same genetic structure as the recipient. Therefore, rejection of the tissue is avoided. If the nation can move past the debate on stem cell research to allow therapeutic cloning, it is conceivable that a person with liver failure could be implanted with a "neo-organ" made of identical liver cells and plastic fibers. Insulin-dependent diabetic patients may one day forego frequent insulin injections because of a semisynthetic pancreas. Synthetic skin is already available in the United States and has saved many lives. These synthetic tissues for organs are known as neo-organs.

Therapeutic cloning is still being developed, however, and is currently not viable for widespread medical application. Research funding for such technology is limited and quite political. Although Congress is presently highly partisan, researchers continue to remind its members that disease knows no political boundaries.

REPRODUCTIVE CLONING

Many said it would never happen. But it did. In February 1997, the first successful mammalian cloning took place in Scotland when a sheep, "Dolly," was cloned. One week later, Oregon successfully produced genetically identical rhesus monkeys through nuclear transfer. To date, cloning has been successful in cattle, rabbits, horses, deer, mice, goats, and pigs. This is called reproductive cloning. It is interesting to note, however, that the health and longevity of cloned animals is sometimes compromised. "Dolly" died prematurely in 2003 after developing arthritis and cancer, yet she was a mother to six lambs bred the old-fashioned way.

Internationally, cloning is controversial. The General Assembly of the United Nations adopted a measure to prohibit all forms of human cloning in August 2005 even though the vote was not unanimous. The basis for the decision was that human cloning was incompatible with human dignity and the protection of human life.

LEGAL AND ETHICAL IMPLICATIONS OF TISSUE CELL RESEARCH

Scientific developments and advances in technology give rise to moral and social issues of considerable complexity. It is difficult to identify all the legal and ethical implications of tissue research. Often there are more questions than answers.

In some cultures, tissue research and certainly human cloning of any form are forbidden. Other cultures and countries are more eager to step into this arena, always pushing science further into the future. Who monitors fraudulent or false research results? Should there be an international advisory group of scientists and ethicists to help determine how tissue research should move forward? If funding for tissue research comes mostly from private entities, who will claim ownership to the results? Should the political climate and leadership in any country determine whether tissue research advances? If tissue research has the potential for curing even one devastating disease, why would we not run as fast as possible toward a successful result? How can ethical guidelines and legal regulations keep abreast of medical technology? One thing is certain; tissue research is both exciting and frightening.

CONSIDERATIONS FOR HEALTH PROFESSIONALS

Genetic screening, testing, therapy, counseling, and tissue research are delicate topics. Because genetic engineering is continually evolving, it is imperative that health professionals remain knowledgeable and up to date on scientific discoveries. For clients to be open and honest about their concerns, all employees involved must demonstrate a professional attitude. Confidentiality must be protected. Informed consent of any procedure or testing is especially important. Employees' personal views on these matters should be fully explored before seeking employment in a facility that actively participates in any procedure related to genetic engineering. Also, those personal views should not be made known to clients during or after any decision-making process.

SUMMARY

Genetic engineering of any kind stimulates a number of legal and ethical issues. Legal guidelines are still limited; both legal and ethical concerns have difficulty keeping up with the medical technology and scientific research. The topics included in this chapter are very personal, intimate, and sensitive in nature. Privacy and confidentiality are imperative. As technology marches on, *compassion* and *care* are watch words for health-care professionals.

Watch It Now! Do you have a role in genetic engineering? at http://davisplus.fadavis.com/lawandethics

Questions for Review

SELECT THE BEST ANSWER

1. The human genome
   a. Is organized in boxlike structures called chromosomes.
   b. Has two sets of 23 chromosomes, one from each parent.
   c. Consists of 300,000 genes.
   d. Includes 12 sets of autosomes.
   e. All of the above.

2. Genetic diseases/disorders
   a. Number about 4000.
   b. Are caused by abnormalities in an individual's genome.
   c. Can be cured or corrected in most cases.
   d. All of the above.
   e. Only a and b above.

3. The NCAA requires all athletes to be screened for
   a. PKU.
   b. Sickle cell trait.
   c. Enlarged heart syndrome.
   d. Hypertension.
   e. Huntington disease.

4. The stem cell research that causes the most controversy are
    a. Adult stem cells.
    b. Umbilical cord stem cells.
    c. Embryonic stem cells.
    d. Amniotic fluid stem cells.
    e. Teenage stem cells.

5. Health-care professionals are expected to
    a. Be up to date and knowledgeable related to genetic research.
    b. Protect clients' confidentiality in all genetic-related matters.
    c. Keep their personal views on the subject to themselves.
    d. Be professional while demonstrating compassion and understanding.
    e. All of the above.

TRUE OR FALSE

T F   6. Eugenics means to improve a species through genetic engineering.

T F   7. Genomics is the study of liposomes and their function.

T F   8. Counseling most likely is a major component of any form of genetic testing and screening.

T F   9. GINA is a law to prevent discrimination based on genetic information in health insurance and employment.

T F   10. About 5% of the human genome is patented by the U.S. Patent and Trademark Office.

CLASSROOM EXERCISES

1. Should genetic screening or testing be mandatory for any disease? Support your answer.

2. Professor Joseph Fletcher, bioethicist and noted author, says, "It is unethical and morally wrong to deliberately or knowingly bring a diseased child into the world, or to turn a cold shoulder on prenatal tests. Never bring a baby into the world with anything more than minimally serious defects or disease." Discuss.

3. Paul Ramsey, professor of religion at Princeton University, says, "We cannot begin by bloodying ourselves with the killing of our own kind because they are defective in the womb, without also going into infanticide of similarly defective born infants." Discuss.

4. On a personal level, identify for yourself what is "normal" and what is "disabled?"

5. In a small group, debate the question, "Who is responsible for the care of severely disabled individuals?" Does the debate bring the group closer to or more distant from support of genetic research?

6. If you were Maryann in the vignette at the beginning of the chapter, would you want to know your genetic risk for Alzheimer disease? Research the genetic relationship in Alzheimer disease, comparing early-onset to later-onset disease. Does this information increase or decrease Maryann's risk?

7. Is adult stem cell therapy more or less ethical than embryonic stem cell therapy? Justify your response.

INTERNET ACTIVITIES

1. Access news and the latest information related to gene therapy at MEDLINEPLUS: Genes and Gene Therapy at **www.nlm.nih.gov/medlineplus/genesandgenetherapy.html.** What new information did you find?

2. Visit **www.cancer.gov** for the latest information on gene therapy in cancer treatment. Identify the cancers that can benefit from gene therapy.

3. Research **www.genetherapynet.com/united-states-of-america.html** to determine how gene therapy is regulated; summarize your findings.

WEB RESOURCES

Alzheimer's Disease Genetics Fact Sheet.
   www.nia.nih.gov/Alzheimers/Publications/geneticsfs.htm

Court Blocks New Federal Funding for Embryonic Stem Cell Research.
   www.foxnews.com

First Human Clinical Trial of Embryonic Stem Cell-Based Therapy Gets Green Light From FDA.
   www.seopressreleases.com

Harold Varmus (*Former Director of National Institutes of Health (NIH); Current Director of National Cancer Institute.) Returns to Politics.
   www.npr.org

Human Genome Project Information, Gene Therapy.
   www.ornl.gov/sci/techresources/Human_Genome/medicine/genetherapy.shtml

National Cancer Institute: Fact Sheet, BRCA1 and BRCA 2: Cancer Risk and Genetic Testing.
   www.cancer.gov/cancertopics/factsheet/Risk/BRCA

National Human Genome Research Institute, Genetic Information Nondiscrimination Act (GINA) of 2008.
   www.genome.gov

Stem Cell Research, National Conference of State Legislatures.
   www.ncsl.org

Who Discovered DNA?
   www.buzzle.com

 DavisPlus | For additional resources please visit http://davisplus.fadavis.com

CHAPTER 15

Reproductive Issues

"I have met brave women who are exploring the outer edge of human possibility, with no history to guide them, and with a courage to make themselves vulnerable that I find moving beyond words."—Gloria

Steinem; American feminist, journalist, social and political activist

KEY TERMS

conceptus General term referring to any product of conception.

heterologous artificial insemination Artificial insemination by donor (AID).

homologous artificial insemination Artificial insemination by husband (AIH).

infanticide A type of homicide consisting of killing the newborn.

mitosis The process by which the cell splits into two new cells, each having the same number of chromosomes as the parent cell.

ovum The female germ cell.

pulmonary surfactant A lipoprotein important in lung expansion in the neonate.

quickening The first perceptible movement of the fetus in the uterus.

spermatozoon The male germ cell.

surrogate A substitute or replacement.

therapeutic abortion Abortion performed to preserve the life or health of the mother.

viable Capable of living, surviving, and developing.

zygote The fertilized ovum; the cell produced by the union of gametes.

LEARNING OUTCOMES

Upon successful completion of this chapter, you will be able to:

15.1 Define key terms.
15.2 Describe female genital mutilation.
15.3 List the many methods of natural contraception.
15.4 Recall prescription contraception methods.
15.5 Identify sterilization for both male and female.
15.6 Discuss the correct use of the terms *abortion* and *miscarriage*.
15.7 Outline the process of fetal development.
15.8 List five theories of when life begins.
15.9 Explain the methods of abortion.
15.10 Discuss the Supreme Court decisions on abortion from 1973 to the present.

15.11   Discuss the "global gag" rule.
15.12   Explain AIH, AID, and IVF.
15.13   Discuss legal and ethical implications of reproductive health issues.
15.14   Identify important guidelines for health professionals in reproductive health services.

COMPETENCIES

CAAHEP

- Identify the effect personal ethics may have on professional performance. (CAAHEP X.C.5)
- Develop a plan for separation of personal and professional ethics. (CAAHEP X.P.2)
- Examine the impact personal ethics and morals may have on the individual's practice. (CAAHEP X.A.3)

ABHES

- Demonstrate professionalism by being cognizant of ethical boundaries. (ABHES 11.b.4)

VIGNETTE

Where Is She Today?

She realized today was her birthday. She wondered what she would be doing. Would she have a party? Would she be traveling? Was she happy and in love with life? Was she as beautiful as she pictured in her mind? Tears filled her eyes. It was difficult to realize that she was not a part of her special day. It was more difficult to realize that when she was born 20 years ago, she could not have been the mother she wanted to be. The decision to give her child up for adoption had been devastating, but even today she knew it had been right—far better than an abortion.

REPRODUCTIVE ISSUES AND RIGHTS OF WOMEN

There are a number of reproductive issues in today's world. Generally, the issues directly affect the lives of mostly women and cover a full range of reproductive health issues. When women's rights to make choices about their lives are threatened, the legal community is called into action. Whenever there is disagreement related to a woman's right to choose, the bioethical debate begins and includes masterful, thoughtful, and passionate opinions on both sides of the issue. Some reproductive issues include, but are not limited to, female genital mutilation, contraception, sterilization as a form of birth control, abortion, antiabortion terrorism, the global gag rule, assisted reproduction, and access to reproductive health information. Each of the many techniques for these topics will first be explored, and then the legal and ethical issues of each are identified.

FEMALE GENITAL MUTILATION

The World Health Organization (WHO) reports that there are nearly 170,000 girls and women in the United States and more than 140 million around the world who have been subjected to female genital mutilation (FGM). Although FGM is currently illegal in this country, the many immigrants from countries where FGM is regularly practiced continue to press legal and ethical boundaries in the United States. The practice is found in several places in African, Asian, and Middle Eastern countries. A mixture of cultural, social, and religious beliefs plays a strong role in the practice.

WHO identifies four major types of FGM, including partial or total removal of the clitoris (female circumcision), partial or total removal of the labia minora and/or labia majora, infibulation (narrowing the vaginal opening by creating a covering seal), and the pricking, piercing, scraping, or cauterizing of the genitals. Rationale given by those performing FGM is to prevent women from engaging in "illicit" sexual practices, thereby preserving the family honor, and to enhance sexual pleasure for men. Meanwhile, the practice severely limits or destroys a woman's capacity for sexual pleasure and can cause serious infections, even death if untreated. The practice can cause problems in urination, persistent urinary tract infections, difficulty with menstruation, chronic pelvic infections, infertility, fibrosis, pregnancy complications, and possible HIV infection.

All forms of FGM imposed on minors are illegal under federal law in the United States, and the practice has been condemned by human rights groups around the world. The Female Genital Cutting Education and Networking Project at **www.fgmnetwork.org** provides helpful and up-to-date information on FGM. The WHO further details the practice in their fact sheet at **www.who.int.** The WHO is particularly concerned about the increasing trend for medically trained personnel to perform FGM. In part, medical professionals have become involved, hoping to provide sanitary conditions and sterile instruments for the procedure in order to discourage the use of common knives, sharp stones, or machetes in very unclean environments. The WHO strongly urges health professionals not to perform such procedures or have any part in FGM.

CONTRACEPTION

There are more issues related to contraception than one might expect. For centuries, women have sought the means to enjoy sexual intimacy with a partner without the fear of pregnancy. In almost all instances and cultures, because the woman is the one who bears a pregnancy, the woman has been the one most responsible for the contraception. Aside from abstinence, which is 100% effective, there are a number of contraception options: fertility awareness (natural) methods, over-the counter methods, prescription options, and permanent methods (Table 15-1).

Fertility awareness methods (FAM) of contraception are neither mechanical nor the result of hormone manipulation. They require that a man and woman abstain from having sexual intercourse during the time when an ovum is most likely to be fertilized by a sperm. FAM requires accurate record keeping, a regular menstrual cycle, and cooperation of the male partner. The ovum is generally released about 14 days before a woman's menstrual cycle. The ovum survives for as long as 3 to 4 days or as little as 6 to 24 hours after ovulation; the sperm can live as little as 48 to 72 hours or as long as up to 5 days in fertile mucus. Therefore, the actual time during which a woman can become pregnant is measured in days or more than a week. FAM is often also used by couples desiring to become pregnant because it can reveal when a woman is most likely fertile and receptive to conception. Although it is not the purpose of this text to fully describe FAM, the Web site **www. medicinenet.com provides detailed information.**

Over-the-counter contraception methods do not require a prescription. They include condoms for both female and male, sponges, and spermicides. All these methods are a barrier form of protection, either covering the penis or being placed within the vagina, and are often used with spermicides. Spermicides come in the form of jelly, cream, or foam and as tablets or suppositories that dissolve. Some forms of spermicide block the entrance to the uterus; all act to disable or destroy the sperm. Condoms are one form of contraception that helps protect against sexually transmitted diseases (STDs) when used properly.

Prescription contraception includes birth control pills, the Ortho Evra Patch, NuvaRing, Depo-Provera shot, intrauterine devices (IUDs), diaphragms, caps, and shields.

The birth control pill is by far one of the most common methods of contraception. There are many brands, with the synthetic forms of hormones of both estrogen and progestin or only progestin. They both work by thickening the cervical mucus, making it hard for the sperm to get through, or in the case of the combination pill, preventing ovulation. There are even extended cycle pills that allow women to have fewer periods a year.

The Ortho Evra Patch, NuvaRing, Depo-Provera shot, and IUDs release synthetic estrogen and progestin, preventing ovulation and providing protection against pregnancy. IUDs are small T-shaped flexible plastic devices inserted into the uterus. Some IUDs can be left in place for as long as 10 years.

TABLE 15-1 Contraception Methods and Effectiveness When Properly Used		
Fertility Awareness Methods	Over-the-Counter Methods	Prescription Methods
70% to 85% effective	85% effective	90% to 98% effective
Calendar rhythm—counts days until ovulation	Male condoms—cover penis during intercourse	Birth control pill; thickens cervical mucus and/or prevents ovulation
Basal metabolic temperature (BMT)—daily measures of temperature to determine ovulation	Female condoms—reverse barrier pouch placed inside vagina	Patch—releases synthetic estrogen and progestin to prevent ovulation
Mucus inspection—cervical mucus produced before ovulation	Sponge—polyurethane foam placed inside vagina, often used with spermicide	Ring—inserted into vagina; releases synthetic estrogen and progestin to prevent ovulation
Symptothermal method; combines calendar, BMT, and mucus inspection	Spermicides—collect and destroy sperm; most effective when used with sponge or condom	Shot—injectable form of progestin; prevents ovulation
Ovulation prediction kits—measure amount of luteinizing hormone in urine		Intrauterine device (IUD)—T-shaped; inserted into uterus; releases progestin to prevent ovulation
Withdrawal—pulling out before ejaculation		Diaphragm and cervical caps—often used with spermicide; cover the cervix preventing barrier for semen
Lactational method—used for 10 to 12 weeks of breastfeeding		

Diaphragms and cervical caps or shields are barrier forms of contraception inserted before intercourse and removed 6 to 8 hours afterward, most often used with a spermicide. According to the Population Center for Research in Reproduction at the University of Washington, men may soon have some contraception options similar to those available for women. The options may include taking a daily pill, having a patch applied to the skin or an implant placed under the skin, or receiving an injection every 3 months for contraception.

EMERGENCY CONTRACEPTION

Emergency contraception (EC) is often referred to as the "morning-after pill." It will either prevent or delay ovulation, block fertilization, or keep a fertilized egg from implanting, depending on where a woman is in her menstrual cycle. EC is not the same as RU-486. (RU-486 is a pregnancy hormone drug used to induce abortion.)

STERILIZATION

Surgical sterilization has become the most popular form of contraception in the world; it is also considered permanent. In certain cases, sterilization can be reversed, but the success of reversal is not guaranteed. For this reason, sterilization is meant for men and women who do not intend to have children now or in the future. Individuals whose genetic testing indicates they are carriers for a serious disease sometimes also consider permanent sterilization.

Sterilization for women is called tubal ligation and involves cutting, tying, cauterizing, or clamping the fallopian tubes so that the ovum will not meet the sperm and pass into the uterus. Tubal ligations are performed abdominally or vaginally. A nonsurgical sterilization method for women is known as *hysteroscopic sterilization*. A long metal coil is passed through the cervix (via a scope) into the uterus and into the openings of the fallopian tubes. In a few months tissue grows over the coils, forming a plug that prevents sperm from fertilizing the ova as it travels from the ovaries to the uterus.

Sterilization for men is by vasectomy. The procedure requires a local anesthetic and a small bilateral incision into the scrotum. Each vas deferens is pulled out and ligated. It is important to check on this procedure to ensure that all the sperm have been discharged before sterility occurs. Two consecutive sperm counts must prove negative before any other contraceptive methods are discontinued.

Case Law

Parents of a minor and incompetent girl, K.M., petitioned through counsel to be appointed guardians of her person and her estate. They also wanted authorization to consent to her sterilization. K.M. has an IQ of 40 with a mental age of 6 to 7 years. Her independent functioning is severely limited. K.M.'s neurologist testified that she would never be able to exercise responsible judgment in sexual matters or in caring for a child. K.M. expressed to a counselor that she did not want to have children, but she may have been parroting what she heard her parents say.

The court ruled that K.M. could be sterilized, and her parents were granted authorization. Authorization was withheld, pending appeal.

Outcome: Upon repeal the decision was reversed and remanded. The court was found in error for not appointing independent counsel for K.M. Juvenile law, case summaries, re the guardianship of K.M., No. 25941-5-1 (Division one), September 16, 1991.

ABORTION

When contraception fails, women (and sometimes, but not always, their partners) can be faced with an unplanned pregnancy. Some couples will adjust their lives and reasons for not wanting a child at that time, embrace their pregnancy, and go on to love and provide for the child born to them. Others will choose a different route. The reasons chosen to terminate a pregnancy are many and varied. They include lack of income to raise a child, lack of a committed relationship, career paths that make a pregnancy particularly difficult, illness or age that is not conducive to childrearing, or even the emotional or physical inability to raise a child.

Abortion, the termination of pregnancy before the fetus is viable, is a highly emotional issue that elicits controversy no matter what the setting. Medically, the terms *abortion* and *miscarriage* both refer to the termination of pregnancy before the fetus is capable of survival outside the uterus. Accuracy related to fetal development is an important issue in understanding the dilemma attached to abortion choices.

Fetal Development

Fertilization occurs when a spermatozoon (sperm cell) unites with an ovum (egg). Normally, this takes place in the fallopian tubes, after which the fertilized ovum, now called a zygote, begins its journey to the uterus (womb). The zygote begins a process of mitosis (cell division) during the approximately 3-day journey to the uterus. Mitosis continues while the zygote floats freely in the uterus and begins to attach itself to the uterine lining. The proper term for this attached ball of cells is a *blastocyst*.

The blastocyst continues development and attachment to the uterus until firmly implanted at the end of the second week. Some authorities refer to the period from fertilization to gestational day 14 as the pre-embryonic period. From the third week until the end of the eighth week, the blastocyst is called an *embryo,* and this time period is referred to as the embryonic period. During this time, organ systems begin to develop, and some features take on a human shape.

At approximately the eighth week, the embryo becomes known as a fetus and is marked by the beginning of brain activity. The term *fetus* is used until the time of birth, usually 9 months after fertilization. Rudimentary formation of all organ systems is complete by gestational week 16. Further maturation of the body systems and organs essential for survival outside the uterus occurs after week 24 when the pulmonary surfactant is formed. The 9-month gestational period is generally divided into three segments, or trimesters. The first trimester is from fertilization to 3 months; the second trimester is from 3 to 6 months into the pregnancy; and the third trimester is from 6 to 9 months (Table 15-2).

WHEN DOES LIFE BEGIN?

Most definitions of abortion refer to the viability of a fetus. *Viability* means capacity for living and generally refers to a fetus that has reached a certain gestational age and weight and is capable of living outside the uterus. The time of viability is changing. In past years it was rare for an infant to

TABLE 15-2	Fetal Development	
End of Week	Size and Weight	Representative Changes
4	$^3/_{16}$ in	Eyes, nose, and ears not yet visible. Backbone and vertebral canal form. Small buds that will develop into arms and legs form. Heart forms and starts beating.
8	$1^1/_4$ in $^1/_{30}$ oz	Ossification begins. Limbs become distinct as arms and legs. Digits are well formed. Major blood vessels form. Size is like a kidney bean.
12	3 in 1 oz	Eyes almost fully developed, but eyelids still fused; external ears present. Appendages are fully formed. Heartbeat can be detected. Body systems continue to develop. Size is a little more than 3 inches.
16	$6^1/_2$-7 in 4 oz	Head large in proportion to rest of body. Face takes on human features, and hair appears on head. Many bones have ossified, and joints begin to form.
20	10-12 in $^1/_2$-1 lb	Head is less disproportionate to rest of body. Fine hair covers body. Rapid development of body systems. Eyebrows and lashes appear.
24	11-14 in $1^1/_4$-$1^1/_2$ lb	Head becomes even less disproportionate to rest of body. Bone marrow begins to make blood cells. Lungs continue to develop, but do not produce surfactant.
28	13-17 in $2^1/_2$-3 lb	Head and body are more proportionate. Skin is wrinkled and pink. Rapid brain development.
32	$16^1/_2$-18 in $4^1/_2$-5 lb	Testes descend into scrotum. Bones of head are soft. Rapid increase in body fat occurs. Body begins storing iron, calcium, and phosphorus.
36	20 in 7-$7^1/_2$ lb	Additional subcutaneous fat accumulates. Nails extend to beyond fingertips. Head hair thickens.

survive if born before 28 weeks of gestation. (A full-term birth is between 37 and 40 weeks of gestation.) Modern technology has made it possible for about a 9.8% survival rate at 22 weeks, 53% at 23 weeks, and 67% at 24 weeks. The term "extreme preemies" is often used to identify those born before 26 weeks of gestation, and these infants often have ongoing health issues.

Five possible considerations of when life begins are commonly identified as (1) at the time of conception; (2) when the brain begins to function, usually at 8 to 12 weeks; (3) at the time of quickening, 16 to 18 weeks; (4) at the time of viability, from 20 to 35 weeks; and (5) at the time of birth (Fig. 15-1).

The religious community often weighs in on the life issue. Judaism, Christianity, and Islam religions use their religious texts, human reasoning, and teaching authorities to make ethical decisions and recommendations. Yet, within these three traditions, there is great variation. Some religious scholars believe that God creates all life and that the embryo is a human being with rights from the moment of conception. Roman Catholics comprise one religious group that claims that life begins at conception because the zygote carries the entire genetic code for a new human being. Abortion is considered a sin against life. Buddhists, who believe in reincarnation, also believe that life begins at conception. This theory is seen in the Chinese and Korean cultures, which count a child as 9 months or 1 year old at the time of birth. A number of religious groups do not take a stand on the status of the fetus and take both the life of the mother and the fetus into account when confronting decisions on abortion.

Another determination for the beginning of life is at the time the brain begins to function. Proponents of this theory believe the fetus cannot be a human without a functioning brain. Because there is strong support for the idea that death occurs when the brain ceases to function, it may be logical to believe that life occurs when the brain begins to function.

Quickening has been determined by some to be the beginning of life. Aristotle believed that before quickening, the human fetus had only a vegetable or animal soul. Another reason for this position perhaps is that women truly feel "life" at the time of quickening.

The idea that life begins when the fetus is viable or can live independently of the uterus is partly based on the premise that if the fetus indeed can live on its own, life has begun. More variation of time is allowed in this theory if you consider that viability may be sometime between 20 and 35 weeks.

Those who believe that life begins only at the time of actual birth believe so because now the being can be seen, can be held, and is perceived as being fully human. Interestingly, the law states that because viability varies so much, each abortion case needs to be considered on its own.

METHODS OF ABORTION

The method of abortion depends to a great extent on the stage of the pregnancy. Both medicinal and surgical methods are presented.

Mifepristone is a pregnancy hormone drug often referred to as RU-486. It has been available for use in the United States to induce abortion since 2000. When a woman discovers she is pregnant,

Figure 15-1. When does life begin?

she may take RU-486 up to 63 days from her last menstrual period. The pill blocks the production of progesterone. Forty-eight hours later, the woman takes misoprostol, a prostaglandin, which makes the cervix dilate and the uterus contract. Mifepristone is often preferred because it is noninvasive, has no risk of infection, requires no anesthesia, is less expensive, and offers greater privacy to women. It can be used in the early stages of pregnancy. Millions of women around the world have used mifepristone since it first became available in the late 1980s in France.

Another combination medication for pregnant women who want a nonsurgical abortion is methotrexate and misoprostol. Studies show these drugs take longer because the woman typically first takes a dose of methotrexate that is followed by misoprostol 2 to 3 days later. Misoprostol is administered either via the inner cheek or gum or vaginally. Most woman abort within 24 hours in what seems like a heavy menstrual flow. A follow-up visit to the provider is made within 7 days after the administration of methotrexate to determine completion of the abortion. Both medicinal methods are 95% to 98% effective.

An approved method of abortion when the pregnancy is less than 7 weeks from the last menstruation is called *menstrual extraction*. In this procedure, a tube with a suction device is inserted through the cervix into the uterus (dilation is usually unnecessary). Within 1 to 2 minutes, the lining of the uterine wall and the conceptus are suctioned out. A woman undergoing this procedure may experience cramping, nausea, and faintness. It is commonly performed in the ambulatory healthcare setting.

To terminate pregnancy between the 7th and 14th weeks, a suction abortion and curettage may be performed. The woman may be sedated or a local anesthetic given while the cervix is dilated to permit suction and scraping of the uterine lining. Cramping, nausea, and vomiting may follow the procedure. The client can go home approximately 2 hours later. These methods of abortion occur in the first trimester up to the end of the 13th week of pregnancy.

A second-trimester abortion, at 14 to 24 weeks, is usually a two-step dilation and evacuation procedure that can take up to 2 days. The cervix is gradually dilated over a period of time. The procedure is accomplished by using a combination of suction, curettage, and manual evacuation of the fetus and placenta. This procedure is more uncomfortable than previous methods identified, often requiring local anesthesia.

A procedure known as intact dilation and extraction (D&X) or partial-birth abortion (not a medical term recognized by the American Medical Association [AMA]) is a controversial procedure, both legally and ethically, that was prohibited by law in 2003. D&X involved an intrauterine decompression of the skull.

Saline-induced abortion is rarely performed today, even though 20 years ago it was the only viable means of aborting a mid-second-trimester pregnancy. In very rare cases, a hysterotomy or hysterectomy is performed to remove the fetus surgically. These latter two procedures usually are performed only in the case of uterine abnormalities.

Generally, the later an abortion of any type is performed, the greater the risk. Most abortion providers are obstetricians and gynecologists, but their numbers have decreased, and medical students can opt out of training for the procedure.

The Centers for Disease Control and Prevention (CDC) maintain statistics in the United States related to abortions (**www.cdc.gov/reproductivehealth/Data_Stats/Abortion.htm**). Reporting is optional, but 46 areas have consistently reported since 1996. The reporting areas are the 50 states and the District of Columbia.

ANTIABORTION TERRORISM

Reflected in the volatility of the abortion issue is the amount of violence expressed by antiabortionists to individuals who perform abortions and to their clinics. Violent acts include arson, bombings, stabbings, and shootings. Eight providers have been shot to death since 1993, and five more suffered serious injuries from gunshot wounds. Offenders justify their acts on the basis that they are preventing the death of unborn children.

These actions are extreme. Other actions may include carrying banners near abortion clinics, approaching clients asking if they can pray for them as they enter the clinics, and distributing print material in opposition to abortion. Some antiabortion groups practice civil disobedience, attempting to disrupt and block abortion clinic activities. These acts have resulted in a great deal of litigation and added to the complexity of the abortion issue.

 In *Schenck v Pro-Choice Network,* 519 US 357 (1997), the U.S. Supreme Court addressed the question of whether an injunction that places restrictions on demonstrations outside abortion clinics violates the First Amendment. Health-care providers and others wanted to restrict blockades and other disruptive activities in front of abortion clinics. The U.S. District Court created a "fixed-buffer zone," prohibiting demonstrations within 15 feet of entrances into abortion clinics, parking lots, or driveways. The court also created a "floating-buffer zone," prohibiting demonstrators from coming within 15 feet of people or vehicles wishing access to abortion clinics. The U.S. Supreme Court held that the fixed buffer zones were constitutional because they protected the government's right to protect public safety. Floating buffer zones were later found unconstitutional because they imposed a greater burden on free speech (First Amendment). ●

GLOBAL GAG RULE

An example of the power of politics in human rights is acutely demonstrated in the global gag rule. In 1984 President Ronald Reagan established a federal rule that blocked U.S. funds being given to international family-planning groups that offered abortion and abortion counseling even if the money was targeted for a different health-care need. President Bill Clinton ended the gag rule in 1993, but it was reinstated by President George W. Bush in 2001. It was rescinded by President Obama very early in his administration—January 2009. Throughout this period, Planned Parenthood of America announced that it would not comply with the gag rule, preferring to do without the funds rather than to change their policies of providing comprehensive services and counseling related to the reproductive rights of women.

ASSISTED REPRODUCTION

Recent scientific and technologic innovations in assisted reproduction have caused rethinking of the concepts of family, parenthood, and human sexuality. The biological concept of family considers those who are genetically related to be a family. However, this does not include the broader cultural customs and kinships that define family.

Societal laws determine the definition of family. There are laws on adoption, artificial insemination, surrogacy, foster placement, custody arrangements, and removal of children from homes where they are neglected or abused. There are, however, few laws related to assisted reproduction. Yet, assisted reproduction raises such complex issues as the right to privacy, the right to make childbearing decisions, the interpretation of any existing statutes that may relate to this issue, public policies regarding termination of parental rights, and the role of financial compensation in assisted reproduction. All of these issues create a continuing challenge to accept and embrace a broader view of human sexuality and family.

Assisted reproduction choices can strain the family unit, the legal system, the health-care team, and the personal values of all involved. Any health-care professional, whether in an ambulatory care setting or a hospital, cannot adequately function without knowledge of these concerns and their legal and ethical implications.

Assisted reproduction is a reality. Artificial insemination, in vitro fertilization, and surrogacy have captured popular attention. The use of semen from either a husband or a donor; the fertilization of the ovum in the laboratory for later transplantation in the uterus, fallopian tube, or peritoneum; the use of frozen sperm and embryos; and the services of a surrogate mother provide alternatives to traditional modes of procreation.

ARTIFICIAL INSEMINATION

Artificial insemination is not a complicated procedure. It is simply the mechanical injection of viable sperm into the vagina, cervical canal, or uterus. This method has been practiced for hundreds of years by breeders seeking to enhance their stock. The first successful artificial insemination in humans occurred during the 1950s but was predated by centuries of scientific study and experimentation. Today, more than 45,000 children are born by artificial insemination each year.

Artificial insemination is described as (1) homologous, artificial insemination by husband (AIH) or (2) heterologous, artificial insemination by donor (AID). AIH might be used when a husband's sperm vitality is too low or a wife's cervical mucus is too hostile to achieve conception. Semen collected and concentrated over a few days often can overcome a low sperm count or a sperm vitality problem. AID might be used when the partner is sterile or carries serious genetic defects. It has also been used by women who want to have children but who choose not to have sexual intercourse with men.

Obstetricians and gynecologists are asked about AIH and AID almost daily. These specialists and their employees should be able to discuss the topic with intelligence and understanding. Women are sometimes referred by their primary care providers to fertility clinics found in most major cities.

IN VITRO FERTILIZATION

The development of in vitro fertilization (IVF) (literally, "fertilization in glass") is the process of fertilizing the ovum in a culture dish, allowing it to grow, and then implanting it in the uterus. It is the most well known of assisted reproduction techniques. Successful IVF and embryo transfer in humans were first achieved in 1978. Today nearly 3 million babies have been born as the result of IVF. One of the creators of IVF in humans, Robert G. Edwards, won the Nobel Prize for medicine in 2010 for his pioneering in IVF.

A benefit of IVF is that it allows many women who are infertile because of blocked fallopian tubes or oviducts to bear children. The woman is given fertility drugs to stimulate the ovaries to produce more eggs. Then the ovum is removed from the potential mother and placed in a dish containing blood serum and nutrients. Sperm is added. Once an ovum is fertilized, it is then transferred to another dish, where for the next 3 to 6 days it divides, creating a cluster of cells called a blastocyst. The blastocyst is placed in the uterus, where it attaches to the wall and development proceeds.

A number of options are available today to assist with IVF, including gamete intrafallopian tube transfer (GIFT), zygote intrafallopian transfer (ZIFT), intracytoplasmic sperm insertion (ICSI), and follicle aspiration (FASIAR). For a more detailed explanation of each, go to **www.IVF-Infertility.com.** Some fertility providers transfer more than one embryo in order to improve the pregnancy success rate. This practice, however, can lead to multiple births. Widespread attention was given to Nadya Suleman, the mother of octuplets born in California in 2009, the result of IVF. The birth of Suleman's babies caused increased discussions related to ethics and limits of IVF.

A test that screens for genetic flaws among embryos fertilized through IVF is called pre-implantation genetic diagnosis (PGD). (Refer to Chapter 14, Genetic Engineering.) With PGD, DNA samples from embryos are analyzed for gene abnormalities that can cause disorders. These results can be used by fertility specialists to select only mutation-free embryos for implantation into the mother's uterus. Before PGD, the only options individuals had for determining whether there were fetal abnormalities were chorionic villus sampling (CVS) in the first trimester or amniocentesis in the second trimester. If abnormalities were found in either trimester, individuals had to determine whether or not to terminate the pregnancy.

SURROGACY

If a woman's eggs and uterus are nonfunctioning, the sperm of her male partner can be injected into another woman's (surrogate) ovum for fertilization. This "surrogate" carries the baby to term. In another scenario, a woman's eggs are retrieved, inseminated by her partner's sperm, and then transferred to the uterus of another woman who is considered to be a gestational surrogate. Also, donor eggs and donor sperm can be used to create an embryo that is placed in the uterus of a gestational surrogate. In a gestational surrogate, none of these individuals is genetically related to the child, and an adoption procedure is recommended for legal parentage.

ACCESS TO REPRODUCTIVE HEALTH SERVICES

Often at issue is the availability of reproductive health services for women. Today, contraception is widely available to any who choose to practice contraception, but that was not always the case. In the not too distant past, condoms and spermicides were kept behind the counter in a pharmacy, and the calendar rhythm method of FAM was not well understood. With the inception of prescription contraception, medical providers became more involved in reproductive health services. Women might have to travel to a larger community where Planned Parenthood clinics could provide a prescription if a country doctor would not.

Sterilization allowed women greater control over their bodies but was originally fraught with much controversy. In some religious communities, sterilization was a far greater sin than the use of contraception. Sterilization was performed by only a few providers, and the written consent of both the woman and her partner was necessary. Tubal ligations, most performed in hospitals, were not allowed in hospitals with religious connections. Today, most sterilizations are performed in the ambulatory care setting, and only the consent of the participant is necessary.

The availability of abortion is just one of the many issues of concern. "Conscience clauses" allow institutions and providers the right to opt out of providing abortion care. Many providers are employees in group practices, hospitals, and health maintenance organizations that prohibit abortion. Catholic hospitals in the United States are even more restrictive, prohibiting sterilization, contraception, condom distribution, fertility treatment, and some emergency pregnancy terminations.

During the past two decades, Congress has debated the limited circumstances under which federal funding for abortion should be allowed. For a brief period of time, coverage included cases of rape, incest, life endangerment, and physical health damage to the woman. However, beginning in 1979, those services were gradually eroded, leaving the states to determine under what circumstances abortions are to be performed for women on Medicaid. To date, the number of states permitting abortions for all or most health reasons to low-income women is limited to 17 (Fig. 15-2). The present version of the Hyde Amendment requires coverage of abortion in cases of rape, incest, and life endangerment. South Dakota legislators have chosen to be noncompliant with the Hyde Amendment. The new Healthcare Reform bill of 2010 says individuals receiving federal subsidy dollars must use their private money to pay for coverage of abortion except in cases of rape, incest, or to save the life of the mother.

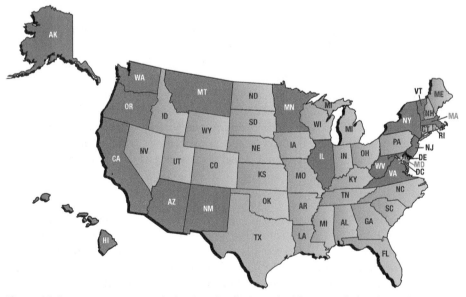

Figure 15-2. Seventeen states permit abortions for all or most health reasons for low-income women.

For the 7.3 million couples in the United States who struggle with infertility, the new health-care bill also carries no mandates to cover the soaring cost of assisted reproduction procedures like IVF and egg donation. Very few private insurers pay for assisted reproduction techniques, either. The cost of one round of IVF can be as high as $15,000, making it out of the reach of even moderate-income families.

Access to reproductive health care or any health care for that matter, is even more difficult in a depressed economy.

LEGAL AND ETHICAL IMPLICATIONS OF REPRODUCTIVE ISSUES

FEMALE GENITAL MUTILATION

As stated earlier, FGM is illegal in the United States under federal law, and Congress is trying to do more to ensure that the practice is completely eradicated. U.S. Representatives Mary Bono Mack, Republican from California, and Joseph Cowley, Democrat from New York, introduced in 2010 the Girls' Protection Act that would make it a crime to transport minors outside the United States for the purpose of performing FGM. This act would amend the federal criminal code and impose a fine and/or 5-year prison term. On April 26, 2010, the bill was referred to the House Committee on the Judiciary. On June 15, 2010, the bill was referred to the Subcommittee on Crime, Terrorism, and Homeland Security. To date, there has been no further action.

Ethically, it is rather easy to oppose such a practice. What is more difficult is to provide adequate and professional reproductive health care to the girls and women who are victims of FGM. Health-care professionals in ambulatory care are most likely to see these women only long after the procedure has been performed. They must be treated with dignity, respect, and compassion with no hint of repulsion. Many may still be living within the family and culture that performed the procedure.

CONTRACEPTION

Contraception is legal in the United States, and most barriers for service have long been lifted. It still is an ethical and bioethical issue in a number of circles, however. The Roman Catholic Church opposes contraception and denies access to it in their hospitals. In the Old-Order Amish tradition, all types of artificial birth control are forbidden, including any variety of natural family planning. Today, however, women in Amish communities are beginning to use contraception, as are many Catholics.

The other issue with contraception comes from the debate, especially in families with teenagers, of the availability of contraception to their sons and daughters. Nearly all parents prefer and support abstinence as the best prevention of unwanted pregnancy. Some parents prefer that contraception not be available to teens; others prefer contraception be used when their sons and daughters become sexually active. The majority do not condone an abortion. Today, many teenagers resort to oral sex as a way to avoid pregnancy, even though it is not a protection against STDs and may even contribute to the increase of STDs.

ABORTION

In the United States, as states turned away from English common law during the late 18th and early 19th centuries, statutory criminal law began to address abortion. In 1821, Connecticut, and then in 1828, New York, passed abortion laws making post-quickening abortion a felony and pre-quickening abortion a misdemeanor. This process continued through to the 1830s and 1850s, respectively. In the 19th century, abortion regulations tightened. By the late 1860s, throughout most of the United States, abortions were prohibited except to preserve the life of the mother. Those laws and subsequent ones remained in place until the 1960s and 1970s, when many states liberalized their abortion laws.

One of the monumental decisions affecting a change of all abortion laws was the 1973 U.S. Supreme Court *Roe v Wade* decision. Jane Roe (a pseudonym) was a single, pregnant woman who took action against Henry Wade, the District Attorney of Dallas County, in 1970. Roe pleaded the 14th Amendment and her "right to privacy," claiming that the Texas antiabortion statute was unconstitutional.

As a result, 3 years later, the Supreme Court held that during the first trimester, pregnant women have a constitutional right to abortion, and the state has no vested interest in regulating abortion at that time. During the second trimester, the state may regulate abortion and insist on reasonable standards of medical practice if an abortion is to be performed. During the third trimester, the state interests override pregnant women's rights to abortion, and the state may "proscribe abortion except when necessary to preserve the health or life of the mother."

Although this court decision did "favor" Roe, many unanswered questions resulted, and states began to apply restrictions. In the 1973 *Doe v Bolton* case, the Supreme Court struck down four pre-abortion procedural requirements: (1) residency, (2) performance of the abortion in a hospital accredited by the Joint Commission on Accreditation of Healthcare Organizations (JCAHO), (3) approval by a committee of the hospital's medical staff, and (4) consultations. It also had a "conscience clause" stating that physicians and medical employees could refuse to participate in abortions without being discriminated against.

Another U.S. Supreme Court decision in 1976 ruled, on constitutional grounds, that spousal and parental consent is not necessary for an abortion. Currently courts tend not to differentiate between minor and adult pregnant women. A 1978 U.S. Supreme Court decision held that a state may not constitutionally legislate a blanket, unreviewable power of parents to veto their daughter's abortion.

In June 1977, three related cases, *Beal v Doe, Maher v Roe,* and *Poelker v Doe,* resulted in Supreme Court decisions affecting abortion laws. The ruling stated "the states have neither a constitutional nor a statutory obligation under Medicaid to provide non-therapeutic abortions for indigent women or access to public facilities for the performance of such abortions."

In 1983, the Supreme Court reaffirmed the *Roe v Wade* decision when it heard *Akron v Akron Center for Reproductive Health, Inc.* In Akron, Ohio, three physicians and the center brought suit against the city, challenging the constitutionality of city provisions that regulated abortion performance. The city had passed an ordinance requiring that (1) second-trimester abortions be performed in hospitals, (2) specific information be given by physicians to patients undergoing abortion, (3) there be a 24-hour waiting period between consent and performance of the abortion, and (4) there be specific procedures about how physicians were to dispose of the fetal remains. The case was appealed to the U.S. Supreme Court, which found all provisions unconstitutional except for the hospitalization requirement for second-trimester abortions.

In a similar case in 1986, the U.S. Supreme Court again reaffirmed *Roe v Wade*. In *Thornburgh v American College of Obstetricians and Gynecologists,* the Supreme Court ruled against the following issues: informed consent and printed information that would have required a physician to provide information 24 hours before the abortion related to available medical assistance benefits; the father's liability for assistance; a description of alternatives to abortion; possible detrimental effects not foreseeable; and medical risks of the abortion, as well as of carrying the child to full term. In addition, the Supreme Court struck down a ruling that would have required physicians to determine whether the fetus was viable and to report to the State Department of Health specific information normally considered private. This information would have included such items as the woman's age, race, number of pregnancies, marital status, and date of last menses. This information was to be open for public inspection without the woman's name. The Supreme Court ruled against physician involvement in postviability care for the child and the requirement for a second physician at postviability abortions.

In 1991, the U.S. Supreme Court upheld the federal rule that banned abortion counseling at federally funded clinics. This ban affected approximately 4000 clinics serving more than 4.5 million women, mostly with low incomes. The result was that these clinics could not mention abortion as an option. What became known as the "gag rule" continues to seesaw back and forth in the political world rather than in the courts.

In July 1992, the U.S. Supreme Court, in *Planned Parenthood v Casey,* ruled that Pennsylvania's requirement that spouses be notified before abortion was an "undue burden." In June 2000, the U.S.

Supreme Court ruled on *Stenberg, Attorney General of Nebraska, et al. v Carhart,* stating that Nebraska's law was unconstitutional. Nebraska law prohibited any "partial-birth abortion" unless that procedure was necessary to save the mother's life. Nebraska held that this was a violation of the law and was a felony. Further related to this issue, however, the Partial-Birth Abortion Ban Act became law in 2003, prohibiting partial-birth abortion. In 2007, the constitutionality of the law was upheld by the U.S. Supreme Court.

In 2003, *Scheidler v NOW; Operation Rescue v NOW,* the U.S. Supreme Court dissolved the 10-year permanent injunction prohibiting protesters from demonstrating outside abortion clinics. In 2006, *Ayotte v Planned Parenthood of Northern New England* challenged the New Hampshire law that requires a parent be notified 48 hours before an abortion is provided to a minor. The Supreme Court held the law unconstitutional because it did not permit an immediate abortion without notifying a parent in medical emergencies that threaten a minor's health.

A number of state lawmakers, disenchanted with *Roe v Wade* and the resultant unsuccessful challenges in the U.S. Supreme Court, have begun to take action on their own. South Dakota banned most abortions in that state, in direct conflict with the U.S. Supreme Court, with the full intention of creating a constitutional challenge. Even though the governor signed the bill in South Dakota, abortions have not stopped and will not stop until the law passes through all the court challenges stacked up against the constitutionality of the act.

IN THE NEWS

As of November, 2011, the Guttmacher Institute reports the following: 36 states require some parental involvement in a minor's decision to have an abortion or allow for an alternative process, such as a judicial bypass procedure or the involvement of a grandparent or other adult relative. Thirty-two of the states that require parental involvement make exceptions either in the case of a medical emergency or in the case of abuse, assault, incest, or neglect (www.guttmacher.org/statecenter/spibs/spib_PIMA.pdf).

In March 2010, the Patient Protection and Affordable Care Act (PPACA) was passed. This act includes the Nelson Amendment, named for its sponsor, Senator Ben Nelson, Democrat from Nebraska. The amendment restricts the means by which insurers can offer insurance coverage for abortion in the state insurance exchanges that will be created by 2014 as part of the National Healthcare Reform Act of 2010.

At least 11 states are considering legislation to effectively limit or ban abortion: Alabama, Georgia, Indiana, Kentucky, Louisiana, Missouri, Mississippi, Ohio, Oklahoma, Tennessee, and Virginia. Other legal challenges continue, and more Supreme Court decisions are expected. The majority of abortion questions arise over the 14th Amendment and the equal protection clause. Every citizen of the United States has "equal protection of the law" and shall not be discriminated against. This includes abortion. The parties are testing the courts on these constitutional issues.

Ethically, there are a number of issues. Is it discriminatory for a woman who has money and insurance coverage to receive an abortion but for a woman who is poor and relies on Medicaid to be denied an abortion? Will this withstand the scrutiny of the court on the issue of discrimination? Another trend in the states is the push to confer personhood status upon fertilized eggs through state constitution amendments, via the ballot measure process. These initiatives have arisen from the Personhood USA movement that realizes the measures "would likely fail if proposed in the legislature" but have a stronger possibility of passing through the ballot measure process. The status of the fetus in any abortion procedure is still most controversial. When does the fetus become a person with the same rights as those who are born?

The abortion issue and abortion law are in a state of flux. Radical changes have occurred during the past 100 years. The political climate, moral attitudes, advances in medical technology, and impact of current abortion laws will influence the next 100 years.

An individual who believes there are reasons to justify a legal abortion likely believes a pregnant woman's right to choose is paramount to the rights of the unborn. Proponents of this theory are often referred to as "pro-choice." Individuals who believe the fetus is innocent, weak, and helpless and that its right to life should be protected at all costs are usually referred to as "pro-life." These individuals often believe abortion is murder and that to allow it is to also condone infanticide. The rights of the fetus and newborn are paramount to the rights of any others. The majority of individuals stand somewhere in the middle of these two theories. These are the advocates who believe that abortion is permissible to save the life of the mother (therapeutic abortion) or in the case of rape or incest.

One may expect that religion offers a solution to the question of when life begins, but there is no consensus or agreement that settles the issue. A few religious groups propose that abortions be performed only when necessary to save the mother's life. Some religious groups determine a time or establish viability of the fetus for performing abortions. All make an attempt to understand the pain and trauma associated with any decision on abortion. Abortion issues are more often based on the following factors: economics, age, health, religion, and culture.

The consideration of how abortions are to be funded is even more complex. The 1977 Supreme Court ruling that said states were not required to fund abortions for indigent women raises the question of fairness and justice in following the law. Essentially, this ruling has the force of denying an abortion to a woman who is unable to pay for one. The right to choose becomes hinged on the ability to pay. This, in effect, denies personal freedom in a free society that has guaranteed equality under the 14th Amendment. The other side of the coin means that opponents of abortion will pay through their taxes in Medicaid funding for those who choose abortion. Persons who object on this basis also must weigh the costs of a funded abortion against the pregnancy, delivery, and welfare costs of the mother and child. One cannot hold that abortions are morally wrong and therefore should not be funded without being an advocate of adequate support that provides for babies born to welfare mothers who will require financial assistance, child care, and health services.

The two highest incidences of "abortions on demand" come from individuals who do not practice birth control because it is not available to them or because it is not convenient. The two groups range in age from 20 to 24 and from 15 to 19, respectively, are white, and are unmarried. There really is no explanation for these statistics other than that sexually active individuals are not using contraception and seek an abortion when they become pregnant. Further data indicate that some of the same women return a second or third time for abortions. It has taken the fear of AIDS to bring this country to the point at which sexuality (and more specifically, contraception) is a topic of national discussion and concern. Yet, for many, this topic is still one of considerable discomfort.

Perhaps the problem has developed because easily accessible abortions have encouraged sexual activity without responsibility. Is sex education, whether in the home or school, adequate? Are parents intentional and realistic about teaching morals? Bringing a new human being into the world is a privilege and a responsibility, and it should not be left to accident as a result of exploitation, fear, or ignorance.

ANTIABORTION TERRORISM

There is little debate here. Terrorism is a crime. It is illegal. The deaths, injuries, and damages caused by antiabortion criminal acts have weakened the influence of those who oppose abortion. To say that the killing of an abortion provider saves the lives of the unborn is to say, "I commit murder to prevent murder." Few would disagree on how irrational that argument is. Those who believe abortion is murder must struggle with the deaths that occur in war, also, or be able to justify why war is any different.

ASSISTED REPRODUCTION

As assisted reproduction methods become more common, legal issues have been increasingly resolved. Informed consent guidelines are to be carefully followed. All procedures should be carefully explained, including their effectiveness and any possible problems. Permission to perform the procedures should be in writing, and confidentiality must be ensured. The primary role of the provider is to inform clients of all aspects of the process. Clients should be allowed to make all necessary decisions while providers facilitate the process.

ARTIFICIAL INSEMINATION BY HUSBAND AND ARTIFICIAL INSEMINATION BY DONOR

AID presents problems separate from AIH. Using the semen of a donor raises the issues of the donor's right to the child and the child's right to know its father, screening for infections and genetic diseases, and when, if ever, a formal adoption is recommended. A federal law that has implications for AIH and AID is the 1973 Uniform Parentage Act (UPA). The 2000 and 2002 amendments to the UPA modernized the law for determining the legal parents of children and methods of testing for parentage. Delaware, Texas, Wyoming, and Washington have adopted versions of the UPA. In Washington, physicians must certify the consent signatures and the date of insemination and file the consent with the registrar of vital statistics, where it is kept confidential and sealed similarly to adoption records. Still, persons seeking AID might be wise to seek legal counsel regarding the legal protection and parentage of their offspring.

For married couples, counseling likely is done to ascertain that both the individuals want AID; however, women can and have received AID without spousal or partner consent. The written consent of the donor is required in all cases to release all claims of paternity. Some fertility clinics have a number of donors who can be called to bring semen when asked and usually are paid a fee for their services. Sperm banks provide another alternative for suitable sperm. For more information, go to **www.spermbankdirectory.com.**

Physicians and clinics using sperm donors must screen them carefully and meticulously. Some considerations include a complete physical and psychological examination, a sperm analysis, a genetic history, and appropriate blood tests, including testing for STDs and HIV/AIDS. Some physicians prefer only donors who have already fathered healthy children. Careful consideration may be given to selecting a donor who has physical characteristics similar to those of the husband or those desired by the woman.

Using frozen sperm for insemination is practiced more commonly. During a 6-month quarantine, the sperm undergoes extensive testing for disorders and diseases, showing a negative result for testing three times every 2 months. Some practitioners who perform AID recommend that the woman seek another practitioner, if she becomes pregnant, for prenatal care and delivery. This precaution may prevent any unnecessary questions regarding paternity of the newborn and may be prudent in states that have not addressed the issue or whose laws are particularly vague.

According to some religions, AID is adultery. Is the child then illegitimate? What occurs in states where no regulations have been enacted? Who monitors physicians practicing AID? Does anyone have the ethical responsibility to prevent the potential marriage of people who have the same father through AID?

IN VITRO FERTILIZATION

The many ethical and legal concerns for AIH and AID apply to IVF. There is, however, the added dilemma of creating life "outside" the normal realm of reproduction, purposely creating more than one embryo to implant hoping for better success, and what to do with those embryos not implanted.

Aside from the religious communities who oppose any assisted reproduction techniques, the greatest conflict arises over the use of the unused embryos. Generally, they are considered the property of the couple for whom IVF was intended. They are cryogenically preserved for future use. A few couples do return for those embryos and have them implanted, resulting in a pregnancy. Others leave them and never return. Some ethicists and scientists say those embryos should be used for stem cell research. That, however, has been denied, generally following political lines. See Chapter 14 for additional discussion on stem cell research. The destruction of frozen embryos after a period of time is viewed the same as abortion for many—it is the destruction of life. For others, it is a fact of scientific technology that occurs every day.

Case Study

A major fertility clinic has a problem. They have a number of frozen embryos stored beyond the recommended 3-year deadline. When the clinic attempted to contact the owners of the embryos, 15% could not be found.

Should the frozen embryos be donated, destroyed, or given for stem cell research?
Who makes these decisions?

Additional specific concerns, more ethical in nature, must be considered in all forms of assisted reproduction. These procedures are most likely not covered by insurance and thus usually performed only for the affluent. Should these procedures be available to all people whether or not they can afford it? Many argue that assisted reproduction is unnatural and an attempt to "play God." Who are the legal parents of an infant born of assisted reproduction? Perhaps equally critical, what rights does the conceptus have? Is selective breeding being practiced?

SURROGACY

Historically, surrogacy received national attention in 1987 when a surrogate mother in Newark, New Jersey chose not to relinquish the infant she bore to the child's biological father and his wife, who had contracted with the surrogate *(Stern v Whitehead)*. The courts ruled in favor of the biological father and allowed his wife to adopt the infant. The decision was appealed to the New Jersey Supreme Court. In what became known as the "Baby M" case, the New Jersey Supreme Court ruled that the child's father, William Stern, could retain custody of the 22-month-old child but that Mary Beth Whitehead-Grould, the surrogate, maintained her rights as a parent.

In California, Crispina and Mark Calvert hired Anna Johnson to gestate an embryo composed of the Calverts' egg and sperm. The Calverts paid Johnson $10,000 and purchased life insurance for her during pregnancy. During the pregnancy, the Calvert–Johnson relationship soured, and Johnson requested her money earlier than agreed on. Before the delivery of the baby, both the Calverts and Johnson brought suits, each side claiming parental rights. The Orange County Superior Court said that a "three-parent, two-natural mom situation" would confuse the child and "invites financial and emotional extortion." The court concluded that Johnson and "the child are genetic hereditary strangers." The judge compared the contract between the Calverts and Johnson to a common foster care arrangement in that Johnson was "providing care, protection, and nurture during the period of time that the natural mother, Crispina Calvert, was unable to care for the child."

The difficulty in surrogacy often arises when the surrogate must relinquish rights to the infant she bore. Some argue that it is similar to buying and selling babies. Others argue that without fees surrogate mothers would have little reason to offer their services. The New Jersey Supreme Court in the "Baby M" case stated that "baby selling potentially results in the exploitation of all parties involved" and that payment in a surrogacy contract is "illegal and perhaps criminal." Funds do exchange hands, however, and can include such items as maternity clothing allowance; a $100,000 term life insurance policy; $150 daily allowance for lost wages, child care, and meals; and attorney fees for the surrogate.

Finally, any time there is a contract, mistrust on the part of one or more parties is a possibility. Significant legal issues include whether contractual arrangements between the parties are legally enforceable and what parental rights, if any, the participants have to the child. Some states with legislation on the issue have declared surrogacy contracts invalid. Other states have no statutes. As long as technology advances further and faster than the legal system can address, these developments and ethical dilemmas will continue.

PROTOCOL FOR HEALTH PROFESSIONALS

Professionals involved in any of the reproductive health issues will want to be comfortable in any of the circumstances identified in this chapter. Individuals who are solid in their own beliefs yet understanding of those whose choices may be different will be most successful. Treating clients in a professional manner, especially with the recognition that providing reproductive health-care services is not a place for slapstick humor, will alleviate clients' anxieties and encourage open communication. All the issues are truly private and extremely personal. Tact and courtesy are essential at all times, and the confidentiality and privacy of those involved must be carefully protected. Care must be taken to preserve the dignity of all involved. Comments made by staff need to be pertinent, informative, helpful, and nonjudgmental.

With any of the assisted reproduction procedures, health-care professionals will want to remember that both men and women may be uncomfortable with the knowledge that several members of the medical staff know of their reproductive issues and that artificial techniques are being attempted. Health-care professionals may have to ask men to manually produce their semen and to explain to women how that semen will be deposited, usually on more than one occasion, in their cervix in the hope of gaining a pregnancy.

Health-care providers and their employees must decide if they will be employed where reproductive services or abortions may be performed. The conscience clause is designed to protect those who choose not to participate. Physicians and employees who understand their own feelings on abortion will be able to make a decision before becoming personally involved. Legally, employees and physicians cannot be forced to participate in abortions against their wishes. The right to refuse, however, does not authorize the right to judge. Health-care professionals must also remember that it is not their place to impose their personal opinions on anyone considering any reproductive health counseling. Even when asked a question directly, the response should be that such a very personal decision can only be reached by the person making it. It is better to select employment outside the arena of reproductive health care when one's personal views conflict with those of the medical practice.

Physicians and employees who participate in any area of reproductive health-care services are advised to adhere to the following:

1. Participate only within the law.
2. Provide medical knowledge to clients on all stages of any procedure.
3. Obtain written, informed consent.
4. Provide counseling as indicated by the situation.
5. Refer as necessary.
6. Keep records confidential.
7. Seek legal counsel when indicated.
8. Be understanding and compassionate.

SUMMARY

The beginning of this chapter introduced reproductive health-care issues and the rights of women. The rights of a partner, the unborn, and in some cases a donor are discussed. There is little if any agreement on many of the issues, even when or if law is in place. Abortion laws, especially, are continually in flux and are constantly challenged. Ethical opinions change, and debate moves on. Abortion is one of the longest debated issues and has become increasingly politicized. Resolutions to any of the reproductive health issues will never satisfy everyone. Health-care professionals will find it difficult to hold a neutral stand. The law grants rights that are to be protected, yet health professionals also must embrace their personal ethics.

Watch It Now! Can you be objective and compassionate when you disagree? at http://davisplus.fadavis.com/lawandethics

Questions for Review

SELECT THE BEST ANSWER

1. FGM
   a. Has been performed in more than 140 million women around the world.
   b. Is illegal when practiced on adult women in the United States.
   c. Is most commonly practiced in South America and Russia.
   d. Enhances both male and female sexual experience.

2. Prescription contraception includes
   a. Ovulation prediction kits.
   b. The female condom and sponge.
   c. Pills, patches, rings, IUDs, diaphragms, caps, and shields.
   d. A law preventing dispensing to teenagers.

3. The most popular contraception method in the world is
   a. *Coitus interruptus.*
   b. Surgical sterilization.
   c. Vasectomy.
   d. The pill.

4. A critical time for the viability of a fetus is
   a. When the brain begins to function.
   b. When the pulmonary surfactant is formed.
   c. The time of birth.
   d. The time of quickening.

5. Assisted reproduction may include
   a. AIH, AID, IVF, and surrogacy.
   b. PGD analysis.
   c. FAM and WHO.
   d. None of the above.

TRUE OR FALSE

T F   6. AID is artificial insemination by husband.

T F   7. A therapeutic abortion is one performed to preserve the life and health of the mother.

T F   8. There are a number of states that deny legal abortions to women on Medicaid.

T F   9. Today many teenagers have oral sex in order to protect themselves from STDs.

T F   10. A conscience clause protects providers and their employees who choose not to participate in abortions.

CLASSROOM EXERCISES

1. Sperm bank donors rely on anonymity when they donate their sperm. With new DNA technology, it is possible to trace ancestry including sperm donors. How will the courts respond when a child has a genetic health risk or disease and needs to know about his or her genetic medical history? Will the courts respond as they did with adoption? Discuss.

2. Should permission of a spouse or partner be mandatory for sterilization or artificial insemination? Explain and justify your response.

3. A couple comes into a fertility clinic for AID. They have determined that the husband's brother should be the donor and already have made arrangements with him. What counseling might be suggested? Discuss the pros and cons of such an arrangement.

4. Katherine is a surrogate mother for a couple living 15 miles away. Katherine, near term of the pregnancy, decides she does not want to relinquish the baby. What she does not know is that the prospective mother was killed in an auto accident 2 weeks ago. Who has the right to the child? How is a decision made?

5. As an individual opposed to all abortions, respond to the following issues:
   a. Pregnancies and resultant births from rape or incest
   b. Unwanted children
   c. Infants with severe birth defects

6. As an individual supporting abortion, respond to the following issues:
   a. Abortion as contraception
   b. A late-term abortion for convenience
   c. The right to life versus the right to freedom

7. Identify where in your community you might refer an individual for the types of reproductive health services discussed in this chapter.

8. Under what conditions can an abortion be performed in your state?

INTERNET ACTIVITES

1. Go to **www.abortionfacts.com.** You will find two sites with opposing information. One has abortion information if you are "pro-choice," the other has information if you are "pro-life." Do these sites help clarify your thinking? Justify your response.

2. Go to the CDC's *Morbidity and Mortality Weekly Report* (MMWR) Surveillance Summary to access the latest report on abortion surveillance **(www.cdc.gov/mmwr/preview/mmwrhtml/ ss5808a1.htm?s_cid=ss5808al_e).** Research your particular state. In which age group is the largest number of abortions performed? How many abortions were performed after 20 weeks?

3. Research Nadya Suleman, the octuplet Mom, on the Internet. Describe your findings. Discuss with a classmate your feelings about Suleman's IVF, identifying both the legal and ethical implications.

4. Research FGM and the Subcommittee on Crime, Terrorism, and Homeland Security to determine whether the 2010 Girl's Protection Act is now law. What additional protection does the law provide?

WEB RESOURCES

Abortion Surveillance—United States, 2006.
   www.cdc.gov/mmwr/preview/mmwrhtml/ss5808a1.htm?s_cid=ss5808al_e

Elective Abortion—eMedicine.
   http://emedicine.medscape.com/article/252560

Encyclopedia of Science and Religion—Abortion.
   www.enotes.com/science-religion-encyclopedia/abortion

Fetal Development/Gestational Age.
  www.nlm.nih.gov/medlineplus/ency/article/002398

National Abortion Federation: Extreme Clinic Violence.
  www.prochoice.org/about_abortion/violence/history_extreme.asp

Planned Parenthood Federation of America Inc.
  www.plannedparenthood.org

State Policies in Brief: Parental Involvement in Minors' Abortions.
  www.guttmacher.org/satecenter/spibs/spib_PIMA.pdf

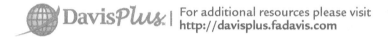 **DavisPlus** | For additional resources please visit
http://davisplus.fadavis.com

CHAPTER 16

End of Life Issues

"Life is not measured by the number of breaths we take, but by the moments that take our breath away."—Author unknown

KEY TERMS

advance directive A state's response to the living will; sometimes called the Natural Death Act; often includes all documents related to end-of-life choices.

code red Medical phrase used to indicate life-or-death emergency.

durable power of attorney An appointed proxy or substitute who makes decisions related to property and finances.

durable power of attorney for health care Sometimes called medical proxy; the legal right to act on another's behalf in making health-care decisions.

euthanasia From the Greek term meaning "good death," willfully allowing death, to keep a person with incurable disease from suffering; more commonly used today to express actively taking one's life.

hospice A lodging, association, or service for those who are terminally ill.

living will Legal document, voluntarily made by an adult, stating what treatment and procedures that person wants done in the event of a terminal illness, especially helpful if the person becomes comatose or incompetent.

Patient Self-Determination Act Federal law requiring institutions giving medical care to inform clients of their option to use such advance directives as living wills and durable powers of attorney for health care.

LEARNING OUTCOMES

Upon successful completion of this chapter, you will be able to:

16.1 Define key terms.
16.2 Describe the living will, advance directive, and durable power of attorney for health care.
16.3 Appraise components of the Patient Self-Determination Act.
16.4 Restate choices an individual might have in death.
16.5 Describe the importance of medications for dying clients.
16.6 Discuss at least three ethical implications of life-and-death decisions.
16.7 Identify and explain at least five psychological aspects affecting dying clients.
16.8 Differentiate among various legal definitions of death.
16.9 Describe two famous court cases and their impact on prolonging life.
16.10 Express possible legal implications of life-and-death decisions.
16.11 Identify and explain at least five physiological aspects affecting dying clients.

16.12 Discuss the stages of dying as defined by Kübler-Ross.

16.13 Describe the services of hospice for dying clients.

16.14 Differentiate between active euthanasia and physician-assisted death.

16.15 Discuss the Uniform Anatomical Gift Act.

16.16 Describe an autopsy and who may authorize one.

16.17 Define the role of the health professional in dealing with clients and families in life-and-death decisions.

COMPETENCIES

CAAHEP

- Identify the effect personal ethics may have on professional performance. (CAAHEP X.C.5)
- Explain how the following impact the medical assistant's practice and give examples:
  Uniform Anatomical Gift Act (CAAHEP IX.C.10.e)
  Living will/advance directive (CAAHEP IX.C.10.f)
  Medical durable power of attorney (CAAHEP IX.C.10.g)
- Develop a plan for separation of personal and professional ethics. (CAAHEP X.P.2)
- Examine the impact personal ethics and morals may have on the individual's practice. (CAAHEP X.A.3)

ABHES

- Use empathy when treating terminally ill patients. (ABHES 5.c)
- Identify common stages that terminally ill patients go through and list organizations and support groups that can assist patients and family members of patients struggling with terminal illness. (ABHES 5.d)
- Advocate on behalf of family and patients, having ability to deal and communicate with family. (ABHES 5.e)

VIGNETTE

What Happened to My Plan?

Ted is 76 years old. He is retired and lives with his wife of 44 years and their adult daughter. As a laborer, he spent most of his working years with heavy equipment and cranes on land, tug boats, and ships. From his home, he sees the Puget Sound and watches the passing ships. Ted has been diagnosed with emphysema and suspected asbestosis. More than 7 years after diagnosis, his breathing is now difficult. His sense of humor, his love of family, his care for others, and his knowledge of the passing ships is as keen as ever.

Ted and his internist are friends. They worship in the same church. When Ted sees his doctor, they tell jokes and swap stories before getting down to the serious business of his illness. Ted refuses using oxygen until he can no longer sleep peacefully. Ted and his wife, Ann, discuss a living will; they talk with their children, and meet with their attorney to update their wills and have the Washington State advance directive executed. Ted shares it with his physician, and they agree on his care management.

On a cold and gloomy December day there is rain and even some snow in the Pacific Northwest. Ted is housebound most of the time now. The weather makes his breathing more labored. He is having severe headaches. When Ann suggests Ted visit his doctor, Ted grumbles that there is nothing more the doctor can do. One evening, Ted is unable to wear even his slippers because his feet and legs are so swollen. The water retention makes his feet feel like water pads. In his humor he comments, "I feel like Jesus—walking on water."

Early the next morning, Ted cannot breathe. He is suffocating. Ann dials 911. In minutes emergency medical technicians are at the door. In their quick assessment, they comment on the strength of Ted's heart but the weakness of his lungs. Ann explains the emphysema and suspected asbestosis. Ted is transported to the hospital, treated in the emergency room, and moved to intensive care. Ann, their daughter, and their son are at his bedside. Although breathing is stabilized, the medical staff inquires about the use of a respirator and his living will. The family responds positively, and the advance directive is supplied to the hospital that afternoon.

Circumstances in the next few days greatly alter Ted's life. Ted's physician suffers his own tragedy and is called to Denmark for a family death. When attempts to remove Ted's excess fluid are not totally successful, a nephrologist is called who orders the placement of a shunt in Ted's shoulder for dialysis. Neither Ted nor the family is anxious to begin dialysis. Ted had watched a close and dear friend suffer greatly, lose a limb, and eventually die after years of dialysis. Ted believes that dialysis will make a "good death" next to impossible. The nephrologist insists and discusses options with the family. "This is just a 'jump start' to get your kidneys going; we will probably only have to dialyze you twice." Ted and Ann discuss dialysis. There is hesitation, but the decision is finally made to go ahead, and the consent for dialysis is signed. Both Ted and Ann are concerned about all the side effects. A chaplain who visits explains why the form has to list all the possible side effects, even though few if any are likely to occur. Dialysis will begin the next morning.

The family goes home for a night's rest before their return to the hospital early the next morning. The weather, however, intervenes; heavy snow falls during the night. The hills of Seattle are clogged with vehicles going nowhere. Freeways are treacherous. Even the streets to the hospital are impassable. Dialysis technicians and portable dialysis machines are delayed. Their load backs up, and patients more critical than Ted wait long past their dialysis time for treatment. Ted's condition worsens. Fortunately, the weather moderates, and the schedule moves forward for Ted's dialysis to begin. It helps little, however. After two treatments, Ted begins to bleed internally, and his laboratory tests indicate that an emergency exists. A surgeon is called in—another stranger to the family, but the "freshest" one available. It seems every surgeon and every hospital is overburdened this Christmas holiday. Emergency surgery is scheduled for 5:00 p.m. The family is at the bedside, but the operating room is full; a code red in the room Ted is to use delays surgery further. Ted's condition is so critical that the surgeon checks nearby hospitals for an operating room. None is available. Finally at 1 a.m., Ted goes into surgery. The family is told that there is only a fifty–fifty chance he will survive.

Ted survives 4 hours of surgery but is returned to the intensive care unit (ICU) on a respirator. There was a bowel perforation, and half his colon was removed. He is critical, but amazingly is able to be weaned from his respirator in 24 hours. By now Ted is receiving food and hydration, blood, platelets, antibiotics, and pain medication intravenously. He cannot speak but is somewhat alert. He is seriously weakened. Urine output decreases, and the question of dialysis returns. At this point, all persons involved in Ted's care meet to discuss treatment; they meet with the family. Each family member is interviewed separately about their wishes and Ted's wishes regarding extraordinary means. Earlier an ICU nurse told the family that if even one of them has any hesitation about treatment, the hospital will not follow Ted's wishes. After completion of the interviews, it is clear that the family intends to follow Ted's wishes. Dialysis will cease. It is only a matter of time now. The nephrologist, however, has other ideas. When she discovers dialysis has been discontinued, she demands to know why. When the family explains, she says, "I was not present for that consultation. I will have to hear it from Ted himself." She goes to Ted's bedside, asks him if he can understand her, and says, "Ted, do you want dialysis?" Ted, in his hospital bed with head and shoulders elevated 10 to 20 degrees, has his arms immobilized at his side for the drip of numerous intravenous (IV) lines. An oxygen mask covers his nose and mouth. His eyes show lack of rest and sleep, fear about what is happening to

Continued

VIGNETTE

him, and concern for his family. Ted shrugs his shoulders and opens his hands palms upward in gesture. The nephrologist is ordering a chest x-ray and dialysis when the family intervenes. An on-call physician and the nephrologist argue outside Ted's room, in earshot of the family. The attending physician indicates that in Ted's condition, dialysis probably will do more harm than good. His body cannot withstand dialysis. The nephrologist disagrees.

When there seems no hope and the family is feeling powerless, their family physician returns and intervenes on behalf of the family. The damage has already been done, however. Ted has suffered not just one but all of the possible side effects the family feared. Ted is now bleeding internally from almost every organ of his body. All IV lines are removed except what is needed to keep Ted comfortable. Every breath is the hardest work his body has ever known. Each member of his family says good-bye and tells Ted how much he is loved. Nurses and doctors, so attentive in the previous 25 days, also stop by. The ICU nurses continue to do what they are best known for—attending to the needs of the critically ill. The primary care physician remains close. The end is peaceful. The end is relief—relief from agony and pain, relief from any more difficult decisions, relief from the disappointment that a loved one's wishes were so hard to carry out.

CHOICES IN LIFE

ETHICS CHECK

Throughout the text, many discussions of rights have surfaced both in the legal and the bioethical context. The dialogue continues in this chapter, taking a closer look at the right to die with dignity.

Choices are continually made about the quality of one's life. How is it decided what health care is received? Is there discrimination in elder care? How can vulnerable populations be protected? People living in dire poverty struggle daily with life issues. An elderly person alone with no transportation and no nearby relatives fears the loss of personal control and independence. Some live with the challenge of decreased mental and emotional capabilities. There are those who respond to life's challenges with grace, strength, and a happy disposition no matter what life gives them. Others may only be able to face life's challenges with awkwardness, difficulties, and depression. All health-care professionals are to be reminded of the vulnerabilities and circumstances of their clients. Understanding and accepting clients and their wishes while providing quality and personalized health care is the challenge, even more specifically when facing death.

Adults have the right to make choices to forego life-sustaining treatments when death is imminent. Life-prolonging technology, however, has pushed death further into the future, and health professionals are often unable to help clients deal with the emotional strain and diminished capacity that often follow. Incompetent adults also need a voice in their choices in dying. These circumstances create an environment for action from the legal community. ●

LIVING WILLS, ADVANCE DIRECTIVES, AND THE PATIENT SELF-DETERMINATION ACT

When health-care professionals found themselves in legal and ethical dilemmas related to end-of-life issues, states began to pass legislation giving clients the specific legal right to forego life-sustaining treatments, nutrition, and hydration. The legislation also provided protection to providers and hospitals carrying out such orders. These directives allow individuals or their appointed agents to make decisions regarding their dying.

California and Washington were forerunners in end-of-life legislation. California's document was the living will; Washington's response to the legal dilemma was the physicians' directive, or Natural Death Act. The intent of both documents was to provide an avenue through which individuals could make choices regarding their death before the event, usually while still healthy. A living will is an advance directive stating an individual's wishes regarding whether to be kept alive through the use of artificial means, such as life support, feeding tubes, and artificial respiration. Advance directives can include the living will as well as powers of attorney and health-care proxies that may be known by other names—medical surrogate, health-care power of attorney, designation of health-care agent, and designation of conservator (guardianship). Each of these documents serves to provide direction and/or name someone to act on an individual's behalf when that individual is unable to convey his or her wishes to others. Today, all 50 states have end-of-life legislation (Fig. 16-1.) ●

In some states, the living will and advance directive documents or appointments are combined into a single form, often called the advance directive. Each state identifies particular stipulations, but the intent is the same: to direct health-care professionals on decisions that are often made before death—if or when to resuscitate and what if any kind of heroic measures are to be performed. In recent years, each of these documents has grown increasingly specific. Individuals can relate if or under what circumstances artificial feeding or hydration is to begin and at what point only "comfort" measures are started. See Appendix II for examples of both a living will and an advance directive.

Another avenue for clients to express their wishes is becoming more popular. The Physician Orders for Life-Sustaining Treatment (POLST) is designed to improve the quality of care individuals receive at the end of life. Not all 50 states utilize the POLST form, but each state that participates has designed its own form. Sections are likely to include information about resuscitation instructions, advance directives, and orders for other life-sustaining orders. See **www.ohsu.edu/polst/programs/state+programs.htm** to see if your state participates and to view a sample form.

In addition, the federal government passed the Patient Self-Determination Act in 1991. This law applies to all health-care institutions receiving payments from Medicare and Medicaid, including hospitals, skilled nursing facilities, hospices, home care programs, and health maintenance organizations. The act requires that all adult persons receiving medical care from such institutions be given written information about their right to accept or refuse medical or surgical treatment. These clients must also be given information about their right to formulate advance directives such as living wills and to designate someone to act on their behalf in making health-care decisions. The Patient Self-Determination Act, however, does not override any state law, allowing a health-care provider to object on the basis of conscience in the implementation of such an advance directive.

DURABLE POWER OF ATTORNEY FOR HEALTH CARE

In addition to living wills or advance directives, many individuals choose to create the durable power of attorney or the durable power of attorney for health care. The durable power of attorney is a legal form that allows a designated person to act on another's behalf, making decisions related to finances and property. Likewise, the durable power of attorney for health care or the medical proxy allows a designated person to make only health-care decisions for another. A person must be competent to sign a power of attorney. Some states require that signers must be able to manage their own property effectively at the time of signing. Signers keep control over the document as long as the person can manage independently. The signed document can be given to a lawyer or a close friend with instructions that it is turned over to the attorney-in-fact only if the need arises. Once signed, the document is in effect until it is revoked. ●

This designated person should know and understand the client's personal wishes to ensure that the person with power of attorney will act on the client's behalf in all instances of health care. This agent is

A

B

C

Figure 16-1. Three legal documents allowing clients to express their choices regarding their health care. (A) Living will. (B) Advance directive. (C) Durable power of attorney for health care.

often a spouse, partner, grown child, close friend, other relative, or someone in whom the person has full confidence. Each state has established rules governing the use of the durable power of attorney. Individuals are advised to periodically update and review their durable power of attorney for health care as well as an advance directive. Also, reviewing each state's laws if moving from state to state is necesssary. Professional legal advice regarding a given state's stipulations may be advisable, but preprinted forms are readily available. See Appendix II for an example of a durable power of attorney for health care.

NATIONAL REGISTRY

Individuals can register their advance directive with a national registry that will electronically transmit a copy of their document to any health-care provider (hospital, doctor, skilled nursing facility, home health agency, provider of home health care, ambulatory surgery center, and hospice). The registry agrees not to release the personal information to any party other than health-care providers, so information is kept private and confidential. The registry provides labels to affix to an insurance card and driver's license, stating that the individual's advance directive is registered. The registrant is contacted annually by mail to confirm that the advance directive has not been changed or revoked and to update personal and emergency contact information. Health-care providers can contact the registry 24 hours a day to gain access to advance directives. See **www.uslivingwillregistry.com** for more information.

 ## CHOICES IN DYING

No one escapes death. From the moment of birth, each day of life moves a person closer to death. Some die suddenly and peacefully, perhaps during sleep. Some die suddenly as a result of an accident or as a victim of crime. Some die slowly and gradually, with bodies that deteriorate and organs that cease to function. Some die with little or no pain or discomfort. Others suffer a great deal. Most want to live, but when faced with death, desire to go quickly, painlessly, and with dignity. However, not all are so fortunate.

In dying, there are choices that can be made. Some face a life-threatening illness and take action to direct their wishes for the time when death is imminent. Others create advance directives when making their last will and testament. There are also a large group of individuals who refuse to think of death, make no plans of any kind, and may leave loved ones to make decisions with a great deal of anguish. Still others live in a culture where discussing or planning for death is forbidden or frowned upon.

Personal attitudes and public opinion have changed through the years regarding death. In 1938 the Euthanasia Society of America was founded. It was a national, nonprofit organization dedicated to fostering communication about complex end-of-life decisions among individuals. The organization invented the living will in 1967. The premise of the organization was to create an atmosphere in which one could take measures to end life, creating a "good death," when threatened with a terminal condition. Euthanasia was identified as passive (allowing death to come naturally, taking no measures to prevent it) or active (the intentional taking of one's life). Now euthanasia is more commonly defined as the latter. Today there are numerous organizations dedicated to choices in dying, such as Compassion in Choices **(www.compassionandchoices.org);** the National Hospice and Palliative Care Organization (www.nhpco.org); the World Federation of Right to Die Societies **(www.worldrtd.net);** and the Death With Dignity National Center **(www.deathwithdignity.org).**

While individuals increasingly seek control over their choices in dying, the almost coercive power of medical technology and medicine to preserve and prolong life may cause many to suffer debility, pain, and perhaps a lesser quality of life. The desire to have choices in dying comes from fears and concerns related to prolonged dying as the result of technological interventions. Most desire the right to be able to refuse treatment or hospitalization. A few might choose assisted death. Generally, individuals do not want to be a burden to significant others. They fear losing their independence and control and want to choose their quality of both life and death.

Every day, medical personnel confront complex issues regarding the meanings of life and death. There is a fine line between helping a person to live and allowing that person to die. When is it appropriate to use extraordinary means to prolong life? What are extraordinary means? What are the legal implications if treatment is withheld or withdrawn? Technological or mechanical intervention has saved the lives of many. Medical technology offers insulin to control diabetes, a cardiac pacemaker or mechanical heart valves for a weak or diseased heart, renal dialysis for kidney failure, angioplasty for clogged arteries, even antibiotics for pneumonia.

Consider the following example from Donald M. Hayes writing in *Between Doctor and Patient:* "Mr. Baker had terminal kidney failure and was comatose. Several tubes came from various places in his body. He was receiving both blood and glucose into his veins. One night he went into cardiac arrest. A team of nurses and physicians responded to a code red and worked vigorously to resuscitate. The attempt was futile, and Mr. Baker died. The memory of Mr. Baker's death was lasting to Mr. Rogers, the recently admitted patient in the same room. He said to his physician, 'Please don't ever let that happen to me. I've tried all my life to live like a man; I want to die like one.' Mr. Rogers underwent surgery that revealed inoperable, widespread cancer. He did not respond well, and a few days later he had a tube in his stomach, a catheter in his bladder, a tube through his nose, and intravenous tubes in both arms. When he suffered respiratory failure, a tracheotomy was performed to save his life. He was given a slate to write on, since a tracheotomy precludes speech. Later one evening, before he managed to switch off this respirator so that he might die peacefully, he wrote on the slate, 'Doctor, remember; the enemy is not death. The enemy is inhumanity.'"

Few turn their backs on the medical technology that has added years of life for so many. Such advances in medicine are heralded by the public and the media; however, if not used judiciously, technology can supplant the quality of life. At some time, every individual is apt to face the issue of how much medical technology to use to prolong life, and hopes, at the same time, for a "good death." Whether or not to prolong life can be a serious problem when the decision is made with little fore-thought or adequate planning. When the cardiologist tells a loved one that a pacemaker is necessary to regulate the heartbeat, the general response is, "When can it be done?"

The decision is more complex, however, when a loved one is hospitalized with a heart condition that is rapidly deteriorating and little can be done. The questions of how much intervention to use and when to intervene are much more serious. When the heart monitor indicates with a buzzing sound and a continuous monotone sound that the heart has ceased to beat, somewhere, someone is going to ask, "Do we resuscitate?" It is at this point that the decisions declared in a living will or advance directive become significant.

SUFFERING IN DYING

It is the fear of suffering more than the actual death that concerns the majority of individuals. Suffering can be short or long term. Short-term suffering presents a set of problems different from those of long-term suffering. Consider the following:

Case Studies

Example 1: A 45-year-old teacher learned in June that acute myelogenous leukemia accompanied by blastic transformation was destroying her body. The prognosis was poor. Hospitalization and chemotherapy followed, with severe side effects and pain. She died 2 months later when remission attempts failed.

Example 2: A 50-year-old electrician was diagnosed with colorectal cancer. Surgery followed, and a permanent colostomy was established. Postoperatively, the client did fairly well and returned to work part-time during chemotherapy. Within a year, cancer metastasized, and complications resulted. Consultation with specialists recommended only symptomatic treatment. Massive doses of analgesics were required to keep him comfortable for the remaining 6 months. The electrician remained home until about 6 weeks before death, when hospice was called.

Consider the variables of time, cost, and dependency in the two examples. Who suffered the most? Where are the greatest costs? Who is most dependent?

The amount of suffering often influences care decisions. Are antibiotics prescribed when a hospitalized person suffering from the last stages of pancreatic cancer contracts pneumonia? Under what circumstances are "do not resuscitate" orders placed in clients' charts? Consider an individual being kept alive by a respirator who has no recognition and no awareness of surroundings. Is the person suffering? Is life being prolonged beyond its natural course of events?

How much pain medication is prescribed to ease the suffering? When sufficient pain medication is prescribed to keep those close to death comfortable, health professionals know the medication provided for pain relief may depress breathing in some clients already so fragile and debilitated that death is hastened. Is this action seen as an act of euthanasia?

USE OF MEDICATIONS

Medications are used to ease suffering and pain, but are also given for many other reasons, including sedatives for sleep and specific medications for the particular disease condition. Antidepressants and tranquilizers also may be prescribed. Medications are to be respected for their intended action and the client's needs. The greatest difficulty arises with pain medications, especially in long-term suffering.

Problems arise when family members, friends, and even health professionals circumvent or question medication orders. This is often disastrous for the client; therefore, it is helpful for all persons close to the client to understand the medication orders. Unless everyone understands that the medication amount is needed to keep the level of pain bearable, the medication amount is often withheld or reduced. Medications may be given in different dosages, frequencies, and combinations for each individual. Age, weight, illness (whether chronic or acute), and the client's threshold for pain all influence a medication choice.

Sometimes health professionals are reluctant to prescribe or administer the known safe dosage of pain medications. In fact, in some cases health professionals will administer less than the prescribed dose because they believe what was prescribed was too much. Some fear the client will become addicted and tend to view opioid orders or prescriptions from a criminal aspect rather than as treatment. The client or family members may push to use less medication than the amount prescribed because of the belief it is too harmful. Clients often wait too long to ask for pain medication, thinking they "can handle it." All these circumstances have the potential of working against the clients' comfort.

PSYCHOLOGICAL ASPECTS OF DYING

Dying clients differ in their psychological experiences. Although basic personalities remain the same, changes occur. A person normally calm and loving may have periods of violence and hostility. A happy person may become severely depressed. An individual who usually is able to accept medical facts may totally deny a life-threatening illness. In fact, a person who is nearly comatose or close to death may be unaware of his or her responses to questions or be unable to make any decisions.

Relationships change. The dying person may reject any close contact or relationships. Some individuals are incapable of continuing a close relationship with a person who is dying. Closest friends may become aloof and distant. Some may fear touching or caressing the dying person. The opposite may also be true. A stronger bond of friendship can develop, and new friendships will be made, possibly from individuals in similar circumstances. Broken relationships may be healed.

Relationships are important because they provide strength and support that may not be available through any other source. The depth of relationships during this time and the degree of acceptance by dying clients may depend on their self-image. When a person is ill, is in pain, lives in a deteriorating body, and possibly is unable to perform the activities of daily living, self-image is fragile. When self-image is lacking, hope is lost; dying clients feel useless, think they are burdens, and have difficulties accepting help. The psychological effect of a poor self-image may even hasten death. Those who are dying worry that they are not fulfilling their usual role in the family and worry about their lack of control.

Personal goals are altered, dropped, or identified. There may be the goal to see a son or daughter graduate or a grandchild born; however, some goals will seem unrealistic to the dying because of limited time. The dying person either gives up or strives to live until a certain event takes place. The total loss of personal goals, no matter how insignificant they may appear, can be devastating to everyone. Indecision is often a psychological dilemma that accompanies lack of personal goals. Individuals close to the dying may be able to recommend goals and provide offers of help in the decision-making process.

Communication may become difficult. Aside from any physiological problems precluding speech or communication, what dying clients are unable to understand or hear may depend on what they choose to hear or are ready to understand. Communication may be complicated further if the client's condition has not been honestly addressed. Of course, the opposite may be true. Some dying clients express the ability to communicate with greater depth because of the urgency of their circumstances.

There is often the question of whether dying clients should be told of their terminal condition. How much information should they be given? Some believe that all clients need to be told the medical facts and treated openly and honestly by all health professionals. They believe informed clients are better able to face death and are less afraid of the truth. Others believe no clients should be told they are dying, or that only those clients who give some verbal or nonverbal indication that they want to know should be told.

In some cultures, only family members rather than the client are told of impending death. Once told some clients may refuse to set goals, give up hope, and wait impatiently for death. Fear is often a traumatic psychological aspect of dying. There is fear of pain, fear of long suffering, fear of losing independence, fear of financial ruin, and fear of death itself. The client's fears are to be recognized and alleviated, if possible. To recognize these fears requires active and passive listening on the part of all people close to the dying individual and a willingness on the part of this individual to express those fears.

Much fear can be lessened if people close to the dying anticipate the fear and provide possible solutions and appropriate resources. Outside help may be sought, if necessary. Social workers, public health nurses, home health aides, clergy, and other health professionals can be valuable resources. Clients' fear should be taken seriously, and reference to their supposed unimportance should be avoided.

The psychological aspects of death are difficult for everyone because they generally are less understood than the physiological aspects of death, but to care for the physical and ignore the psychological is to treat only half the client. As Norman Cousins said, "Death is not the greatest loss in life. The greatest loss is what dies inside us while we live."

PHYSIOLOGICAL ASPECTS OF DYING

Medicine has numerous treatments for some of the physiological problems of suffering and pain experienced in the dying process. Sometimes the treatments are sufficient; at other times, they barely address the problem. Untreated or undiagnosed physiological problems can cause or enhance psychological difficulties. Separating the psychological from the physiological is difficult. For example, pain and suffering, if untreated by therapy or medicinal means, may prove to be a psychological barrier for clients, their families, and health professionals.

Loss of communication skills as seen in the aphasic or the comatose client may be frustrating and unbearable. If clients are indecisive or suffer from dementia because of physiological changes, they may not be able to participate in the decision-making process of their life-threatening illness. Family members then may need to assume greater roles in talking for clients and making decisions.

Other common physiological problems encountered include loss of bodily functions; inability to move or ambulate; inability to eat or drink; and inability to tolerate medications, treatments, light, or sound. In some settings, these symptoms may be treated without much difficulty. However, if clients choose to die at home, professional help or training may become necessary. If clients become severely disabled physically, they may be reluctant to go anywhere, even to the ambulatory health-care setting. Family members may become exhausted caring for their loved ones and may be unable to administer some of their treatments. The more severe these physiological problems, the more difficult daily existence becomes.

Physiological difficulties may hinder sexual identity and involvement, altering sexual expression. The physiological and psychological aspects of sexuality are so intertwined that cause and effect are difficult to determine. It may be difficult or impossible to have sexual intercourse, so other ways to express love, caring, or the relief of sexual tension are sought. A discussion of the expression of sexuality and related client problems ought to be initiated by the health professional but rarely is.

 ## HOSPICE

The first hospice, lodging for the dying, was formed by Cecily Saunders in London in 1965. Hospice provides care for the terminally ill at home, in a hospital, in a skilled nursing facility, or in a special hospice facility. The main objective of care is to make clients comfortable, "at home," and close to family. Treatments, such as cardiopulmonary resuscitation, intravenous therapy, nasogastric tubes, and antibiotics, are discouraged. Treatments are given in light of the client's personal and social circumstances.

Death is seen as "all right." A balance is kept between human needs and medical needs. Children are encouraged in the hospice as a reminder that life is an ongoing process. Clients might share a cup of tea with staff and each other rather than receiving an intravenous solution during their last hours.

An advantage hospice offers is that death is managed with dignity, and experienced staff members want to care for the dying. The expense is generally less than acute care costs and may be covered by insurance. In a special hospice facility, the dying client is not isolated behind curtains but rather is surrounded by others. An empty bed remains empty for at least 24 hours to allow adjustment by everyone. In addition, survivors are helped to deal with the death. If the hospice care is at home, clients are in familiar surroundings, may have their favorite foods, and are close to loved ones.

 ## STAGES OF GRIEF

Elisabeth Kübler-Ross defines five stages of grief or responses to dying. There is no set period for any one stage, nor will every dying person go through every stage. Some believe that no real grief work begins until passing through all five stages. Some may stay in denial until death; others may manage denial and bargaining and stumble in depression. Still others may move back and forth from one stage to another. Some may move through some or all of the stages several times. There is no set or acceptable pattern. However, the stages do offer information on how to relate to clients and their families who will experience similar stages.

Elisabeth Kübler-Ross defines five stages of dying and death: (1) denial, (2) anger, (3) bargaining, (4) depression, and (5) acceptance.

DENIAL

Clients deny their life-threatening or terminal illness or go through periods of disbelief. Clients commonly say, "This is not happening to me" or "I'll go for another opinion." Denial generally is a temporary defense and offers therapeutic meaning to clients. Health professionals should listen to clients during this stage. Trying to contradict clients or force them to believe what is happening to them will be to no avail. Encourage clients to talk about death. Listen, listen, and listen.

ANGER

Clients suddenly realize "It is me. This is happening to me. Why me?" They may become "problem clients" and are envious and resentful. Anger may be dispersed in all directions, at people and toward the environment. Rage and temper tantrums can occur. Professionals and family members will want to remember that the anger is truly not directed toward them and will want to be understanding no matter how angry the client becomes. Listening to clients is important, allowing them to vent their own feelings.

BARGAINING

During this stage, clients try to make deals with their provider, God or a higher being, or family, usually for more time or for a period of comfort without pain. Clients tend to be more cooperative and congenial. Common responses include the following: "Please let me see my homeland again." "Dear God, I'll never…if you make me well." Health professionals can listen to dying clients' requests, but are not to become a party to the bargain. Some bargaining is associated with guilt. Bargaining can give the client the hope and stamina to reach a desired goal. It is OK to mourn and cry. Allow for silences.

DEPRESSION

The dying client's body is deteriorating, sometimes rapidly; financial burdens are likely increasing; pain is unbearable; and relationships are severed. All can lead to depression. The dying are losing everything and everyone they love. Dying may be a time of tears, and crying may allow relief. Professionals who appear happy, loud, and reassuring will not provide much help to depressed clients. Clients may need to express their sorrow to someone or merely have someone close. They may have little need for words at this stage. Simple tasks may be impossible. Helplessness is real.

ACCEPTANCE

The final but perhaps not last stage is when clients are accepting of their fate. They usually are tired, weak, and able to sleep. They are not necessarily happy, but rather at peace. Professionals will be aware that clients may prefer to be left alone and not bothered with world events or family problems. Family members usually require more help, understanding, and support than clients in this stage. Touching and the use of silence may prove helpful.

Case Study

Relate the five stages identified to any death or grieving experience you have had. Did you pass through all the stages? What was/is most difficult for you?

Following a death or the experience of loss, there will come a time when friends and neighbors stop calling, "closure" has occurred, and everything slowly gets back to normal. Some say this is when the real and the very difficult grief work begins. A common definition of grief work is summarized by the acronym TEAR.

T = To accept the reality of the loss
E = Experience the pain of the loss
A = Adjust to the environment of what was lost
R = Reinvest in the new reality

LEGAL DEFINITIONS OF DEATH

 An early legal definition of death was the cessation of the heart and lung. The two were so interrelated that the cessation of one leads to the cessation of the other, followed by the cessation of all cognitive activity, all other brain functions, and all general responsiveness. The cessation of the heart and of breathing has been the simplest to identify and the easiest test of life, and it became the acceptable definition of death. Today, the majority of deaths in the United States are still determined by this traditional definition of death. ●

With medical technological advances, resuscitative devices, increased complexities of life, and the increased demand for organ transplants, the heart–lung definition of death was found insufficient in some cases. Death is a continuum, and different parts of the body die at different times. As long as there is any heartbeat to pump oxygenated blood to tissues, cells thrive. Even when an irreparable brain injury does not support life and life support is removed, the heart continues to beat for a short time. However, when the blood it pumps is no longer oxygenated, tissues and cells die. Approximately 3 to 4 minutes pass before there is irreparable brain death. Once the brain dies, all the other body organs die at various intervals.

Subsequently, the concept of brain death was presented by the Harvard Ad-Hoc Committee, chaired by Henry Beecher. The criteria follow: An individual appears to be in deep coma. The condition can be satisfactorily diagnosed by the following points: (1) unreceptivity and unresponsivity, (2) no movements or breathing, (3) no reflexes, and (4) a flat electroencephalogram. Each of these tests is to be repeated at least 24 hours later with no change. This definition of brain death does not cover cases such as Karen Ann Quinlan, who was in a persistent vegetative state, or people who are in comas but do not meet other accepted criteria. ●

In 1983, President Ronald Reagan formed a commission to discuss the ethical implications of dying and death. The commission recommended that all U.S. jurisdictions accept the Uniform Determination of Death Act developed with the guidance of three organizations: the American Bar Association, the American Medical Association, and the National Conference of Commissioners on Uniform State Laws. The act "established that the irreversible cessation of all circulatory and respiratory functions, or irreversible cessation of all functions of the entire brain, including the brain stem" is the criterion of death.

Some believe that this higher brain death definition addresses all purposes. Whatever the state's legal definition of death, the declaration of death will be made by medical standards as defined in the Uniform Determination of Death Act. This means that as technology changes and medicine advances, laws will not necessarily change; rather, good medical practices will determine what counts as good evidence that the legal definition of death has occurred.

LEGAL IMPLICATIONS

Most legal rulings on life and death center on "Who makes the decisions?" Prolonging life by artificial means usually poses few legal problems. Federal laws state that clients with failing kidneys have the right to funding and the use of kidney dialysis machines. Some means of prolonging life artificially, such as insulin administration, are so easy, inexpensive, and widely practiced that there is no controversy about their use. On the other hand, some procedures, such as dialysis, are so expensive that federal legislation was necessary to ensure that every citizen has the right to such treatments.

Choices in dying, however, are complex and controversial. Consider landmark case law in the following two circumstances. In seeking greater choice in the process of dying, the courts appear to be regulating in a more restrictive manner. The fear of litigation is the reason in some cases why health-care professionals and institutions are hesitant to abide by clients' choices in dying.

Case Law

Karen Ann Quinlan: The litigation over the case of Karen Ann Quinlan was widely publicized. Quinlan was a New Jersey woman who, at age 21, was taken to the hospital in a comatose state by friends after a birthday party. No one is sure exactly what happened to Karen on Tuesday, April 14, 1975, but the world soon began to follow her life closely. Her case was a newsworthy first. Karen's condition deteriorated. On July 31, her parents asked her physicians to take Karen off the respirator and signed a letter to that effect. The physicians disagreed with the decision on moral grounds and refused to take Karen off the respirator. Legal action ensued.

Continued

On September 12, the attorney for Joseph Quinlan, Karen's father, filed a plea with the superior court on three constitutional grounds: (1) the right to privacy, (2) religious freedom, and (3) cruel and unusual punishment.

Judge Robert Muir ruled against Joseph Quinlan, who then appealed the decision to the New Jersey Supreme Court. The court's decision was in Joseph Quinlan's favor and set aside any criminal liability for removing the respirator. It further recommended that Karen's physicians consult the hospital ethics committee to concur with their prognosis for Karen. Weeks later Karen was weaned from the machine. She lived until 1986.

Theresa (Terri) Schiavo: Terri Schiavo suffered cardiac arrest in February 1990, probably due to an eating disorder that may have caused a serious electrolyte imbalance diagnosed when she was admitted to the hospital. She was without oxygen 5 to 7 minutes longer than medical experts believe is possible without irreversible brain damage. Her husband, Michael, insisted she be intubated, given a tracheotomy to breathe, and placed on a respirator. Without these actions, she would have died. Terri lived in a coma for 2 months and then was repeatedly diagnosed as in a persistent vegetative state. She was removed from the respirator and kept functioning with an artificial feeding and hydration tube. She could breathe and swallow her saliva, but could not drink or eat. What happened in the next 15 years is almost unimaginable.

Terri's husband and her parents struggled for a few years, but conflict arose when Michael and her parents disagreed about removing the feeding tube so that Terri could die peacefully. Terri had no living will. Twice courts ordered the feeding tube to be removed, but Terri's parents fought to have it reinserted. The Florida legislature passed a law known as "Terri's Law" to give the governor the prerogative of reinserting the feeding tube and required a special guardian ad litem be appointed. Later, the Florida Supreme Court ruled Terri's Law unconstitutional, and the U.S. Supreme Court refused to overturn that decision. Just a week before Terri's death, the U.S. Congress passed legislation to move the case from Florida to the federal courts. The Florida Federal District Court, the 11th Circuit Court of Appeals, and the U.S. Supreme Court refused to review the findings of the lower courts.

By this time and through all the court battles, Michael and Terri's parents were estranged and could no longer be civil toward each other. In testimony, Terri's parents said that even if Terri had a living will, they would have fought to have it voided. Michael became even more determined to carry out the wishes he believed Terri would have had. In the last few days of Terri's life, private citizens, religious leaders, and news media lined up on both sides of the issue outside the hospital to witness a most public death. Michael's wishes finally prevailed, and Terri died March 31, 2005, 14 days after the feeding tube was removed and 15 years after her cardiac arrest.

Both cases provoked discussions about end-of-life issues and medicine's limitations. Both Quinlan and Schiavo were alive when their cases were brought before the courts. The question in both cases was whether each woman should be kept alive, one by use of a respirator, the other by artificial hydration and nutrition. It was not whether they were legally dead. There are questions to be asked. Should the two women have been allowed to die earlier? Is vegetative existence better than death? What impact does medical technology have on these decisions? Who pays for the exorbinate fees incurred in these cases? Who should decide? Is it more difficult to remove hydration and nutrition than a respirator?

ETHICAL CONSIDERATIONS

ETHICS CHECK

Life-and-death choices are numerous. The many factors to consider include the following: Who makes the decision? What role do politicians and the courts play in making decisions? What is the influence of economics? Do circumstances influence decisions? What is ordinary and extraordinary treatment?

The burden of such decisions is heavy. If a decision is required in an emergency life-and-death matter, those in closest proximity to the client will decide. In health-care facilities, the law may determine who decides. If there is any question, consideration is given to the wishes of the client, the wishes of the family, the recommendations of the provider, and perhaps the recommendations of a professional team of individuals (ethics committee) whose purpose it is to make a decision—not necessarily in that order.

The problem arises over whose right is paramount in a decision. At times it is obvious. If a client is unable to decide, others are involved. The family has an influence, but the cases of Karen Ann Quinlan and Theresa Schiavo demonstrated that the influence of family is not decisive. In the case of Theresa Schiavo, the governor of Florida, the 11th Circuit Court of Appeals, the Florida Supreme Court, the President of the United States, Congress, and the U.S. Supreme Court were all involved.

The same often is true of a client's wishes. Even if clients are able to express their wishes to physicians and health-care providers, circumstances may override them, as was so clearly demonstrated in the vignette at the beginning of the chapter.

Many circumstances influence decisions. Age is a factor. Resuscitation may be started on a 16-year-old and not on an 89-year-old. Cost is also a factor. Triple cardiac bypass surgery may be performed for someone of substantial means more readily than for the indigent derelict. Health is a factor. A pacemaker may be inserted for the elderly client whose general health is good, but it may not be used if the client's health is poor and other severe physical difficulties exist. The availability of resources is a factor. With only one kidney and four needy persons, three will have to do without.

Other factors include region, personal philosophy of life, the amount of pain one can endure, whether a client is comatose, and what the client's feelings are about a good life versus a good death. Yet, all these factors are relative. Some are old at age 55; others are young at 90. Some can endure great pain, and others have a low threshold for pain. What is poor health to one person may seem to be good health to another. The relativity of the factors complicates the decision and mandates that each decision be considered individually on its own merits.

CULTURAL VIEWS

Cultures view life and death differently. For example, people of Jewish heritage strive to appreciate each day and live it as though it is their last. Death is seen as a part of the life cycle. Mexicans also view death as a natural part of life and the will of God. In the Filipino culture, planning one's death is taboo; hence, discussing advance directives and living wills is difficult. Many Chinese believe their spirits do not rest unless living descendants care for the grave and worship the memory of the dead. In the Japanese culture, family members want to be by the dying person's bedside, and traditionally the eldest son has decision-making responsibility at this time. There is, however, a taboo against the discussion of serious illness and death. Cultural and religious differences exist in cases of organ and tissue donation. For example, many Hmong immigrants from Southeast Asia believe that organ donation prevents the person from experiencing reincarnation; for this reason, the Hmong also resist autopsies. Many Native Americans often oppose organ donation because of their enormous reverence for the body, which is considered both the residence and the manifestation of a person's essence.

Health-care professionals will want to be sensitive to, understand, and appreciate cultural preferences. Being aware of a client's cultural perspective and asking questions related to his or her wishes is better than assuming everyone thinks and believes alike.

ASSISTED DEATH

Some people believe that assisted death weakens the moral fiber of the country and has far-reaching consequences. If death is justified for one individual to prevent further suffering, why not for infants with severe disabilities who have no possibility of a "normal" life? Consider the circumstances of an infant born with severe congenital defects and no possible chance of survival. The parents may choose not to begin measures to preserve the infant's life. This can mean watching a tiny infant gradually deteriorate over a period of days. The ordeal can be terrible. Parents may be some protected from this experience if the infant remains in the hospital, but the medical staff is not. Many physicians and health professionals ask, "Would it not be more merciful to inject the infant with a lethal dose of medication that would hasten death and prevent the suffering?"

Perhaps even more personal and difficult questions are raised related to death. "How do I want to die?" "What kind of lifesaving measures do I want?" "Might I choose assisted death?" "Can I stand to suffer?" "Do I have any control over my own death?" "What do I want health professionals to do for me?"

Questions arise about whether assisted death or euthanasia should be endorsed. It is considered assisted death when the physician provides a dying individual with a lethal dose of medication to be self-administered; it is considered active euthanasia when a physician administers a lethal dose to the client. In physician-assisted death, the client acts last, whereas in active euthanasia, the physician acts last.

Just as California and Washington were forerunners with their living wills and natural death laws, they were forerunners in legislation to give people the option to seek "aid in dying from physicians to end life in a dignified, painless, and humane manner." These laws are much broader in their scope than any living will or advance directive. In 1994, Oregon passed the Death With Dignity measure that was later challenged by the courts. In 1997, the act was reaffirmed by the Oregon voters. Oregon became the nation's first state to allow a physician to prescribe a lethal dose of medication when asked by a terminally ill client. The four safeguards in this measure are as follows: (1) The attending physician must truly convey informed consent, which must include all feasible opportunities, such as pain management, hospice, and palliative care. (2) The attending physician's diagnosis and prognosis must be confirmed by a consulting physician. The latter physician must verify that the client has made a voluntary and informed decision. (3) If either physician thinks the client might have depression that might impair judgment, a counseling session must be attended. (4) The client making the request must do so both orally and in writing. The law details specific time lines and a waiting period for the client before receiving the lethal medication. The request must be witnessed by at least two people who can verify the client's capacity to make a decision and that the decision is voluntary. There were 59 individuals who exercised their right to end their lives under the Oregon Death With Dignity Act in 2009 according to the state's department of health. That number appears to be average for each year since the Act became legal. ●

In fall 2001, U.S. Attorney General Ashcroft determined that the government would step in to revoke the licenses of any physician who prescribed controlled substances to clients seeking physician-assisted death in Oregon. By a 6-to-3 vote the U.S. Supreme Court ruled that Ashcroft exceeded his authority when he tried to block the Oregon law to help terminally ill clients die. The Supreme Court decision opened the door for other states to legalize physician-assisted death.

In 1997, the U.S. Senate passed a bill barring the federal government from financing physician-assisted death. The vote was 99 to 0. The same measure previously cleared the House of Representatives by a vote of 398 to 16. Medicare and Medicaid are prohibited from funding physician-assisted death. In June 1997, all nine Supreme Court justices refused to grant assisted death as a fundamental liberty for the terminally ill.

On November 4, 2008, the state of Washington passed Initiative 1000, the state's Death With Dignity Act, which became law on March 5, 2009. This act allows terminally ill adults seeking to end their life to request lethal doses of medication from medical and osteopathic physicians. These individuals must be Washington residents who have less than 6 months to live. Details of the Washington Death with Dignity Act can be found at **www.doh.wa.gov/dwda.**

States with current legislation related to assisted death are California and Montana. In California, the Right to Know End-of-Life Options Act became law January 1, 2009 (AB 2747—Berg;

Chapter 683 Statutes). The act is the first in the nation to provide those with a life-threatening illness full disclosure of, and counseling about, all legal treatment options, including the right to refuse unwanted treatment. Proponents of the bill believe it ensures that clients will receive the necessary information and power to influence the manner of death. It shifts client–physician communication on the subject from a physician-oriented decision to a cooperative one. A duty to share information enables clients to work with their physicians in determining the option that matches their values and desires. Montana's Supreme Court ruled on January 31, 2009 that end-of-life decisions are a matter of personal liberty solely between client and physician. In both states, there was high opposition and the fear that the rulings opened the doors for assisted death legislation.

Legislation on physician-assisted death continues to be controversial, contradictory, confusing, and as emotional as legalization of abortion has been in the United States. In fact, many right-to-life organizations oppose assisted death legislation based on the principle that abortion and assisted death are the same as murder.

UNIFORM ANATOMICAL GIFT ACT

The legal definition of death identified earlier is particularly important in the area of organ transplantation. All 50 states have some form of the Uniform Anatomical Gift Act. Persons 18 years or older and of sound mind may make a gift of all or any part of their body to the following persons for the following purposes:

1. To any hospital, surgeon, or physician for medical or dental education, research, advancement of medical or dental science, therapy, or transplantation
2. To any accredited medical or dental school, college, or university for education, research, advancement of medical or dental science, or therapy
3. To any organ bank or storage facility for medical or dental education, research, advancement of medical or dental science, therapy, or transplantation
4. To any specified individual for therapy or transplantation needed by him or her

The gift may be made by a provision in a will or by signing, in the presence of two witnesses, a card. The card is generally carried with the person at all times. The card method may be the best because advance directives may not be readily available until it is too late for donation of organs or tissues. Donated organs include heart, lung, kidney, pancreas, liver, and intestine; tissue includes eyes, skin, bone, heart valves, veins, and tendons. There is no cost to the donors or their families. See Figure 16-2 for the steps followed in organ donation. ●

Steps to organ donation:

1. Irreparable brain damage occurs; life support is to be suspended. Individual's signed donor agreement is presented; family agrees.
2. Transplant surgical team is notified; ethics dictate that transplant surgeons not be present when life support is removed.
3. Life support is removed (usually a ventilator); heart continues to beat and pump deoxygenated blood to tissues and cells.
4. If heart continues to beat more than 1 hour, organs are unfit for transplant due to the lack of oxygen; transplant is called off; if the heart ceases to beat in less than an hour, transplant moves forward.
5. Transplant team must wait 120 seconds to make sure heart does not start to beat again; if it does, the team waits—back to step 4.
6. Once heart has stopped for the 2 minutes, death is announced; transplant team arrives to harvest donor organs for waiting recipients.

Figure 16-2. Steps taken before organ donation.

It is illegal to sell body parts in this country; however, the practice is common in some developing countries. It is becoming increasingly popular to find compatible donors for transplant organs on the Internet. Many clients needing a transplant organ are telling their life stories on their own Web sites, making electronic pleas for willing donors. One such example reports of a 32-year-old man suffering with liver cancer who took out newspaper ads, set up a toll-free number, and bought space on two billboards along busy highways to appeal for a liver donor. In just a few months, he was rewarded with a liver from a deceased donor. Another example tells of an individual on a waiting list for a kidney for 5 years who paid monthly fees to have his profile posted on **www.matching-donors.com.** He received 500 offers for a donation, found a match, and is expected to pay his donor $5000 in transportation costs and other expenses incurred. Currently more than 100,000 Americans are on lists for organs, mostly kidneys and livers. As many as 7000 will die waiting because less than 20% of American adults are registered organ donors and only 50% of families agree to donate organs of their deceased loved ones when asked. Bartering for organs is apt to continue.

Persons may place conditions on their organ donation, and donors are carefully screened before their body parts are used. The physician and hospital may be found negligent, so there are strict standards for donor screening.

AUTOPSY

An autopsy is an examination of a dead body to determine the cause of death. Statutes generally state who can authorize an autopsy and under what circumstances. Coroners or medical examiners may give such authorization. Others include, in order of priority, the following:

PRIORITY AUTHORIZATION FOR AUTOPSY

1. The surviving spouse
2. Any child of the deceased who is 18 years of age or older
3. A parent of the deceased
4. An adult sibling of the deceased

Autopsies may be complete or partial. In other words, a pathologist may perform an autopsy on the entire body and examine every part and organ or do an autopsy only of the thoracic cavity or the brain. The extremities rarely are involved unless indicated by trauma, prior surgical procedure, or vessel involvement. No parts of the body can be retained for any reason without family consent. If the autopsy is done properly and in a professional manner, the body can be viewed by survivors or at a death ritual.

Some circumstances require an autopsy to investigate the cause of a suspicious death. Autopsies also offer valuable information for medical science and research. Knowledge gained from an autopsy may prevent another person from suffering similar circumstances. Refer to Chapter 7, Public Duties, for further information on autopsy.

ROLE OF HEALTH PROFESSIONALS

Health-care employees will make life-and-death decisions in personal relationships with their families and friends, but rarely in any professional capacity. They often, however, may be involved in conversations with clients or their families who are struggling with the question. They also may be sounding boards to providers involved in the decision-making process. Certainly the law should be followed, religious and cultural practices considered, and the clients' rights protected when possible, but no clearly established guideline is available.

Clients who willingly and openly discuss their beliefs and wishes concerning their own deaths should be encouraged to complete living wills, advance directives, and durable power of attorney documents. Legal counsel should be recommended to people if appropriate. Clients should not be made to feel ashamed or guilty because of their feelings about death, no matter how much they differ from your personal feelings.

Understanding and compassion are important. Every attempt must be made to respect the feelings of clients and their families. Families should be allowed to express any guilt they may feel in making decisions. A clear picture of the circumstances, explained by the provider in words clients can comprehend, can alleviate much of that problem. Clients who have strong feelings about having their lives prolonged should be encouraged to make their wishes known.

When health professionals are confronted with situations or questions they cannot handle, consultations and referrals should be sought. Attorneys may be called, and medical societies may offer assistance. Hospital ethics committees may be valuable. Hospital chaplains, staff psychiatrists, and social workers are specially trained to help others with these personal issues and processes involved.

SUMMARY

Choices about dying are best made while living whenever possible. Legal documents should be executed and shared with loved ones, family members, and health professionals in order to ensure that personal wishes are followed. These choices are not easily made unless there is a willingness to discuss the issue of death and what measures are to be taken when dying. If death can be viewed as another stage in life, even if the final one, it will be easier to have this discussion. Health professionals are bound to abide by the wishes of their clients within legal parameters.

Watch It Now! Are you familiar with end-of-life issues? at
http://davisplus.fadavis.com/lawandethics

Questions for Review

SELECT THE BEST ANSWER

1. An advance directive
   a. Is quite different from the living will.
   b. Is a release made by parents for children.
   c. Expresses end-of-life issues.
   d. Replaces the Patient Self-Determination Act.
   e. None of the above.

2. Durable Power of Attorney for Health Care
   a. Appoints an agent to act on the behalf of another.
   b. Makes decisions related to finances and property.
   c. Is executed at the time of death.
   d. Must be recorded in the National Registry.
   e. Only a, b, and d above.

3. Euthanasia
   a. Is defined as murder.
   b. Means bad death.
   c. Is a term not often used today.
   d. Literally means "good death."
   e. Only c and d above.

4. Assisted death
   a. Is illegal.
   b. Is supported by the American Medical Association.
   c. Is legal in Washington and Oregon.
   d. Is under consideration in a number of other states.
   e. Only c and d above.

5. The five stages of grief
   a. Are identified by Kübler-Ross.
   b. Spell the acronym TEARS.
   c. Are passed through in sequence.
   d. Apply only to the dying.
   e. Only a and c above.

TRUE OR FALSE

T F   1. A national registry is available to electronically store and send advance directives to any chosen health-care provider.

T F   2. Family members and friends often circumvent prescription or medication orders.

T F   3. Pain and suffering enhance self-image.

T F   4. A common definition of grief work is summarized in the acronym FEAR.

T F   5. Most individuals have a greater fear of suffering than of dying.

CLASSROOM EXERCISES

1. If you knew you would be put in the same situation as Karen Ann Quinlan or Terri Schiavo, what would you wish? Why?

2. Identify procedures that prolong life that you would be willing to have. Identify those you would not choose and justify your responses.

3. A family member comes to the ambulatory health-care setting. She is angry because the hospital "won't stop the endless testing" and "keeps trying the impossible with my husband." What is your response?

4. In the case of Ted, in the conflicts that arose among Ted, the family, and the medical professionals, who held the power? Was the comment made by the ICU nurse regarding the advance directive dilemma appropriate? Explain your answer. Discuss your personal reaction to Ted's case. What went right and what went wrong?

INTERNET ACTIVITIES

1. Research the Web site "Choices in Death Chronology." What is your reaction? What surprises you the most?

2. Research the living will and/or advance directive appropriate for the state in which you live. Print the form and fill it out. What difficulty do you have in doing so? Discuss with a family member or a loved one.

3. Research artificial feeding and artificial hydration. Describe the difference. What makes the choice a critical one in the death process?

4. Research the Internet to determine the criteria necessary to be placed on a list for a donor kidney.

5. After Internet research, identify the requirements for an autopsy in your particular state.

REFERENCES

Hayes, D. M.: *Between Doctor and Patient.* Valley Forge, PA: Judson Press, 1977, pp. 9–11.

Munson, R.: *Intervention and Reflection: Basic Issues in Medical Ethics.* Belmont, CA: Wadsworth, 1992, p. 147.

WEB RESOURCES

Compassion and Choices.
  www.compassionandchoices.org

Death With Dignity National Center.
  www.dwd.org

National Hospice and Palliative Care Organization.
  www.nhpco.org

Scientific American Special Issue.
  www.scientificamerican.com

Washington Death With Dignity Act.
  www.doh.wa.gov/dwda

World Federation of Right to Die.
  www.worldrtd.net

DavisPlus | For additional resources please visit http://davisplus.fadavis.com

Have a Care

CAROL'S NOTE

As a colleague, friend, confidant, and receiver of Marti Lewis's resilience throughout the many years of our friendship, I never heard her ask, "Why me?" and never did she come close to giving up.

When Marti and I wrote the first edition of this text, she did not talk much about her illness. "Have a Care" came about because Marti's story told more poignantly about the importance of being sensitive and compassionate toward your clients than any advice we could possibly have given.

After you read her story, I think you'll understand why.

MARTI'S STORY

It's early December, many years ago. I hurt. I can't function at home or at work. The pain in my back is so bad I can't lift my 5-month-old infant without excruciating pain. It hurts to shower and turn the steering wheel of the car. I go to bed before my husband, and then I can't move. Terrible spasms awaken me. I am so tired and have no energy.

I'm not really afraid. I trust my doctor. I know he'll find out what is wrong, fix it, and I'll be back to normal. I have to take time from work to see my doctor. It is inconvenient, but I can do it. No one does my job while I'm gone; it waits for my return. I expect action from my doctor today, and I don't want sympathy.

Fortunately, I don't have to wait long in the clinic. The pain is a little less; probably from the addicting psychological release from knowing I'll soon be better. But I put up a front, too. I won't cry or tell the doctor how really bad the pain is. The assistant's greeting is cheerful, but I could use some help with my clothes in the exam room. I can hardly get them off. The bra is terrible, and the pantyhose are worse.

My physician is quiet, professional, and concerned. I feel better just seeing him. His smile is warm. I can tell he cares. The examination is not too difficult. He finally says, "It looks serious. We have to run a lot of tests. It is going to take time to get to the bottom of this." Laboratory tests and x-rays are ordered. The doctor says that physical activity is allowed until it causes pain. I don't tell him how hard that will be. He tells me to bring my husband with me the next visit. I have to get dressed and go to the laboratory. The awful bra and pantyhose again, and it hurts to tie my shoes.

The atmosphere is sterile in the laboratory—cool and too professional. My mind is racing while I wait. I'm in torment. "What is it? What about my baby? Will I be able to take care of her? I've waited 36 years for her.

The laboratory technician withdraws the blood, and I give the laboratory a urine specimen. The awful pantyhose again! "Collect a 24-hour urine." They hand me this weird, antifreeze-like container with an opening like a vinegar bottle. It is white and has large black letters: "For 24-Hour Urine Only." I also am told to collect some feces. I'm handed three unfolded cardboard containers and some tiny spatulas. No instructions.

As I leave, I wonder, how long before I know what is wrong? I'm exhausted. I want to get home and see my husband. I need to talk to someone. Oh, the pain is bad. I hurt.

A telephone call a week later from my physician tells me the progress of the tests, but no indication of a diagnosis. His conversation is very general.

Christmas is a blur. There is no change in my condition. Questions from family and friends are not helpful. They don't understand. Neither do I. I hide my true feelings.

I'm back in the doctor's office a few weeks later with my husband. He had to take time from work. The receptionist seems surprised that my husband is with me. I wonder if she thinks I can't handle this. Well, guess what, I can't!

The consultation is hard. My physician is open and honest—he tells us that a metabolic bone disorder is rampant. I hear him tell my husband that I can have no physical activity. I must take off work. I cannot drive. To fall would be disastrous. My bones are like a loaf of bread. "You know what a loaf of bread is like when it is smashed." I cannot lift anything, even my baby. I'm not supposed to bend over. My husband asks, "Should we have outside help come into the home?" The doctor says, "Yes." Immediately I think about the expense. The doctor describes the medications I'll be taking. But the final blow comes when he says, "That is not all; something else is wrong." He hopes more tests will reveal what.

A month passes. I hate having someone do my work. A temporary replacement is hired for my job. I don't ask for help easily. I can't even get my own groceries. I'm terrified of falling. I can't vacuum my floors. I can't lift my baby to change her. If she cries, I can't pick her up. When no one is looking, I do lift her. I do carry her. And I do make my condition worse. This creates conflict with my husband. Life is not good.

During this time, there are more tests. More referrals. More doctors. I feel so inhuman. The worst tests are the small bowel biopsies. My physician tells me that they will put a tube in my mouth and pass it through to the small intestine. He says it is painless and won't take very long.

My husband takes me to see the specialist and have the test. He is told I'll be finished in about 1 hour. They will call him. In the examination room, I'm partially disrobed, and I put on a full-length gown that opens down the back. I can keep my slacks and shoes on. The gastroenterologist passes the tube through my mouth into my stomach. There is no pain, but it is awful. I gag over and over again. I must try not to. I tell myself to breathe slowly, to concentrate on not vomiting. When the gastroenterologist finishes, the LPN says, "Let's go to x-ray."

To my horror, she hands me a box of tissues and an emesis basin, drapes my coat over my shoulders, takes my elbow, and says, "Be careful not to fall." I bite on the tube in my mouth and try to stabilize it with my free hand as we walk through a large, crowded reception area, out the front door, and across two office parking lots covered with early morning frost. While I am still in disbelief, we walk into the lowest floor of a multiple-office building where the x-ray receptionist tells us the radiologist is still at the hospital making rounds. I snarl through my teeth, "Get that doctor here now."

In the x-ray waiting area, I sit for 30 minutes, still trying not to gag. The tears come, first haltingly, then freely. The saliva flows from my mouth and nose. I'm finally able to get a hold of myself. I stop crying. I don't want to ruin the test. Finally the doctor appears. He looks at me. In my revulsion at the situation and him, I whisper, "You son of a —!" His response is, "What's wrong with you?" How can I tell him? I still have the tube in my mouth. He checks the placement of the tube in the small intestine several different times. When he verifies that it is in place, he calls another LPN to take me back. Over the same route. I pray to God no one recognizes me. I am in a state of shock about my circumstances.

Upon returning, the biopsy is taken. The doctor pulls the tube. I sigh with relief. In a few minutes, he turns to me and says, "We didn't get it." The instrument to snatch a piece of the intestinal wall didn't grab properly. The same procedure must be done again. The tube goes back in, across the parking lots; check the tube, back across the parking lots. This time, the biopsy is successful.

This whole time my husband is trying to call the office and wondering what has happened. They tell him only that there is a problem. He is not allowed to speak to anyone else. Four-and-a-half hours later, they call to tell him I'm finished.

***

For more than 30 years Marti lived with the metabolic bone disorder, which gradually improved. The intestinal biopsy helped to diagnose celiac disease, which Marti was able to control with diet that she religiously monitored. Her activities were somewhat limited, and she could not lift anything heavy or participate in any sport other than swimming. She took a lot of medication, some experimental, and lost 5 inches in height as her bones disintegrated. She suffered a profound hearing loss, but learned to read lips and fooled most of the people most of the time. She never was totally free from pain. Sometimes the severe spinal pain struck like lightning, stealing her breath away. She might wake up screaming, unable to move because of pinched nerves. Her fear was that one day she might be paralyzed and confined to a wheelchair.

Through it all, Marti believed she was blessed. She continued to teach, co-authored two books, and witnessed her daughter's completion of graduate school and the purchase of her first home. Marti became a much admired administrator at Olympic College where her teaching career began. Marti lived in the here and now. She practiced a healthful lifestyle and willingly shared a priceless sense of humor. She enjoyed life to the very fullest, and so loved being an author of this book. Her family and friends gave her strength. In turn, she gave everyone she met strength and encouragement, both personally and professionally.

She enjoyed retirement and the beach condominium in Oregon. She lived for the professional football season, and knew the names of the players and coaches of all the teams. She loved music, good movies, and good books. She loved chocolate.

FINAL NOTE FROM CAROL

We ended the last edition of this book with the following:

Together now, we walk along the beach and river. Sometimes it is shallow, rocky, and hard. We wade in together, holding onto each other. Sometimes the river is deep, sweeps us off our feet, and we float freely in warmth and peace. Sometimes there are bends in the river, bends we can't see around, and it scares us. But we go on. We are reminded constantly (thank you, Judy Collins) that:

> "In the valleys, we look for the mountains.
> In the mountains, we've searched for the rivers.
> There is nowhere to go. We are where we belong.
> We can and do live the life we dreamed."

We did not know then that in 2 years, Marti would be diagnosed with acute myelogenous leukemia. She was given two options. She could choose treatment, hope for remission, and have a couple good more years. Or, she could choose no treatment and have only a few good weeks. She chose treatment.

The treatment was no picnic. She grew weaker every day, became very fatigued, lost her appetite for all the foods she enjoyed and soon was unable to eat much of anything. In just a few months she could not hold a paper or a book to read, she could not drive or get her e-mails at the computer.

We wrote about death and dying and end-of-life issues, but what we learned during these last few months together is that we didn't have a clue about dying. There is nothing more personal than death; it must be done alone, no matter how many friends and loved ones rally around. Marti was not afraid to die, but she was oh so sad to leave those she loved so much.

Marti is now gone from this earth, but she lives on—in every former student, in her family, in her co-author, in the hundreds of medical assistant and nursing students who will share funds from a scholarship in her name, and, lastly, in every reader of this story.

Our final words for you have not changed.

This story is shared with you because we care. We hope that by sharing Marti's story you'll be better able to share your own compassion. Remember to be loving, gracious, human, and able to put yourself in the place of your clients. Remember that the client is more than someone with an illness or injury. Clients are people with responsibilities, families, and personal and emotional needs.

Please, throughout your career as a health-care professional, do your clients and yourself a huge favor: Have a care!

Carol Tamparo
Marti Lewis (2/18/44–5/02/09)

APPENDIX 1

Codes of Ethics

1. Hippocratic Oath, Classical and Modern Version
2. American Association of Medical Assistants (AMAA)
3. Principles of Medical Ethics: American Medical Association

1. HIPPOCRATIC OATH, CLASSICAL VERSION*

I swear by Apollo Physician and Asclepius and Hygieia and Panaceia and all the gods and goddesses, making them my witnesses, that I will fulfil according to my ability and judgment this oath and this covenant:

To hold him who has taught me this art as equal to my parents and to live my life in partnership with him, and if he is in need of money to give him a share of mine, and to regard his offspring as equal to my brothers in male lineage and to teach them this art if they desire to learn it without fee and covenant; to give a share of precepts and oral instruction and all the other learning to my sons and to the sons of him who has instructed me and to pupils who have signed the covenant and have taken an oath according to the medical law, but to no one else.

I will apply dietetic measures for the benefit of the sick according to my ability and judgment; I will keep them from harm and injustice.

I will neither give a deadly drug to anybody if asked for it, nor will I make a suggestion to this effect. Similarly I will not give to a woman an abortive remedy. In purity and holiness I will guard my life and my art.

I will not use the knife, not even on sufferers from stone, but will withdraw in favor of such men as are engaged in this work.

Whatever houses I may visit, I will come for the benefit of the sick, remaining free of all intentional injustice, of all mischief and in particular of sexual relations with both female and male persons, be they free or slaves.

What I may see or hear in the course of the treatment or even outside of the treatment in regard to the life of men, which on no account one must spread abroad, I will keep to myself holding such things shameful to be spoken about.

*From Ludwig, E.: The Hippocratic Oath. Baltimore: Johns Hopkins University Press, 1943; and Lasagna, L.: A modern version of the Hippocratic Oath. Tufts University Medical School, 1964. Available at: www.medterms.com

If I fulfil this oath and do not violate it, may it be granted to me to enjoy life and art, being honored with fame among all men for all time to come; if I transgress it and swear falsely, may the opposite of all this be my lot.

HIPPOCRATIC OATH, MODERN VERSION

I swear to fulfill, to the best of my ability and judgment, this covenant:

I will respect the hard-won scientific gains of those physicians in whose steps I walk, and gladly share such knowledge as is mine with those who are to follow.

I will apply, for the benefit of the sick, all measures which are required, avoiding those twin traps of overtreatment and therapeutic nihilism.

I will remember that there is art to medicine as well as science, and that warmth, sympathy, and understanding may outweigh the surgeon's knife or the chemist's drug.

I will not be ashamed to say "I know not," nor will I fail to call in my colleagues when the skills of another are needed for a patient's recovery.

I will respect the privacy of my patients, for their problems are not disclosed to me that the world may know. Most especially must I tread with care in matters of life and death. If it is given me to save a life, all thanks. But it may also be within my power to take a life; this awesome responsibility must be faced with great humbleness and awareness of my own frailty. Above all, I must not play at God.

I will remember that I do not treat a fever chart, a cancerous growth, but a sick human being, whose illness may affect the person's family and economic stability. My responsibility includes these related problems, if I am to care adequately for the sick.

I will prevent disease whenever I can, for prevention is preferable to cure.

I will remember that I remain a member of society, with special obligations to all my fellow human beings, those sound of mind and body as well as the infirm.

If I do not violate this oath, may I enjoy life and art, respected while I live and remembered with affection thereafter. May I always act so as to preserve the finest traditions of my calling and may I long experience the joy of healing those who seek my help.

2. AMERICAN ASSOCIATION OF MEDICAL ASSISTANTS (AAMA)**

The Code of Ethics of the AAMA shall set forth principles of ethical and moral conduct as they relate to the medical profession and the particular practice of medical assisting.

Members of AAMA dedicated to the conscientious pursuit of their profession, and thus desiring to merit the high regard of the entire medical profession and the respect of the general public which they serve, do pledge themselves to strive always to:

A. render service with full respect for the dignity of humanity;

B. respect confidential information obtained through employment unless legally authorized or required by responsible performance of duty to divulge such information;

C. uphold the honor and high principles of the profession and accept its disciplines;

D. seek to continually improve the knowledge and skills of medical assistants for the benefit of patients and professional colleagues;

E. participate in additional service activities aimed toward improving the health and well-being of the community.

Creed

I believe in the principles and purposes of the profession of medical assisting.

I endeavor to be more effective.

**American Association of Medical Assistants, Chicago, IL, 1996-2011. Reprinted with permission.

I aspire to render greater service.

I protect the confidence entrusted to me.

I am dedicated to the care and well-being of all people.

I am loyal to my employer.

I am true to the ethics of my profession.

I am strengthened by compassion, courage, and faith.

3. PRINCIPLES OF MEDICAL ETHICS: AMERICAN MEDICAL ASSOCIATION†

Preamble

The medical profession has long subscribed to a body of ethical statements developed primarily for the benefit of the patient. As a member of this profession, a physician must recognize responsibility to patients first and foremost, as well as to society, to other health professionals, and to self. The following Principles adopted by the American Medical Association are not laws, but standards of conduct that define the essentials of honorable behavior for the physician.

Principles of Medical Ethics

I. A physician shall be dedicated to providing competent medical care, with compassion and respect for human dignity and rights.

II. A physician shall uphold the standards of professionalism, be honest in all professional interactions, and strive to report physicians deficient in character or competence, or engaging in fraud or deception, to appropriate entities.

III. A physician shall respect the law and also recognize a responsibility to seek changes in those requirements which are contrary to the best interests of the patient.

IV. A physician shall respect the rights of patients, colleagues, and other health professionals, and shall safeguard patient confidences and privacy within the constraints of the law.

V. A physician shall continue to study, apply, and advance scientific knowledge, maintain a commitment to medical education, make relevant information available to patients, colleagues, and the public, obtain consultation, and use the talents of other health professionals when indicated.

VI. A physician shall, in the provision of appropriate patient care, except in emergencies, be free to choose whom to serve, with whom to associate, and the environment in which to provide medical care.

VII. A physician shall recognize a responsibility to participate in activities contributing to the improvement of the community and the betterment of public health.

VIII. A physician shall, while caring for a patient, regard responsibility to the patient as paramount.

IX. A physician shall support access to medical care for all people.

†From the American Medical Association, adopted by the American Medical Association's House of Delegates June 17, 2001. Reprinted with permission from American Medical Association, Code of Medical Ethics, Copyright 2001.

Sample Documents for Choices About Health Care, Life, and Death

DURABLE POWER OF ATTORNEY FOR HEALTH CARE AND HEALTH CARE DIRECTIVE

Available at http://www.wsma.org/patient_resources/advance-directives-qa.cfm

DURABLE POWER OF ATTORNEY FOR HEALTH CARE

Notice to Person Executing This Document

This is an important legal document. Before executing this document you should know these facts:

- This document gives the person you designate as your Health Care Agent the power to make MOST health care decisions for you if you lose the capability to make informed health care decisions for yourself. This power is effective only when you lose the capacity to make informed health care decisions for yourself. As long as you have the capacity to make informed health care decisions for yourself, you retain the right to make all medical and other health care decisions.

- You may include specific limitations in this document on the authority of the Health Care Agent to make health care decisions for you.

- Subject to any specific limitations you include in this document, if you do lose the capacity to make an informed decision on a health care matter, the Health Care Agent GENERALLY will be authorized by this document to make health care decisions for you to the same extent as you could make those decisions yourself, if you had the capacity to do so. The authority of the Health Care Agent to make health care decisions for you GENERALLY will include the authority to give informed consent, to refuse to give informed consent, or to withdraw informed consent to any care, treatment, service, or procedure to maintain, diagnose, or treat a physical or mental condition. You can limit that right in this document if you choose.

- When exercising his or her authority to make health care decisions for you when deciding on your behalf, the Health Care Agent will have to act consistent with your wishes, or if they are unknown, in your best interest. You may make your wishes known to the Health Care Agent by including them in this document or by making them known in another manner.

- When acting under this document the Health Care Agent GENERALLY will have the same rights that you have to receive information about proposed health care, to review health care records, and to consent to the disclosure of health care records.

1. Creation of Durable Power of Attorney for Health Care

I intend to create a power of attorney (Health Care Agent) by appointing the person or persons designated herein to make health care decisions for me to the same extent that I could make such decisions for myself if I was capable of doing so, as recognized by RCW 11.94.010. This designation becomes effective when I cannot make health care decisions for myself as determined by my attending physician or designee, such as if I am unconscious, or if I am otherwise temporarily or permanently incapable of making health care decisions. The Health Care Agent's power shall cease if and when I regain my capacity to make health care decisions.

2. Designation of Health Care Agent and Alternate Agents

If my attending physician or his or her designee determines that I am not capable of giving informed consent to health care, I _____, designate and appoint:

Name _____ Address _____

City _____ State ___ Zip _____ Phone _____

as my attorney-in-fact (Health Care Agent) by granting him or her the Durable Power of Attorney for Health Care recognized in RCW 11.94.010 and authorize her or him to consult with my physicians about the possibility of my regaining the capacity to make treatment decisions and to accept, plan, stop, and refuse treatment on my behalf with the treating physicians and health personnel.

In the event that _____ is unable or unwilling to serve, I grant these powers to

Name _____ Address _____

City _____ State ___ Zip _____ Phone _____

In the event that both _____ and _____
are unable or unwilling to serve, I grant these powers to

Name _____ Address _____

City _____ State ___ Zip _____ Phone _____

Your name _____

DURABLE POWER OF ATTORNEY FOR HEALTH CARE

3. General Statement of Authority Granted

My Health Care Agent is specifically authorized to give informed consent for health care treatment when I am not capable of doing so. This includes but is not limited to consent to initiate, continue, discontinue, or forgo medical care and treatment including artificially supplied nutrition and hydration, following and interpreting my instructions for the provision, withholding, or withdrawing of life-sustaining treatment, which are contained in any Health Care Directive or other form of "living will" I may have executed or elsewhere, and to receive and consent to the release of medical information. When the Health Care Agent does not have any stated desires or instructions from me to follow, he or she shall act in my best interest in making health care decisions.

The above authorization to make health care decisions does not include the following absent a court order:

   (1) Therapy or other procedure given for the purpose of inducing convulsion;

   (2) Surgery solely for the purpose of psychosurgery;

   (3) Commitment to or placement in a treatment facility for the mentally ill, except pursuant to the provisions of Chapter 71.05 RCW;

   (4) Sterilization.

I hereby revoke any prior grants of durable power of attorney for health care.

4. Special Provisions

_____

_____

_____

_____

DATED this_____day of _____, _____.

                                                           (year)

                            GRANTOR _____

STATE OF WASHINGTON   )

)ss.

(COUNTY OF_____)

I certify that I know or have satisfactory evidence that the GRANTOR, _____ signed this instrument and acknowledged it to be his or her free and voluntary act for the uses and purposes mentioned in the instrument.

DATED this _____ day of _____, _____.

                                                                 (year)

                                      _____

                                      NOTARY PUBLIC in and for the State of Washington,

                                        residing at _____

                                        My commission expires _____

                                        NOTE: Washington state does not require this directive to be notarized or witnessed. Since some states do require it to be notarized; you may want to do so in the event you travel out-of-state.

HEALTH CARE DIRECTIVE

Directive made this _____ day of _____, _____.

(year)

I, _____being of sound mind, willfully, and voluntarily make known my desire that my dying shall not be artificially prolonged under the circumstances set forth below, and do hereby declare that:

(A) If at any time I should have an incurable and irreversible condition certified to be a terminal condition by my attending physician, and where the application of life-sustaining treatment would serve only to artificially prolong the process of my dying, I direct that such treatment be withheld or withdrawn, and that I be permitted to die naturally. I understand "terminal condition" means an incurable and irreversible condition caused by injury, disease, or illness that would, within reasonable medical judgment, cause death within a reasonable period of time in accordance with accepted medical standards.

(B) If I should be in an irreversible coma or persistent vegetative state or other permanent unconscious condition as certified by two physicians, and from which those physicians believe that I have no reasonable probability of recovery, I direct that life-sustaining treatment be withheld or withdrawn.

(C) If I am diagnosed to be in a terminal or permanent unconscious condition, [*Choose one*]
I want _____ do not want _____
artificially administered nutrition and hydration to be withdrawn or withheld the same as other forms of life sustaining treatment. I understand artificially administered nutrition and hydration is a form of life-sustaining treatment in certain circumstances. I request all health care providers who care for me to honor this directive.

(D) In the absence of my ability to give directions regarding the use of such life-sustaining procedures, it is my intention that this directive shall be honored by my family, physicians, and other health care providers as the final expression of my fundamental right to refuse medical or surgical treatment, and also honored by any person appointed to make these decisions for me, whether by durable power of attorney or otherwise. I accept the consequences of such refusal.

(E) If I have been diagnosed as pregnant and that diagnosis is known to my physician, this directive shall have no force or effect during the course of my pregnancy.

(F) I understand the full import of this directive and I am emotionally and mentally competent to make this directive. I also understand that I may amend or revoke this directive at any time.

(G) I make the following additional directions regarding my care:

_____

_____

_____

_____

Signed _____

The declarer has been personally known to me and I believe him or her to be of sound mind. In addition, I am not the attending physician, an employee of the attending physician or health care facility in which the declarer is a patient, or any person who has a claim against any portion of the estate of the declarer upon the declarer's decease at the time of the execution of the directive.

Witness _____

Witness _____

What To Do With These Forms

The attached Health Care Directive and Durable Power of Attorney for Health Care forms are all legal documents once they are completely filled out and signed with the appropriate signatures. Signed copies of the completed directives should be included in your medical record, given to any person to whom you give your durable power of attorney—including any alternate people you may have named—and to your personal attorney. Originals should be kept by someone you trust and who can obtain them in an emergency.

Washington's Online Living Will Registry

Washington residents can now register their advance planning documents with the Department of Health (DOH) on the online Living Will Registry. The Registry allows physicians or other health care providers to quickly access a patient's documents via a secure website.

Registration is free and easy; fill out a registration form available at www.doh.wa.gov/livingwill and then mail or fax it and your documents to the DOH. Those who register will receive a wallet card and a sticker to place on their driver's license. For more information, go to the Washington State Living Will Registry website at www.doh.wa.gov/livingwill, or call the DOH's Consumer Hot-line toll free, 1-800-525-0127.

For Further Information

These forms have been provided as a public service by the Washington State Medical Association. You are encouraged to discuss the directives with your physician. Any legal questions you may have about the use and effect of these directives may be answered by an attorney.

ORGAN DONATION FORM

ORGAN DONATION FORM

I, _____, of _____, give my organs, tissues, or parts as directed below. This Anatomical Gift will take effect upon my death.

I give: (initial one of the three options)
_____ any needed organs, tissues, or parts.

_____ any needed organs, tissues, or parts except:

_____ the following organs, tissues, or parts only:

I give my organs, tissues, or parts indicated above to be used for: (initial one of the two options)
_____ any purpose authorized by law.
_____ the following purposes only: (initial all that apply)
    _____ transplantation
    _____ research
    _____ therapy
    _____ education

Limitations or special wishes, if any:

If any provision in this document is held to be invalid, such invalidity shall not affect the other provisions which can be given effect without the invalid provision, and to this end the directions in this document are severable.

Date Signed _____

Donor _____

Signature _____

Donor's Date of Birth _____

I witnessed that this document was signed in my presence by the Donor. I am signing in the presence of and at the direction of the Donor and in the presence of the other witness.

Witness _____

Signature _____

Witness _____

Signature _____

ORGAN DONATION CARD

Available at http://www.vtethicsnetwork.org/forms/donorcard.pdf

Limitations or special wishes, if any:

or education.

for the purpose of transplantation, therapy, medical research,

(specify the organs or parts)

(b) —— only the following organs or parts

I give: (a) —— any needed organs or parts,

marks below indicate my desires.

if medically acceptable, to take effect upon my death. The word and

In the hope that I may help others, I hereby make this anatomical gift,

(Print or type name of donor)

of ——

UNIFORM DONOR CARD

- - - - - FOLD HERE - - - - -

UNIFORM DONOR CARD

Signed by the donor and the following two witnesses
in the presence of each other

Signature of Donor   Date of Birth

City and State   Date Signed

Witness   Witness

This a legal document under the Uniform Anatomical Gift Act
or similar laws. For further information, contact the New England
Organ Bank 1 800 446-NEOB or the Center for Donation and
Transplant 1 800 803-6667.

Index of Resources

REFERENCES

American Association of Medical Assistants: "What is a Medical Assistant" http://www.aama-ntl.org/

Beauchamp, T. L., & Walters, L.: *Contemporary Issues in Bioethics*, 4th ed. Belmont, CA: Wadsworth, 1994.

Blanchard, K., & Peale, N.V.: *The Power of Ethical Management*. New York, NY: Wm. Morrow, 1988.

Department of Social Work, Wright State University, 2005. www.rcgd.isr.umich.edu/prba/perspectives/fall2000/mbaker.pdf

Fletcher J. *The Ethics of Genetic Control Ending Reproductive Roulette*. Buffalo, NY: Prometheus Books, 1988.

Furrow, B., Greaney, T., Johnson, S., et al. *Health Law: Cases, Materials and Problems*, 6th ed. St. Paul, MN: Thomson West, 2008.

Harris, D.M.: *Contemporary Issues in Healthcare Law and Ethics,* 3rd ed. Chicago: Health Administration Press, 2008.

Harris, G. "More Doctors Giving Up Private Practices." www.nytimes.com

Medical Insurance Exchange of California: "Managing Your Practice," Advisory Number 2. 2000.

Hayes, D. M.: *Between Doctor and Patient.* Valley Forge, PA: Judson Press, 1977, pp. 9–11.

Munson, R.: *Intervention and Reflection: Basic Issues in Medical Ethics.* Belmont, CA: Wadsworth, 1992.

Purnell, L.D., & Paulanka, B. J.: *Transcultural Health Care: A Culturally Competent Approach,* 3rd ed. Philadelphia: F.A. Davis, 2008.

INDEX

Page numbers followed by f indicate figure
Page numbers followed by t indicate table